Rich Symonds

Fitness, Health,
and
Work Capacity

Fitness, Health,
and
Work Capacity:
International Standards for Assessment

**International Committee for the
Standardization of Physical Fitness Tests**

Leonard A. Larson, Editor

MACMILLAN PUBLISHING CO., INC.
NEW YORK
COLLIER MACMILLAN PUBLISHERS
LONDON

Macmillan Publishing Co., Inc.
866 Third Avenue, New York, New York 10022

Collier-Macmillan Canada, Ltd.

LIBRARY OF CONGRESS CATALOGING IN PUBLICATION DATA

International Committee for the Standardization of
  Physical Fitness Tests.
  Fitness, health, and work capacity.

  1. Physical fitness—Testing. I. Title.
  [DNLM: 1. Physical fitness—Congresses. 2. Sport
medicine—Congresses. QT260 I56f 1972]
GV436.I57   613.7   72-90543
ISBN 0-02-359750-X

Printing: 1 2 3 4 5 6 7 8   Year: 4 5 6 7 8 9 0

Preface

Fitness, Health, and Work Capacity: International Standards for Assessment is an outgrowth of work by the International Committee for the Standardization of Physical Fitness Tests. The committee was informally organized in Tokyo in 1964 and formally structured in Tokyo in 1965. The committee and its objectives are the result of an invitation by the officials of the Congress of Sport Sciences, held in Tokyo in 1964 as a part of the Olympic Games program, to continue work toward standardization of assessment on an interdisciplinary basis. The request had its origin in the presentations made at the Tokyo Congress and represents the first organized and systematic program of standardization for the assessment of work capacity and physical fitness, utilizing resources and research from the disciplines of medicine, physiology, physique and body composition, and human performance.

The contributions toward an understanding of physical fitness from within these disciplines were well known in 1964. What was unknown were the relationships among the various disciplines and the relative worth of each in the assessment of work capacity and physical fitness as they relate to various tasks or work levels. Now, after some ten years of work by the committee, the foresight of the congress and that of the members of the committee is clearly apparent. No single discipline can make a full assessment of work capacity and physical fitness. Each makes an important contribution, and the significance of each contribution will vary with the physical task. This book includes the work of the committee over these years, including that of authors who have devoted a lifetime to assessing work capacity and physical fitness. The book covers the research literature and presents experiences that can be applied with confidence to people in all walks of life.

Standardization required research. An evaluation of the existing literature and an analysis of the assessment procedures and tests being applied in the various laboratories represented by the committee membership were needed. In order to advance the work on standardization, the committee members agreed to meet yearly at some designated institution that sponsors an ongoing research program on work capacity and physical fitness. Nine meetings have been convened since 1964. The first two were in Tokyo, then at Sandefjord, Norway (1966), Magglingen, Switzerland (1967), Mexico City, Mexico (1968), Tel Aviv, Israel (1969), Oxford, England (1970), Magglingen

(1971), and Cologne, Germany (1972). During these years, a research program on standardization was planned and is now operational in institutions throughout the world.

The full range of the research program is covered and presented in five phases. The research program began with the standardization of assessment procedures and was followed by the application of these procedures to population groups in various countries which have different environmental settings. The program is now advancing throughout the world. The factors under study concern basic differences within the populations. Included are social and sex differences, occupations, types of sport and performances in them, along with other factors of importance in understanding the people and their health and fitness status and changes.

Phase One. Possibly the most significant decision made by the committee was that research on standards should be interdisciplinary. Its members recognized that several disciplines were actively involved with research directed toward the determination of man's ability to do work and to withstand the stresses of the physical and social environments. In the past relatively few studies have been interdisciplinary. This is possibly due to the relative independence of the various professional groups. It was the committee's strong opinion that each discipline could make a significant contribution to understanding and assessing work capacity and physical fitness. An interdisciplinary approach is particularly important when dealing with an understanding of the *total* organism at work. This should include an evaluation of all organs, systems, and functions related to work along with the instruments and standards needed to assess their contribution to work and physical activity in settings of varying intensities, durations, and frequencies.

Research programs to prepare standards for the assessment of work capacity and physical fitness were the first goal of the committee. The programs included the scientific and medical disciplines that have contributed to this goal. The work required a number of years of research within each of the selected disciplines. The major portion of the work was completed in two years, but refinements from reviews have continued to the time of the publication of this text. This text includes both the standards and the scientific rationale that provide an understanding of the standards. The sources of information and research were derived from (1) medicine, which was concerned with the preparation of a medical examination to serve as a prerequisite for participation in physically stressful activities; (2) physiology, which dealt with the assessment of the physiological responses of man in work activities that placed physical stress on the various systems and organs; (3) the physical and biological sciences, which considered the assessment of physique and body composition correlated with physical work and the functioning of the human organism; and (4) sports, athletics, and physical education, which were concerned with the assessment of human abilities in physical activities of various types that would reflect work capacities and levels of fitness for physical performances. It was the judgment of the committee that standards developed from these resources would yield information about the human organism that would be sufficiently reliable and valid to make the results useful in assessing the capacity of the organism for work and physical activity.

Phase Two. It was agreed by the committee in 1964 that the first phase of the research program on standardization should include a survey of the assessment procedures and instruments utilized in the selected disciplines. Dr. T. Ishiko agreed to be responsible for this survey. His findings, which were reported at the meetings in 1965 and 1966, provided the empirical data needed to start the process of standardization.

Phase Three. Following the survey, the first set of standards was prepared. The committee reached agreement on these tentative standards at Sandefjord, Norway, in 1966. The report on these standards was then distributed to all members of the committee for review. The comments and recommendations made by its members served as the basis for discussion at Magglingen, Switzerland, in 1967. The standards drawn from the disciplines in the sciences and medicine were classified into four categories on the basis of their contributions to an understanding of work capacity and physical fitness, and on the basis of the uniqueness and specificity of the contributions.

The *medical examination* is designed to serve as a prerequisite for an individual's participation in stressful activities and work and not as a general health examination, except in those instances where the items are common to both. The items of the medical examination are classified into four categories: personal history, athletic history, medical examinations, and laboratory tests. In each instance, items were included only if they were valuable as prerequisites for stressful physical participation. And, of course, the items vary in worth according to the nature of the activity and the intensity and duration of physical participation.

The *physiological* measurements and indices were selected by applying the principle that work capacity and physical fitness are based on the direct relationship between the capacity to perform maximum work for periods of several minutes and the capacity of the cardiovascular-respiratory systems to deliver oxygen to the active tissue. The capacity for short duration maximum work is not generally related to "physiological" physical fitness because individual variations in oxygen debt capacity, a predominant factor in sprint type efforts, are not a factor of importance in physical performances of long duration.

The selection of physiological items is guided by two principles: (1) that testing procedures must be basically the same for investigations both in the laboratory and in the field and (2) that all testing procedures should permit the direct measurement or the indirect estimation of the maximum oxygen intake capacity, which is the most meaningful basis for judging physiological physical fitness. For example, under laboratory conditions the aerobic capacity will be directly assessed through the use of sophisticated procedures, whereas in the field aerobic capacity will be indirectly assessed from fewer or restricted physiological measurements.

The basic physiological instruments are the treadmill, the bicycle ergometer, and the stepping ergometer. These are primarily laboratory instruments that make it possible to directly assess oxygen capacity. The indirect measurements are heart rate, arterial blood pressure, and blood properties, including postexercise blood lactic acid, hematocrit, and hemoglobin. Indirect measures also include systolic, diastolic, and pulse pressures.

The *physique and body composition* measurements and indices are the basic skeletal and external measurements, body composition determinations, and age and maturation indices. The basic determinations include somatotype and anthropometric measurements of weight, height, chest circumference, and abdominal circumference. Additional anthropometric measurements are length, width, girth, and adipose tissue. The body composition measurements are total body fat, the ultrasonic method of assessing body fat, and total body water. Skeletal age and puberty ratings are measures of age and maturation.

The *performance* instruments are the physical skills and abilities that directly represent the various elements in work capacity and physical fitness. Tests are selected to measure each ability. These abilities are muscular power, strength, the general endurance of the body as indicated by the power of the respiratory and circulatory systems, flexibility and change of direction, and the ability of the individual in speed performances. The items selected were judged to be adequate measures of the ability to sustain hard physical work of both short and long durations.

Phase Four. At the 1967 meeting in Magglingen, pilot studies were planned and designed to gather data on the standards. These pilot studies, which used various population and age groups, investigated the proposed testing procedures and assessed the reliabilities and validities of the proposed test items. The results of the studies and the continuation of the work led to the final approval of the standards at the 1971 meeting in Magglingen. These are the standards presented in Part VII of this text.

Phase Five. This phase represents the ultimate goal of the committee as recognized at its inception in 1964, which is international research in work capacity and physical fitness that deals with all important aspects of people throughout the world. This program was approved at Oxford in 1970 and is now in the process of being implemented in institutions in many countries. The objectives of the research program include continued work on standardization; a comparison of groups across national, discipline, and specialty lines; studies on the effects of the environment, social groups, training, experiences in physical activity, occupational work, and so on; relationship studies involving various items of measurement and different types of sports, designed to yield a more complete understanding of the dynamics of work capacity and physical fitness; and descriptive studies which would provide information about the levels of work capacity and fitness of people living under many varying circumstances.

The research program deals with population characteristics such as nationality (e.g., European, Asian), environmental conditions (e.g., geography, altitude, climate), racial groups (e.g., caucasian, negroid), social groups (e.g., tribal, peasant, laborer), sex differences, age, physique types, ability differences, types of sports, and personal status (e.g., education, religion). The details of this program are presented in Part VII.

This text and program are the results of the efforts of the Committee on Standardization. In the constitution approved in 1965, committee membership was designated as *regular* and *corresponding*. The authority in the committee rests with the regular members. The purpose was to give security to the proposed ongoing program through agreement of the regular members to contribute their services to the achievement of the committee's goals. These goals have been realized by the committee over a relatively few years of continuous work. The results represent the first set of interdisciplinary standards for the assessment of work capacity and physical fitness and a planned international research program.

The authors of the text are recognized authorities in some aspect of work capacity and physical fitness and have contributed their services. Their work will lead to an improved understanding of the physical organism and will provide the tools and instruments that can be used in widely varying circumstances to assess health and fitness and to aid people in the improvement of both.

This text represents the collected effort by members of the International Committee for the Standardization of Physical Fitness Tests. Their contribution to the development of this text and to the ongoing research program is a recognition of their high dedication to an improvement of health and fitness levels of people throughout the world. Agreement on measurement instruments and procedures and an understanding of the basis for health and fitness were viewed by the committee as the first needs. Work in the future will result in a very rapidly growing research program. The assessment findings to be derived from this research will serve as the basis for implementing programs to improve the human condition.

The work involved in the preparation of the text for publication includes research conducted at the authors' institutions and at the University of Wisconsin. Editorial reviews were made by the section editors and by individuals at the University of Wisconsin. In the latter instance editorial services were rendered by Mr. James Frances and Mr. Tom Grogg, as research assistants, and by university faculty members, who reviewed sections of the text against editorial criteria for publication. They were Dr. Allen J. Ryan, University Sports Physician, Dr. Bruno Balke, University Physiologist, and Mr. Donald E. Herrmann, Executive Secretary for the American College of Sports Medicine.

The committee acknowledges with deep appreciation Mrs. Martha Fisk and Mr. Tom Grogg for their editorial services and the work of Mrs. Helen Ringgenberg, whose administrative services were essential in meeting the schedule requirements for publication.

LEONARD A. LARSON

Contents

Introduction

Little doubt exists in the minds of scientists in sports medicine that wide differences in work capacity and physical fitness exist among individuals living under varying cultural and physical environmental conditions throughout the world. General observations and clinical examinations yield support for this judgment. Unfortunately, the specifics are not known and judgments to a great extent are limited to broad generalizations. This observation was possibly the major reason for the founding and the subsequent work of the Committee for the Standardization of Physical Fitness Tests. It was the early judgment of the group that preparing the necessary instruments for research was clearly the first order of business. Thus, we have the beginnings of the work by a group of scientists to gain specific knowledge and understanding about different groups of people in the world. Research studies and programs that develop out of their efforts will contribute to one facet of personal health and human welfare—the ability to do hard physical work and participate in physical activities of all kinds with the potential for obtaining favorable physiological and medical results. The current need for physical activity can then be demonstrated by empirical findings from various groups of people within the world population.

The content of this text is designed to present scientific and medical rationales and facts about the work capacity and physical fitness of man that permit him to participate vigorously in various daily requirements and, of equal importance, the ability to participate in physical activity in order to sustain and develop the functions of the body needed for good health and fitness.

The seven parts of the text and the appendices are designed to give knowledge and understanding about work capacity and physical fitness; of even greater importance, however, this text provides instruments and procedures for their assessment. The text therefore presents both the rationale and the techniques that will provide information needed by an individual if he is to obtain favorable results from direct participation in physical work and physical sports activity. The individual's work capacity and physical fitness potentials can be positively and favorably developed, but unwise use of physical work and physical activity can be destructive and negative. Judgments must be based on empirical data derived from the sciences and medicine. Each participant must be examined for physical capacities, abilities, and potentialities. This text is an attempt to provide the professional resources, instruments, and techniques for accomplishing these objectives.

1

Possibly the two major contributions derived from the work of the committee have been (1) the presentation of what is considered to be work capacity and physical fitness, which can serve the scientist in judging the participant's performance in a full range of physical work and physical activities (to accomplish this goal the resources of several disciplines were required); and (2) the development by committee members of both a theoretical understanding and a practical application of techniques for making assessments ranging from highly sophisticated laboratory procedures to field operations where practitioners are without the resources of such sophisticated equipment. One major value of the interdisciplinary work of the committee was that it provided an understanding of the validity of the assessments according to disciplines and the applied instruments and techniques.

Part I. These chapters are designed to present an overall view of work capacity and physical fitness. The content includes the full range of work and physical activity; it deals with the organs, systems, and functions of the human organism that are involved in work of varying intensities, durations, and frequencies. Before assessment procedures and techniques can be developed or applied, one must understand the human organic requirements for each physical task.

Part II. The value of, and the requirements for, the medical examination that should precede participation in physical work and physical activity is presented in these three chapters. What systems, organs, and functions should be examined, how they can be measured and assessed, and the worth or importance of the information are topics that are considered. The chapters also deal with the varying need for a medical examination according to the person's physical fitness and the severity of the participation requirements. Needless to say, a great variance exists.

Part III. Body physique and composition are closely related to work capacity and physical fitness. The structure of the body is a significant component of work capacity, particularly in sports at the higher levels of performance. It is most difficult, if not impossible, to become a world champion without a body structure that contributes significantly to performance and work capacity. Physical fitness, as a performing phenomenon, is also directly related to the tissue composition of the human organism. The chapters in this part present the content and relationship between structure and composition as they correlate with work capacity and physical fitness.

Part IV. The capacity of the organism for physical work and participation in sports activities can be assessed internally by physiological examination of certain organic systems. The basis for adequate performance in many work activities lies in the potential of certain systems and functions of the organism. Physiology, therefore, is basic to an understanding of all human performances, but particularly for those performances that require general endurance abilities. Assessments are made principally of the circulatory-respiratory potentials because they are central to adequate functioning of the human organism. The essential basis for training and preparation programs for physical work lies therefore in knowledge of the physiological characteristics of each participant.

Part V. The most commonly utilized procedures and techniques for the assessment of work capacity and physical fitness involve the direct measurement of human performance. Knowledge of theoretical relationships (interdisciplinary) increases the value of these procedures. Direct performance assessments are the most practicable for judging an individual in his day-to-day preparation for work and for desirable levels of physical activity. These measures do represent human resources but fail to provide the broader information that can be gained by applying instruments utilized in other disciplines.

Part VI. The chapters in this part view work capacity and physical fitness as a human developmental phenomenon. They consider questions concerning the capacities of the organism and how far they can be developed. Work capacity and physical fitness potentials vary widely with each individual, and the patterns for the development of each potential require understanding and special programs. The content of these chapters will aid the practitioner and the participant in determining levels of work capacity and physical fitness suitable for individual capabilities and in setting goals that are reachable and desirable.

Part VII. This portion of the text contains the standards for the assessment of work capacity and physical fitness. The descriptive content also makes it possible for the professional worker to actually apply the procedures used in making the assessments. Procedures by which one can measure work capacity and physical fitness have been derived from the contributions made by researchers in each discipline. Because work capacity and physical fitness are generally specific to each work task, it becomes a function of the professional practitioner to select the items, content, or procedures essential for judging the status of each individual from each of the four disciplines representing the resources of this text. In most cases, all the disciplines will be involved in one fashion or another, but in some instances the procedures used will come essentially from a single discipline.

The Future and Goals

This text represents the fulfillment of the two major objectives of the Committee for the Standardization of Physical Fitness Tests. The ultimate goal was to initiate and operate an international research program dealing with the work capacity and physical fitness of people from all parts of the world. However, before this goal could be realized, it was necessary to determine the nature of work capacity and physical fitness within the context of conditions that exist in various parts of the world, and then to select and standardize research procedures, instruments, and techniques among the relevant disciplines so as to yield reliable and valid results. These two goals have been accomplished over a period of ten years of international work. The content of the text can now be applied to research programs in all countries involving all the various population groups within each country. Of course, adaptations are needed and can be made for special circumstances and for individuals requiring services deviating from the normal.

The Human Organism at Work

Part I

SECTION EDITOR:
T. ISHIKO
Juntendo University

The Organism at Work

1

Leonard A. Larson
The University of Wisconsin
Madison, Wisconsin

Physical activity is one of the basic essentials in sustaining life. It is classified along with the other essentials, such as food, sleep, and rest, which constitute the daily needs of human beings. In addition, physical activity is a basic essential in human development. Without it, the body would retrogress and bodily functions would be impaired. The human organism is dependent upon physical activity or physical movements. For levels of activity beyond the day-to-day needs, physical activity is required to develop or improve the functioning of organs and systems so as to permit higher levels of action—physical, emotional, and intellectual.

Physical activity is not only a basic need in sustaining life, but it also has amazing potential in social and cultural life. Physical activity, in the form of sports and athletics, is a miniature society containing all the requirements for organization and direction that are found in the larger society. The team contains the elements of democratic human relations, ranging from respect for the individual personality to group self-government. Physical activity, in an organized team form, is a person-to-person, group-to-group, social and interpersonal phenomenon. The individual as a social being is influenced by the stresses of hard, vigorous play or competition. The personal qualities of cooperation, dignity, and equality are only some of the social and personal concepts being applied. The individual is constantly adjusting himself to others and to the physical environment. All these qualities are contained in physical activity. The influence of sports and athletics in the development of highly desirable levels of adjustment is strong. Matters of race, religion, ethnic origin, and nationality are resolved through the process of respect for the teammate who drives toward improvement and contributes his abilities to the success of the team.

No attempt will be made in this presentation to identify the complete role of physical activity in the life of the people. Rather, this chapter will consider the social and cultural aspects of life in order to judge the place or the relationships of physical activity to it. The approach will involve the classification of physical activity into its various applications. We hope the results will yield some understanding of the role of physical activity in the life of the people. This analysis will provide a basis for better understanding the presentation of the scientific and medical rationales of physical activity as it contributes to the development of the human organism in terms of work capacity and physical fitness. The fitness of man is also considered in the context of life's demands found in the social and cultural conditions of the family, community, and nation, as well as the world.

Classifications of Physical Activity

In order to study or analyze any field of knowledge it must be defined, conceptualized, and organized into a meaningful structure. It is not possible to study or to apply single concepts systematically without viewing them in all possible relationships and contexts. The only exception might occur when one is interested in the analysis of the single concept itself rather than the relationships, references, or applications it might have. Conceptualizing a body of knowledge, however, is always an excellent starting reference. It provides for larger understandings even when only minute details become the objective.

Human physical activity or the movement of the organism in all its daily tasks is a most complex phenomenon. It involves all the joints of the body, the limbs utilized in movements of the joints, and sections of the body, when movements require more than joint or limb action. The latter are the patterns or systems of human movements applied in work, play, or in meeting daily needs.

The systems or patterns of human movement display an infinite number of combinations and strategies in games, sports, athletics, recreational activities, and other forms of physical activity that have meaning, value, and direction. Classification, therefore, has at least three references for consideration—the basic joint movements, the patterns or systems of human movement derived from the potential range of joint movements, and then the various combinations of strategies in games, sports, and other organized forms of physical activity. Classifications of all forms or applications of physical activity start with these three basic references.

It is a most difficult task, but an essential one, to prepare a conceptual structure and an organizational framework that will include all the movements of man and a structure that will include all possible applications. Even if all the details in the organizational framework are not complete, it would be most helpful for further study to have the overall structure complete so as to establish a classification reference. Such a structure will provide an understanding of physical activity that will be useful in all its scientific or professional applications. With an organizational structure, the study of physical activity will become more meaningful.

The most basic movements of the organism involve limb articulations along with their anatomical capacities. These movement potentials represent the capacities of muscular contractions around the joints of the organism (see Table 1-1). Regardless of the size or the intensity of human movement, limb articulations constitute the basic element. Movements of the fingers, hands, feet, or toes are examples. As physical activity becomes more complex, so does the involvement of the human organism in meeting activity requirements. Human movement can also be viewed from workload or caloric requirements. When movements include only the hands, feet, or the smaller segments of the body, the energy costs are low. When the total body is in action, and if the action is intense, the costs will be considerably higher. This represents another basis for the classification of physical activity.

Fundamental movements of the limbs, originating from the joints of the body, can be advanced to more complex fundamental systems or patterns of the total organism (see Table 1-2). These are the systems or patterns of locomotion (e.g., running), nonlocomotion (e.g., stretching), rhythm (e.g., dancing), gravity (e.g., jumping), friction (e.g., sledding), and patterns of manipulation with both light objects (e.g., precision) and with heavy objects (e.g., pulling).

A third context for the classification of physical activity involves its application in strategies of organized movement patterns or systems (see Table 1-3). The classification also provides for activities in their most basic forms. The strategies include applications within several professional, scientific, or administrative frameworks. There are eleven categories, each having special meaning and application. For example, the classification "Organizational Type" has special value in planning administratively for physical activity. The organizational type of activity will indicate the administrative requirements (space, time, equipment, and so on) needed for the activity. Activities classified under "Developmental Potentials" will be helpful in planning activities designed to achieve developmental objectives for the individual.

Because the classification of physical activities by strategies represents physical activity in its social, cultural, and professional contexts, the nature of the applications will be briefly reviewed.

Classification by Organizational Type

Classification of physical activity on the basis of systems or patterns for performance or participation is the most common form. It is probably traditional because of the applications of physical activity in instructional programs. When considering an activity for instruction, the nature of the activity itself is probably the most immediate consideration, that is, whether

[*Text continued on page 16.*]

Table 1-1 Basic Human Movements

Flexion[1]	Extension[2]	Abduction[3]	Adduction[4]	Circumduction[5]	Rotation[6]	Gliding[7]
Hip	Hip (little hyperextension)	Hip	Hip	Hip	Hip	Knee (patellar)
Touching toes	Standing	"Snow plow" in skiing	Skiing	Trunk rotation	Twists in diving	Running
"Tuck" position	Jump for height	Leg splits	Crossing legs	Shoulder	Knee (slight)	Intertarsal
Knee	Back handspring	Shoulder	Shoulder	Cricket bowling	Swimming "whip kick"	Running
Walking	Knee (no hyperextension)	"Iron cross" in still rings	Moving arms to side from the horizontal positon	Wrist	Shoulder	Elbow
Squatting	Sprint start	Holding arms out at sides when balancing	Wrist	Rope skipping	Gymnastics, ring work	Throwing
Ankle	Climbing stairs	Wrist	Gymnastics—work on the rings	Elbow	Elbow (except at radioulnar joint)	
Walking	Ankle	Gymnastics work on the rings	Fingers	Rope skipping	Badminton stroke	
Running	Basketball rebounding	Fingers	Bringing fingers together	Ankle	Wrist	
Toe	Toe	Spreading fingers as in a handstand	Spine	Ankle circling exercise	Throwing	
Running	Walking	Spine	Straightening after side-bending		Spine	
Sprint start	Running	Side-bending exercise			Turning the head	
Shoulder	Shoulder					
Arm swing in running	Arm swing in running					
Elbow	Gymnastics—horizontal bar work					
Biceps curl	Elbow (no hyperextension)					
Wrist	Throwing					
Throwing	Pushups					
Fingers	Wrist					
Throwing	Throwing					
Spine	Fingers					
Back dive	Throwing discus					
	Spine					
	Trunk "curls"					

[1] Occurs when the angle between two body parts decreases. "Bending" refers to this action. Foot flexion is generally called dorsiflexion. Flexion is fundamental to the majority of sports, dance, aquatics, and gymnastics, as well as to daily tasks.

[2] Occurs when the angle between two body parts increases. This action is often called "straightening." It is the opposite of flexion and occurs whenever flexion takes place. Included in the meaning of extension is hyperextension—continuation of movement past straight alignment. Extension of the foot is generally termed plantar flexion.

[3] Occurs when there is lateral movement away from the central plane of the body. Abduction takes place most often at the hip and shoulder joints in sports.

[4] Occurs when there is movement inward toward the central plane of the body. It is the opposite of abduction and takes place whenever there is abduction.

[5] This is actually a combination of flexion, extension, adduction, and abduction. Circumduction occurs when the end of a body segment describes a circular pattern.

[6] Occurs when a body segment moves around its own longitudinal axis and is often called turning or twisting. The body part may be rotated medially or laterally (inward and outward). Supination and pronation refer to upward and downward turning of the palm, respectively. Similarly, eversion refers to outward rotation of the plantar surface of the foot and inversion to inward rotation.

[7] Occurs when the contour of one bony surface glides more or less freely over the cartilaginous covering of its neighbor.

SOURCES

King, Barry G., and Mary Jane Showers: *Human Anatomy and Physiology.* Philadelphia, W. B. Saunders, 1963.
Munroe, A. D.: *Pure and Applied Gymnastics.* London, Arnold, 1959.
Schurr, Evelyn: *Movement Experiences for Children.* New York, Appleton-Century-Crofts, 1967.
Scott, Gladys M.: *Analysis of Human Motion.* New York, Appleton-Century-Crofts, 1963.

Table 1-2 Basic Movement Systems

Locomotion[1]	Rhythm[2]	Gravity[3]	Friction[4]	Manipulation of Light Objects[5]	Manipulation of Heavy Objects[6]	Swimming[7]
Walking	Dancing	Jumping	Sliding	Precision	Pushing	Strokes
Recreational walking	Social dancing	High jump	Basketball defense	Basketball shooting	Football block after contact is made	Free style
Golf	Women's floor exercise	Long jump	Baseball	Typing		Back crawl
Running		Diving	Starting	Throwing	Pulling	Aquatic games
Baseball		Springboard diving	Sprinting	Baseball	Tug of war	Water polo
Tennis		Trampolining	Football	Discus	Throwing the hammer	Games of low organization
Hopping		Vaulting	Stopping	Catching		
Triple jump		Pole vaulting	Tennis	Football	Lifting	
Children's play		Horse vaulting	Dodgeball	Baseball	Weight lifting	
Skipping			Landing	Striking	Carrying	
Children's play			Jumping	Handball	Hiking with pack	
Movement education			Vaulting	Soccer		
Galloping			Changing direction			
Children's play			Football			
Movement education			Ski slalom			
			Balancing			
			Gymnastics			
			Football			
			Skating			
			Speed			
			Hockey			
			Skiing			
			Cross-country			
			Downhill			

[1] Emphasis is on moving the body through time and space. The simplest form of locomotion, walking, is likely to be the most efficient act in which the human being engages. The principal joint movements are flexion and extension at the hip, knee, ankle, and toe, and inward rotation of the hip. Running, hopping, skipping, and galloping involve essentially the same joint movements.

[2] Emphasis is on moving the body according to arbitrary patterns of time divisions described by voice, drum, and so on. Although there is no doubt much of human movement is rhythmical to the eye, rarely is movement in sport conducted according to arbitrary patterns. Of course, almost all basic movement systems can be adapted to rhythm patterns.

[3] Emphasis is on exploiting gravity. The "in the air" phase of jumping and diving generally consists of rotation around the body's transverse axis or longitudinal axis. In vaulting, especially pole vaulting, elbow extension is often a main propelling force.

[4] The nature of the surface upon which one performs is the major environmental factor. Emphasis, then, is on exploiting the nature of the surface.

[5] Emphasis is on skill in producing effects on objects in the environment. In most of these patterns the hand is the main functional unit; flexion and extension of the fingers are the principal movements.

[6] Emphasis is on use of maximal or near maximal force in affecting objects in the environment. Elbow flexion and extension and knee extensions are probably the most important basic movements.

[7] Swimming is unique because it is conducted in the medium of water where buoyancy counteracts the pull of gravity. Because water offers resistance, progress is difficult and swimming is among the least efficient of man's activities in terms of energy input/work output.

13

Table 1-3 Strategies of Movement Systems

Organizational Type[1]	Developmental Potentials[2]	Professional Applications[3]	Objectives[4]	Applications as an Academic Discipline[5]	Administrative Requirements[6]
Low organization activities	Muscular power	Sports and athletics	Individual health	Biology	Outdoor facilities
Playing catch	Long jump	Golf	Jogging	Endurance	Hiking
Shooting baskets	Sprinting	Hockey	Calisthenics	activities	Soccer
Tag	Kicking	Baseball	Swimming	Adapted	Skating
Individual	Muscular strength	Leisure and	Effective	activities	Resident camps
activities	Weight training	culture	utilization of	Cross-country	Swimming
Swimming	Isometrics	Hiking	human	running	Canoeing
Archery	Gymnastics	Bowling	organism in	Sociology	Riding
Gymnastics	Muscular	Camping	work, play,	Group games	horseback
Dual activities	endurance	Education	and rest	Team games	Indoor facilities
Fencing	Push-ups	Dance	Walking	Outdoor living	Basketball
Wrestling	Handstands	Life-saving	Standing	Psychology	Gymnastics
Tennis	Running	Football	Relaxation	Competitive	Circuit
Team activities	Flexibility	Health	techniques	sports	training
Baseball	Bending	Weight lifting	Knowledge,	Individual	Recreation
Basketball	exercises	Jogging	understanding,	sports	buildings
Water polo	Gymnastics	Walking	and apprecia-	Team sports	Dance
Group activities	Twisting	Institutions	tion of the	Physical	Badminton
Calisthenics	exercises	Swimming	human	sciences	Relay games
Tag games	Accuracy	Dance	organism and	Running	Stadiums and
Relays	Dancing	Fitness	the process	Kicking	fieldhouses
Aquatics	Batting	activities	essential for	Jumping	Basketball
Diving	Bowling	Dance	development	Philosophy	Football
Swimming	Balance	Folk	and	Sports	Indoor track
lengths	Ball on nose	Social	maintenance	Games	
Synchronized	Handstand	Jazz	Distance running	Physical	
swimming	Skating	Preventive	Weight training	education	
Conditioning	General endurance	medicine	Hiking	History	
exercises and	Bicycling	Jogging	Social efficiency	Sports	
activities	Skating	Calisthenics	Team games	Games	
Weight training	Swimming	Walking	Dance	Physical	
Distance running	Speed	Recreation	Camping	education	
Calisthenics	Sprinting	Outdoor living	Democratic		
Remedial activities	Throwing	Dance	qualities of		
Weight lifting	Punching a bag	Skiing	leadership and		
Jogging	Agility	Rehabilitation	fellowship		
Swimming	Obstacle course	Walking	Team games		
	Football half back	Running	Outdoor living		
	Dodge ball	Calisthenics	Community		
	Coordination	Sports medicine	projects		
	Skipping	Treadmill	Individual as a		
	Catching	running	self-adjusting		
	Kicking	Fitness training	organism		
	Alertness	Jogging	Self-testing		
	Basketball		Cross-country		
	Tennis		running		
	Baseball		Team games		
	Steadiness				
	Fowl shooting				
	Putting				
	Shooting a gun				
	Timing				
	Passing				
	basketball				
	High jumping				
	Breaking into				
	clear in soccer				
	Rhythm				
	Modern dance				
	Floor exercise				
	Ballet				
	Reaction time				
	Boxing				
	Wrestling				
	Football line				
	play				

Physical Environment [7]	Age Requirements [8]	Maturation Requirements [9]	Environmental Settings [10]	Energy Expenditure [11]
Land	Birth to 3 years	Infant (first year)	Geographic location	Light (2.5–5 kcal/min)
Running	Play	Gross motor	Arctic—snowskiing	Bicycling 5 mph
Skiing	Gross motor	movement	Temperate—tennis	Shining shoes
Walking	movement	Begins fine motor	Subtropical—golf	Mowing lawn
Water	Fine motor	movement	Tropical—shuffleboard	Ping pong
Water skiing	movement	Play	Climate	Moderate (5.1–7.5
Swimming	3–5 years	Early childhood	Hot wet—walking	kcal/min)
Water polo	Jungle gym	(first to sixth	Hot dry—baseball	Push ball
Air	Slides	year)	Cold wet—bowling	Digging with pickaxe
Sky diving	Swings	Jungle gyms	Cold moderate dry—	Bicycling 10 mph
Jumping	6–7 years	Climbing	skating	Heavy (7.6–10 kcal/min)
Aerial trapeze	"It" games	"It" games	Moderate wet—	Touch football
	Relays	Late childhood (sixth	handball	Horseback riding at a
	Throwing and	to tenth year—	Altitude	gallop
	catching balls	boys)	0 ft—sprinting	Karate
	8–9 years	Team games	+ 6000 ft—golf	Very heavy (10.1–12.5
	Tag games	Ball games	+ 12000 ft—high	kcal/min)
	Cowboys and	Rough and tumble	jumping	Basketball games
	indians	Adolescence (twelfth	Urbanization	Bicycling 15 mph
	Baseball	to twentieth year	Rural—horseback	Exhausting (12.6+
	10–11 years	—boys)	riding	kcal/min)
	Soccer dodge ball	Fitness activities	Urban—handball	Ice hockey
	Mass volleyball	Game 'skills	Industrial—bowling	Running at 7.5 mph
	Baseball	Swimming	Sociocultural	Cross-country skiing
	12–13 years	Postadolescence	Primitive—hunting	at 6 mph on hard
	Softball	(twentieth to	transitional—baseball	snow
	Tennis	twenty-fifth year)	Modern—scuba diving	
	Volleyball	Golf		
	14–15 years	Tennis		
	Swimming	Running		
	Conditioning			
	exercises			
	Tennis			
	16–17 years			
	Distance running			
	Badminton			
	Dance			
	18–22 years			
	Swimming			
	Ice skating			
	Golf			
	22–45 years			
	Canoeing			
	Tennis			
	Bowling			
	46–65 years			
	Jogging			
	Golf			
	Calisthenics			
	65+ years			
	Walking			
	Swimming			
	Calisthenics			

[1] Classification is according to the degree and type of organization required to conduct the activity; degree of organization ranges from almost none—such as in low organizational games when there are few rules and when a variable number of players can participate—to highly structured team athletics. Knowledge of the number of participants required (one, two, four, team, or variable) enables administrators to organize equipment, and so on.

[2] Appropriate physical activity, conducted correctly, can contribute to the development of the human organism in a variety of ways. Developmental potentials, then, are those dimensions of human physical performance that may be enhanced by activity. Although what should comprise these components is frequently argued in the literature, the above is intended to be an all-inclusive classification.

[3] This classification refers to the facets of physical activity where professional personnel—those who devote their occupational careers to the pursuit of excellence in the activities—are to be found. These may range from the professional athlete to the scientist working in the field of exercise physiology.

15

it is organized as a team sport, dual activity, individual sport, or otherwise. Classification of physical activity by organizational type is highly related to plans for instruction, leadership requirements, space needs, facilities, and time schedules. This classification is basically for *administrative* considerations and is concerned with the *structure* of the activity itself, not with the worth of the activity for human development or other possibilities or potentials.

Classification by Developmental Potentials

Strategically structured physical activity (the most common application) can be classified in terms of the potentials of the activity for the development of the human organism. It should be noted that physical activities will vary considerably in their potentials for human development (see Table 1-3). Classification of physical activity according to the development criterion gives understanding about an activity that cannot be obtained when activities are classified by "Organizational Type." Information about the developmental potential of physical activity has many values, among the most important of which is instruction geared toward the achievement of goals for human development. This classification provides an excellent basis for the scientific study of physical activity in its role in human development. It also represents a starting point for programs of physical activity in which human development is the goal. Development should be the object for all instructional programs and, in fact, for all people. Physical activity should be con-

---

[4] Although there may be a variegated range of objectives for physical activity (e.g., making money could be one), the above list refers to physical education in the broad sense of the term. Objectives and claims for physical education have proliferated for decades and are often the subject of dispute; however, the present list encompasses those most frequently advanced.

[5] With the human organism in movement as the focus of attention, the above broadly conceived disciplines seek to understand man in motion from their special vantage points. Due to the current tendency to investigate human movement within nearly every discipline in the academic spectrum, attempts to delineate the body of knowledge comprising the study of movement have proved difficult and, not surprisingly, little agreement has been reached.

[6] This classification refers to the administrative requirements—in terms of facilities required to conduct various physical activities—for a community. Ideally, then, to provide for the activity needs of all its citizens, a community will have all the above facilities. The facility, of course, often determines the type of activity that can be conducted.

[7] Man in motion can be characterized by the environment in which he moves: land—with its subclassifications of grass, snow, cement, dirt, sand, and so on; water; and air. Outer space could be a fourth and, assuredly, will receive greater attention in the future.

[8] Educational and recreational institutions attempt to build their activity programs on types of movement most appropriate to the age of the participants—physically, psychologically, and socially—although chronological age does not always accurately reflect physical, psychological, or social level, it appears to be the most efficient indicator currently available, although this state of affairs is certainly changing.

[9] Certain "minima" of muscular activity are necessary for normal growth and for maintaining the integrity of tissues during the years of physical maturation. Thus, human beings must literally move to stay alive. In addition, beyond these minima, heavy exercise during the growing years can dramatically affect muscle tissue and, apparently, favorably affect the growth in weight and diameter of bone tissue.

[10] A complete list of environmental settings would be endless; the present one refers only to the physical and sociocultural environment. Environmental variables, obviously, may affect physiological performance. They also help determine what types of activity are suitable and, indeed, possible. For example, the residents of urban ghettos do not tend to play tennis since the required facilities, and perhaps motivation, are generally absent.

[11] Energy expenditure can be measured in terms of oxygen consumption or caloric cost. The classification of energy expenditure given above is based on number of kilocalories (kcal) used per minute. Tasks that require less than 2.6 kcal/min are not classified since their cost is little more than that of basal metabolism. The examples listed are for the 154-lb man—average for North America.

sidered as an important factor in the advancement of individual health, fitness, and general well-being.

Classification by Professional Applications

Physical activity is applied professionally for a number of purposes. Activities can therefore be classified according to professional objectives. There are at present at least ten organized professions that utilize physical activity as their basic program (see Table 1-3). In some instances the total professional program is physical activity, for example, athletics. In some cases it forms only a part of the professional objectives and program, for example, recreation.

It is amazing to note the wide scope in the professional values of physical activity. The point, to a large extent, is *how* the activity is applied to meet professional goals or objectives. There are some wide differences in this regard, for example, between the professions organized around the dance and those organized around athletics. The goals of each are quite different.

The United States is one country where physical activity is applied most extensively in education. It forms a part of the programs designed to achieve educational goals. When athletics are a part of school programs, the goals are educational; when athletics are a part of professional sports, the goals are economic. The same physical activities constitute each program to a very large degree, but some have more public and others have more commercial appeal.

A proper classification of physical activity according to professional worth is of considerable importance. The classification will aid in clarifying the confusion that could and does exist in understanding physical activity itself and, of more importance, in directing this activity toward meeting specific professional goals.

Classification by Objectives

Physical activities can be classified by the objectives that can be accomplished through participation. Developmental potentials vary with each activity; therefore, it is desirable to classify activities according to the objectives that determine which activities should be selected to reach specified goals (see Table 1-3).

The physical activities are classified by six objectives (Larson, 1970)—individual health, the effective utilization of the human organism, understanding of the human organism, the individual as a social being, the individual as a democratic leader-follower, and the self-group adjusting individual. These objectives can be achieved by the proper selection of activities and, of course, through proper leadership and participation. The classification will serve as an aid toward the fulfillment of purposes.

Classification by Academic Disciplines

Physical activity can be classified in terms of disciplines. As a discipline, activity is studied and analyzed to determine its contribution to human development and its relationship to human traits and characteristics. Activity is studied to determine its inherent characteristics in order to understand better the nature of the activity itself. The ultimate purposes are knowledge and understanding of physical activity.

Study and analysis, of course, must have a starting point. In the case of physical activity, this starting point is in the established disciplines of the sciences and philosophies. These are represented in Table 1-3 by physiology, psychology, sociology, history, physical sciences, and philosophy. The bases for study stem from the knowledge and understanding established in these basic disciplines. Facts and principles are then applied to physical activity to establish the nature of physical activity as an applied discipline. Physical activity has been studied in reference to all six disciplines; however, the most intensive analysis is in physiology where there is a span of many years of research.

Recent developments in the application of the disciplines include research in the psychology and sociology of physical activity. Future developments in physical activity will include increased emphasis on the disciplines of history, sociology, psychology, and philosophy. The result will be a scientific and philosophic understanding that will make physical activity more meaningful professionally for the teacher and the participant.

Classification by Administration

Physical activity is classified by administrative requirements in Table 1-3. It is most useful to know the type of facility needed by an activity prior to selection. This is certainly necessary for instructional purposes and possibly is equally important for recreational purposes. The administrative classification of activities in no way reflects their developmental value or worth. The classification simply places activities into categories according to facilities required.

Classification by Physical Environment

Facility requirements for physical activities include various environmental settings (see Table 1-3). Physical development will result when the individual attempts to overcome the forces provided by these settings. When physical activity is selected for educational purposes, the environment is provided under simulated conditions. The ultimate benefit to the individual is obtained from activity under natural environmental conditions, utilizing the mountains, the lakes, and all of nature as a laboratory for human development and particularly for the enjoyment of physical activity along with nature itself.

The medium for human development through physical activity is found in both the physical and social environments. Instructional programs simply simulate these environments for the sake of time and efficiency, but the objective is physical activity in the natural settings. The results achieved using the natural environment are more complete and satisfying than those achieved with a simulated environment where physical activity is the only objective.

Classification by Chronological Age

Participation in physical activity has an age requirement. The classification of physical activity by age therefore provides information on the appropriateness of the activity for a given chronological age (see Table 1-3).

Classification by chronological age is a common practice for professional workers applying physical activity for educational, recreational, or other purposes. Of course, when the individual does not have the skill or the physical resources required for an activity, successful or satisfactory participation cannot result.

The age classification has a sequential structure. When followed for human developmental purposes, participation results in the improvement of human abilities that make it possible to advance to higher performances in physical activity. These sequences continue until finally only a few (possibly one) persons can reach the ultimate level for a given age (for example, a world champion).

Age classification for physical activity is usually the starting point for both the professional worker and the participant. Regardless of the goals, the individual cannot achieve them without the ability (set by growth during the early years) to meet activity requirements.

Classification by Maturation

The maturation of the individual is probably the most valid reference for the proper fit of an activity. This is classification according to physiological age not chronological age. The difference can be significant. During the early years of growth, and up to maturity, the differences between chronological age and physiological age are noteworthy. With an increase in chronological age, the differences can become larger. Upon maturity, differences continue but for different reasons. It is then not a matter of physical growth (along with development) but of personal qualities, environmental influences, and particularly personal life practices.

The maturation levels during the growing years are generally described as prepubescent, pubescent, and postpubescent. Identification of these periods is possible. In this report the periods are categorized as infant, early childhood, late childhood, adolescence, and postadolescence (see Table 1-3). After the postpubescent or postadolescent period, classification is not a matter of maturation but of human development and the effects of aging. The most common classifications are young adult, mature adult, and the periods when aging itself will have significant influences.

Each period represents the physiological status of the organism that is reasonably or significantly descriptive of the group and the individual and, therefore, constitutes important references for the adaptation of physical activities to fit the individual's potential resources.

Classification by Environmental Setting

The classification of physical activity by both the social and physical environments has many useful purposes. One is for the adaptation of activity to the normal life of people. The individual lives in his environments. Human success or failure in health and development will be largely influenced by these personal settings. In addition, classification provides a more complete understanding of the activities as they fit the individual in his environments (see Table 1-3).

Participation in physical activity can be individual but, if so, it is still related to the physical environment. This can be hot-wet, hot-dry, cold-wet, and so on (see Table 1-3). Physiological processes are affected by the physical environmental conditions; selection, therefore, must be appropriate to the physical environment. That is, people live in a particular physical environment that is reasonably permanent. Activities must be adapted to the environment so that physical conditions are conducive or favorable to them and so that the full range of possible activities are available and encouraged for the people.

In addition to the physical environment, consideration must be given to participation with other individuals. This can be between two people or in small or large groups. Activities should be appropriate for the social environment as an individual or as a group. People generally form into some social group (family, club, and so on), and seek activities in this setting. Additional strength for the setting is obtained when the activities are appropriate—that is, if they fit the group.

Classification by environment is, therefore, most desirable and valuable.

Classification by Caloric Costs

Physical activities differ in their potential energy requirements. It is possible and most desirable, therefore, to classify activities by their caloric requirements in order to provide a basis for the adaptation of physical activities to the developmental needs of the individual. Classification provides a guide for planning physical activity programs designed to balance caloric utilization between input and output. The information is especially helpful for someone attempting to maintain acceptable body weight.

Classification is by caloric expenditure when participating during a defined unit of time and at a specific intensity. A five-group classification is provided ranging from activities that are "light" in costs to those that are "exhausting" (see Table 1-3).

The human body maintains itself through energy resources derived from food intake and through physical activity, which is made possible only by the release of energy from foods. Each person will differ in his caloric requirements; age, maturation, and body structure are some of the factors causing these differences.

Sociocultural Applications of Physical Activity

Physical activity is a part of a society and an integral facet of any culture. It varies in each nation, community, and within each group. Physical activity is and has been a part of the life of all people extending from the earliest years, when it was primarily a part of survival, to the highly developed current period of sports, athletics, and physical recreation. International sports have enhanced the importance of physical activity as a part of the life in many nations, and thus they are now a very strong integrating force in the world.

Physical activity and its organized forms (sports and athletics) as they are practiced and applied by the people will influence a society and its culture. Likewise, the social and cultural interests of the people will influence the nature and kind of physical activity in which they participate. Some of the most powerful forces that influence physical activity are found in social institutions such as government, school, military, the church, industry, and so on.

The individual, as a citizen, is responsible for the conditions that exist in a society. The cultural mores are determined by man. If man desires a setting that is conducive to the growth, development, and adjustment of the people, then he begins with the physical environment, practices, and life style of the people in this setting. What is desirable for the people must be determined, and social procedures enacted to accomplish the desired ends.

The only purpose of sport, and the various other forms of physical activity, as a social institution is to achieve goals that are important to the individual and are most desirable for a society. Optimal health and well-being cannot result from a sick society, and a sick society must be corrected. Positive individual development will upgrade a society, and it is advanced by social and physical environments that aid in the process of human development and adjustment.

The growth of sports, athletics, and physical activity in the lives of the people has been more rapid during the twentieth century than at any other period in history. The increase in the United States in professional sports alone has reached a level unpredictable only 25 years ago. The applications of physical activity to the personal life of the people, in industry, in religious institutions, and in colleges and universities are only some examples of its growth. The potential of physical activity as a social force is beyond the imagination of most people, in general, and of the scientists, in particular, who have only recently begun serious systematic studies.

Government

Society must have the interest and participation of all people in the affairs of the community, not only in social life but also in government. A citizen is obligated to be concerned and take action to maintain acceptable social conditions. The range of concern is from the physical conditions of the environment to the social life of the people, "as it is" to "what it should be."

The processes of industrialization and urbanization have increased rapidly over the past few years. The result is a more centralized government with greater powers, which therefore assumes increasing responsibilities for the welfare of the people. This responsibility includes the leisure life of the people. Recreational sports are increasingly becoming the responsibility of governments at all political levels. In the United States this responsibility has been manifested in some instances by direct operations (state and federal parks), and in most instances by strong supporting sponsorships. It is the recognition of the impact of urbanization and automation, with the resulting loss of physical activity, that has led governments to give strong support to outdoor recreation by procuring land, providing bicycle trails, and clearing the lakes and streams. These concerns and actions have been manifested not only in the United States but also on a worldwide basis.

Society, the general public, and governments have given strong support to programs oriented to sports, athletics, and physical activity. In many nations these activities are part of school programs (as physical education), community programs (as physical recreation), hospitals (as physical rehabilitation), commercial enterprises (as professional sports), and numerous other forms having support and sponsorship. The action comes from the people— through governments, private agencies, or through private sponsorship or private enterprise.

The most basic outcome of government support, involvement, or sponsorship for physical activity is a gain in strength for the government itself. Physical activity sustains the government by a development of the people to higher levels of life and living through desirable citizenship practices and activities. Sport and physical activities, because they are meaningful aspects of the culture, can contribute significantly to the management of people through democratic principles. Such principles are fundamental processes in sports participation. The principles of respect for the human personality, equality of opportunity, cooperation in the resolution of conflicts, the use of reason and intelligence for the solution of problems, and self-discipline as a basis for responsibility and self-government are integral parts of the sports participation process; in fact, these principles are so basic that sports could hardly exist without the fundamental democratic tenets of human relations.

Professions

Physical activity is basic in a number of professions. There are professional organizations developed around physical activity and devoted to accomplishing purposes concerned with these activities. It is amazing to note the professional potentials and flexibility of physical activity in terms of its services.

The next large section of this chapter will be devoted to the professional roles of physical activity. Only a brief review, therefore, will be made now. Currently in the United States, and in most other countries, there are ten established types of professional societies or organizations developed, structured, and operating with physical activity as their principal program or as a large part of the function of the organization. The purposes or reasons will differ with each type of organization.

The dance is an art form of physical activity or movement directed toward human expression. It is the communication of ideas, moods, and feelings through human movement. It is expression through and in the physical. There are several highly organized dance professions or groups dealing with various potentials or forms of physical activity.

One of the well-established professions concerned with physical activity is *education*. The educational profession attempts to achieve certain educational goals through and in physical activity. A number of the *health* professions also organize and administer physical activity for the accomplishment of health goals. A significant number of *social institutions* (YMCA, boys' clubs, sports clubs, and so on) program physical activity for social institutional reasons. In these instances physical activity is the medium for the accomplishment of goals for their clientele.

Other social institutions or organized professional groups also employ the medium of physical activity. The *leisure and culture organizations* (clubs, societies, fraternities, and so on) program physical activity as all or part of their services.

Practitioners in *preventive medicine*, as a part of their professional activities, program physical activity. *Recreation* professions are highly organized both publicly and privately with physical activity as one of the major facets of their programs. *Rehabilitation* has a very strong dependence on physical activity for social, emotional, and physical reasons or purposes. *Sports and athletics* are probably the most prominent in the development of physical activities with purposes ranging from pleasure by participation to spectator interests. *Sports medicine* has several professional groups organized to study and supervise physical activity to give protection and to provide positive results from participation in all forms of physical activity.

Disciplines

Physical activity as a facet of culture and society is developed as part of scientific disciplines. The objective is to understand the nature of the impact of physical activity on the human organism within the context of a discipline. The process involves the study of physical activity utilizing concepts and knowledge from the basic disciplines—physiology, psychology, sociology, history, physical sciences, and philosophy.

In physiology the empirical research is concerned with determining the physiological effects of physical activity of various types and intensities on the functions, organs, and systems of the body. Such studies have valuable professional applications. In psychology, the basic psychological concepts that have been theoretically defined and experimentally tested are applied to the individual within the context of participation in physical activity. The number of these studies, over the world, is rapidly increasing.

A more recent development has occurred in the discipline of sociology where physical activity has been studied under the rubric of "sociology of sport." The sociological nature of the individual participating in physical activity is now being rapidly advanced as a unique discipline.

The disciplines of history, physical sciences, and philosophy have produced studies of physical activity in many different forms. These disciplines are very necessary, indeed, to provide full understanding of physical activity and the effects of individual or group participation.

Labor and Industry

The second industrial revolution, which followed World War II, brought about tremendous changes in industry and labor. It has become commonplace knowledge that the world is experiencing a scientific and technological revolution. These changes are referred to as the "knowledge revolution," "second industrial revolution," or "automation revolution" by people the world over. These technological advances have caused serious social and economic problems for both labor and industry. On the positive side, the advances in technology have given man more leisure and have extended his control over the environment. Properly used, advanced technology could favor man both socially and economically.

Leisure is directly related to the advances in science and technology, which have provided increased free time and have reduced the physical work of man. Both increased free time and reduced workload are fundamental social-cultural matters and become problems if they are neglected. The constructive use of leisure and an increase in the physical activity of man are both essential for health, physical well-being, and certainly for an acceptable society.

The very rapid increase in physical activity programs—sports, athletics, commercial recreation, and health clubs—is a direct result of industrial and labor changes during the past 50 years. The end is not in sight as these activities have become one of the largest cultural components in society. The sport pages of the newspapers, televised sports, the increase in community swimming pools and golf courses, plus many other physical activity programs in community life are a few examples. It is most difficult to estimate economically the part that these activities play in the culture. Individually, a considerable part of the 16-hr waking time is spent on physical activity, either as a spectator or as a participant.

Education

The role of education in a society and as a part of the culture is profound. In the United States, education accounts for the largest part of the budget at the state level. In addition, the federal government is increasing its support for education.

Physical activity has always been an integral part of the education program in the United States, as it is in many other countries the world over. In all instances, physical activity in its many forms constitutes a large part of the culture of the people. This role is supported because of the positive contributions made to the life of the people, a very important educational objective.

There are many reasons why physical activity and sports have become important parts of educational programs—contributions to the health and fitness of the people, preparation for an active role during leisure time, the potential of sports in social integration, and contributions to the social and cultural life of a community. The efforts of educators are directed toward improving and increasing the contributions made by the physical activity medium.

It is highly desirable that physical activity become a part of education, more so today than at any time in history. In addition to the educational potentials, it is necessary to prepare people for the physical activity part of their life. Skills and interests in physical activity must be developed and thus carefully planned. Instruction is needed. In the United States instruction reaches all children because all are required to attend school. It is the time and place to establish desirable cultural and social patterns. Physical activity, in the form of sports, should be a part of community life that is an important addition to the school and the home. Cultural interests can be sustained and developed through community programs. The school and the home will play vital roles. The school also represents facilities that are part of the community.

Communications

The role of newspapers, magazines, popular books, films, radio, and television in modern societies and cultures goes beyond the imagination of the people. The communications media have the power to shape the social patterns and the cultural practices of the people. In fact, much has already been accomplished, although some is most undesirable.

The space devoted to sports in the newspapers, the time allocated on radio and television, the books written on sports and exercise programs, and the films on sport are examples that indicate the influence of the communications media in modern societies. In fact, productions involving sport and physical activity in a society represent a large part of the programming time and space of communications media. From a strictly commercial point of view, this practice has increased the interest of the people in the various sports. They are popular. The use of famous athletes for commercial advertisements attests to the popularity of sports.

The introduction and practice of sports and physical activity by all people are significantly supported by the communications media. Personal participation, in addition to viewing, is thereby increased. This is very evident from exercise programs that range from running to sport clubs in nearly all communities. The benefits of physical activity are recognized by the people.

Leisure

Technological developments have liberated man from routine and drudgery. They have given him mastery of time and space; they have given him the leisure that he has desired over many years.

One of the most important considerations for leisure concerns what man does or should do with his time. It could be spent very naturally in inactivity; man can rest, watch, do nothing. Such practices will lead to retrogression of the physical organism and the human personality. Man must be involved in social and cultural affairs that include physical activity.

Basically, man longs for struggles. He enjoys a struggle to master. He loves competition. Work alone does not provide this outlet and, certainly, unused leisure does not. Sports, athletics, and physical activity, in general, have become large parts of man's life. These activities, which provide an acceptable form of struggle, add to enjoyment, personal satisfaction, health, and well-being. Such personal practices should be encouraged by society and should be a part of the cultural setting for all people.

Health

The health of the people is a social and cultural desire of everyone. The struggles of a society are almost directly determined by the health and physical resources of the nation or the society.

The health potential of physical activity is probably the most important reason for engaging in it. Good health has a physical base because the body is a biological organism. The daily practices of man in all aspects of life will determine the effects on the physical organism, and these effects will establish the health and fitness levels. In this connection, to a very large degree, the destiny of man is determined by what he does daily.

Physical activity plays a major role in setting the health levels of the individual. Health is not only a question of a disease-free organism but also a condition that makes possible enthusiastic and vigorous living. From 60 to 70% of the American people are unfit for energetic living. Certainly this is evidence of poor health. Others who are physically active have developed resources of physical energy that sustain them on the job, with reserves remaining to enjoy leisure. Whether leisure interests are social or physical, one is unable to participate if exhausted.

During the past few years research has demonstrated the health worth of physical activity. The evidence is most convincing. It ranges from the ability to perform feats of skill and strength to proof that physical activity sustains the cardiovascular system in a normal functional state and helps prevent cardiac failure.

Physical activity has a large role in society with regard to sustaining the health and fitness levels of the people. A social and cultural life of inactivity, resulting from technological discoveries, must be compensated for by physical activity. The losses in activity that come from the elimination of physical work must be added to the life of man in leisure. Sports, along with enjoyment, add to one's physical health.

Religion

The moral and spiritual life of a society and a culture is highly correlated with the strength and the quality of living in the society. Religion contributes directly toward this end.

The church is a social institution functioning in a culture in a manner similar to the school, the home, and other social institutions. The concerns and goals are much the same—an acceptable society with desirable social and cultural practices. It is possible, and most desirable, for the church and religious institutions to become concerned with human behavior, social practices, and attitudes without interfering with or compromising the fundamental concepts in the various religions. The moral and spiritual values stemming from religious teachings tend to have common meanings to a society and culture.

The role of physical activity and sports has increased significantly, becoming a part of church programs during the past several years. The gymnasium, swimming pool, playgrounds, and recreation rooms in church buildings are designed for physical activity under church auspices. The gains in human development of youth have been most noteworthy. The role is an important one for the church, and thus the use of physical activity will probably increase. Such qualities as integrity, dignity, honesty, loyalty, and fair play are moral values that can be achieved through physical activity under church leadership and auspices.

Ethnic, National, and Racial

The social and cultural integration of people toward common human understanding is a community and world problem of the first order. Differences that appear unsolvable exist due to color, race, and nationality, yet these differences have no basis in fact. The place of sport and physical activity in contributing to the solution of these social problems has received extensive special reviews and test applications over the past quarter century. The results appear favorable to the use of sports by social institutions and governments as a medium for human understanding and communication.

Sports and athletics have been most successful in social integration. The motivation for success of the team is stronger than attitudes about the races. The acceptance of human skill and achievement as a basis for understanding is also stronger than biased attitudes and feelings. These are the results of sports largely since World War II. It is safe to say that integration (including ethnic and national) made its first significant strides in the United States through sports. It is only within the past few years that integration has been emphasized in other social, cultural, and vocational activities. Sports represent an ideal beginning because of the common goal held by all players—the strong desire to win.

The increase in international sports has been rapid only within the past few years. Ease of transportation is one positive factor, but the emphasis on international understanding is another. It is most pleasant to observe the Olympic Games. Youth from all over the world mingle in a setting of friendship and hard competition with only a few instances in which unfavorable attitudes and behaviors are displayed. Success in the Olympic Games has stimulated competition among countries throughout the world.

The strength of sport as an integrating force has been satisfactorily observed in the past few years. Its place in the social and cultural practices of each nation has been well established. And, the influence of sports will increase in future years when economic conditions permit transportation of teams on a worldwide basis.

Professional Applications of Physical Activity

Physical activity has professional potentials. It has been used as a base for several well-established professional organizations; athletics is only one example. As a profession, physical activity is organized to meet objectives established by the professional groups and represents the medium for all actions and accomplishments. Professions are structured with regulations that define membership, dues, leadership requirements, and officers along with conditions necessary for the efficient accomplishment of objectives. Established professional organizations employ personnel to operate the organization. In athletics, for example, there are a number of professional organizations. The National Collegiate Athletic Association and the American Football Coaches Association are both examples, along with numerous others developed for specific sports to give direction to the sport and the personnel associated with it.

A brief review will be presented on the professional applications to physical activity. The presentation will include ten aspects of professional concern with physical activity that are now considered to represent established professions. Within these ten categories there are numerous subgroups or professional associations to give specific direction to a phase of the total program. The coaches' associations, for example, are generally part of a larger parent professional structure.

Athletics and Sports

Physical activity, organized as athletics or sports, has many established professional organizations. They are international, national, regional, state, local, and institutional in scope. These organizations range from physical activities as athletics organized collectively (e.g., Olympic Games) to individually structured sports (e.g., American football). They also range from high-level commercially planned sports (e.g., National Football League) to locally organized sports developed largely for recreational purposes. All, however, are organized with varying degrees of structure and regulations, some on an informal basis but others highly regulated by paid leadership, regulated programs, membership dues, and a constitution that defines all procedures.

It is most difficult to judge the scope of organized athletics and sports in countries throughout the world. They represent a major aspect of the national culture and are practiced at a rapidly increasing economic rate in each society. Sports, as recreation, are widely enjoyed by people in most countries. Facilities are provided in nearly every city for sports for all age groups.

When judging any aspect of physical activity, the part organized as athletics and sports is most likely the largest and probably the most dominant in each social order. Organized sports and athletics have significant effects on nearly all individuals and play a large role in the culture of the people.

Culture and Leisure

Physical activity in a leisure or cultural context is common to all nations of the world. The activities are not structured as they are in commercially organized sports, but still represent a significant part of the lives of each person. In nearly all communities, facilities are provided, such as playing fields, parks, and swimming pools, on the premise that physical activity should be a part of the lives of people in the community.

The scope of physical activity within a culture can be easily ascertained by observing the planned activities of the various social institutions—the schools, community recreation programs, the churches, social groups, newspapers, radio and television, industrial leagues, community sports, and home facilities—organized or simply informal. Opportunities for physical activity (bicycling paths and so on) are available for everyone.

The growth of physical activity as a part of individual lives has been rapid during the past two or three decades. The loss of physical effort in work is one reason why physical activity is needed for each person. The scope is worldwide and applies to all individuals.

Dance

The dance is widely practiced and organized in various forms of physical activity. It is to a large extent organized in artistic forms for human expression. The range is from professional to personal, from ballet to social, from commercially organized entertainment to personal forms for recreational purposes. Dancing is a constituent part of the total professional organization of physical activity. Dances are forms of physical activity from the most vigorous to activities involving precision and grace.

The dance is a part of the culture of each nation. The naturalistic types represent the people of the nation; their traditions and mores are incorporated in the expressions of the dance. Physical activity in the dance is unique indeed. It is within the context of the culture and the social practices of the people. It is in close relationship with the people and their traditions.

Education

In the United States, and in many other countries, physical activities are organized as a part of the educational programs. They are planned specially to contribute to the total goals of education. The potentials of activity and the processes applied by specially prepared leaders will determine the possibilities for the development of the individual toward the goals set by the various educational programs. In the United States in particular the scope of educational institutions goes beyond the required school years for children. The programs of physical activities are planned in other social institutions, such as the churches and private social clubs. The activities also vary; athletics, sports, formal gymnastics, club sports, winter sports, and others are organized to aid the individual toward development as set by educational goals.

When the goals for education are within the total context of desirable citizenship, the contributions that can be made by physical activity are most significant. Values or qualities such as improved health, improved skill in the movement of the organism, knowledge about the human body and its care and development, and social qualities for adjustment of self and others are some of the potentialities.

Physical activity applied in educational programs is classified as "physical education." It is the education of the individual "in" and "through" physical activity. In the United States, it represents one of the largest professional organizations of qualified leaders. The profession is well-established with regulations and constitutions that provide direction for physical activity toward educational purposes or goals.

Health

Physical activity is part of a number of health professions in the form of programs for the improvement of personal health. These professional groups include all health education professions, health science professions, and professions that include the environmental influences on the health of the individual. Probably the most common application of physical activity is for the improvement of physical health. It plays an essential role in the development and maintenance of personal health.

There are many health professions and they are organized with specific objectives and structured to achieve their objectives efficiently. In education alone, a number of professional groups are well-organized; the American School Health Association is one example. Others are organized around school, university, and community agencies having health objectives. The role of physical activity varies in each instance but is a program, in part, for the accomplishment of professional objectives.

Institutions

Numerous social institutions include physical activity as a part of their total programs. The YMCA, for example, utilizes physical activity (about 60% of the total program) as a medium for the accomplishment of its goals. Other social institutions provide physical activity for other purposes. For example, industry plans organized sports to deal with problems of morale and to develop the well-being of employees. The number of social institutions are many, including clubs, societies, fraternities, churches, and social groups.

In a number of instances, professional organizations are formed from those employed as physical activity personnel in institutions. The YMCA Physical Recreation Society is one example; the Industrial Recreation Society is another.

It is most difficult to approximate the number of professional groups now established through physical activity in institutions. Because of the basic purposes and direction of the institution, the profession is developed around institutional aims, for example, the Boys Club of America. Each provides professional requirements and programs designed to upgrade institutional practices and objectives.

Preventive Medicine

The growth of professional interest in preventive medicine has been rapid in recent years. The role of physical activity is very much a part of preparing or rehabilitating the organism to avoid loss of normal functions. The efforts are particularly important when attempting to eliminate or reduce the effects of factors that will lead to the deterioration of functions or the breakdown of the body systems. Being overweight, lack of physical activity, tensions and stresses that are emotional in nature, and inabilities to meet stressful conditions in daily work are some of the conditions that lead to deterioration. Physical activity can aid in preparing one, in part, to avoid such deterioration. Poor physical condition of the organism is a great risk factor leading toward organic breakdowns.

There are a number of professional organizations that devote part of their programs to preventive medicine: physicians who devote work to this end, trainers of athletic teams who prepare the organism for stressful team play, sports physicians who treat injury, and others concerned with the organism and its preparation.

The role of exercise as an aid in preventive medicine has had major emphasis during the past three decades. It has been clearly demonstrated that exercise is a deterrent to conditions of the organism that lead to malfunctions and, in many cases, to loss of life.

Recreation

A large part of the programs of the various professional organizations in recreation involve physical activity as sports, games, athletics, camping, hiking, and as many other forms as there are personal interests. Professional recreation associations range from the international level to an infinite number in local communities. They are organized around interest groups related to the highly structured and well-established national and international organizations. The National Recreation Association is an example in the United States of an organization that has advanced recreation programs for many years. There are many others with paid leadership, organized by constitutions and regulations, with membership that pay dues and other financial activities to sustain the organization economically.

The recreational application of physical activity is most popular. It touches the lives of nearly everyone from the spectator to the active participant. Recreational physical activity is now a major aspect of each culture and is rapidly growing in need and popularity.

Rehabilitation

The professions of physical rehabilitation have had rapid growth during the past quarter century. Programs that began after World War II following injury and loss of functions gave emphasis to the applications of physical activity in restoring functions or in compensating for the loss of functions. The programs have been most successful. The growth of many professional groups has followed with programs planned in hospitals, schools, universities, and in various social agencies.

Programs dealing with social and emotional rehabilitation are specifically designed for each person. The range is from social disorders to specific activity designed to strengthen a muscle group, all with the objective of preparing for improved performance or an adaptation of the organism to a desired level of performance.

Sports Medicine

Professional organizations in sports medicine are relatively recent. The International Federation of Sports Medicine originated in Europe some five decades ago. In the United States, the American College of Sports Medicine was founded about twenty years ago. The professions deal with the medicine and science of the human organism in sport and physical activity. The objectives are prevention, protection, and correction of injuries, and preparation for physical activity in its full range of intensity.

The professions of sports medicine and sport sciences utilize the basic disciplines of the sciences, particularly physiology and psychology, and the various aspects of medicine correlated with the requirements of physical activity. The scope is large indeed—from physicians who give supervision to local sport groups to researchers in universities studying the effects of physical activity and the factors and conditions for improved performance and protection in performance.

Physical Activity in a World Setting

Physical activity in its basic form (as simple means of exercise) and in its applied combinations (as sports, athletics, recreation, and so on) assumes a large role in the cultures of the modern world. Hardly a person or a social institution is not influenced by physical activity either directly or indirectly. The range is from employers dealing with personal health and fitness of their workers to professions and scientific work concerned with determining the value of activity in achieving professional goals. Research programs in the science and medicine of sport and physical activity have increased rapidly within the past 50 years, with numerous social institutions and people being involved.

Physical activity within a society has always had a large place in the past. During recent years (since World War II) the growth of the influence of sports and physical activity on each person and on society has been rapid. Their importance in television, radio, newspapers, individual time, facilities, and space all give evidence of this increasing influence.

Sports, athletics, and physical activity in many forms are integrally woven into the culture of all nations. The nature of physical activity and its many possible combinations vary within each country. The traditions, ways of life, and mores will influence its nature and place. The effects on the people are far reaching socially, politically, and economically.

Social

The social interests and practices of people within a culture have an infinite number of variations. The combinations will differ to some degree in each culture with overall differences among the various social groups within a nation and among nations. In some instances, the social and political differences are highly influential.

All human behavior represents interrelationships between and among the elements and forces of the environment—both social and physical. These are the conditions that the individual lives with each day. The most powerful force is the social institution of the family. It is the basic and fundamental unit of society. During the twentieth century, the American family has undergone many changes in mores, location, stability, work schedules, economics, and, probably of greatest value to each person, in additional leisure and free time from work. This latter freedom is highly related to sports, athletics, and physical activity of all kinds and types.

The part that sport and physical activity plays in the modern life of man is large indeed. This is true whether the individual is a participant or a spectator. The very rapid growth of professional sports in the United States gives evidence of increased spectator interests.

The place of sports and physical activity within the social context of a society has greatly increased and is increasing. It is most difficult to judge the amount of daily time, space, thought, and action sport plays in each person's life, but it is very large indeed. Sport and physical activity are large and integral parts of the social life of each person, not only in the United States but in countries throughout the world. They are an influential social force.

Economic

Not only have sports, athletics, and physical activity become important factors in the culture for fitness and health reasons but also for economic reasons. Commercial sport is now big business. In the United States professional football, basketball, and baseball are all well-established economically. They are professions for the player and, certainly, for management. Physical activity as physical education represents one of the largest and most expensive parts of the school budget. Some of these funds are returned to the school through commercialization of sports. In universities and colleges, an attempt is made to cover all costs of intercollegiate athletics from gate receipts. In the United States the program in colleges and universities involves a number of sports, physical facilities, and paid coaches—representing staggering economic amounts when viewed nationally.

Without question, sport, athletics, and physical activity have entered into the economic world in the United States. Similar conditions are found in many other countries. This trend is now rapidly increasing on an international level and becoming a large force in the economy of each country. Involvement with all forms of physical activity is one of the largest social practices of the individual. Services to provide for the interest of citizens in physical activity require professional workers and economic support.

Political

Sport and athletics are large factors in the politics of a culture and of a nation. They have many involvements—in governmental operations, in the management of people, in providing desirable activities for people, in advancing the fitness and health status of the citizens, and many other political facets.

Probably the most powerful political worth of sport and athletics is its potential for the development of desirable citizenship. The team represents a miniature society. It contains all of the political elements needed for a good society—respect for the human personality, equality of opportunity, use of reason and intelligence for problem solving, and self-government, along with other political-democratic elements. These potentials represent one of the reasons for including athletics as a part of the school programs in the United States. Athletics, properly taught and organized in the schools, will prepare the individual for an understanding of democratic principles as they can be practiced in the home and the community. Similar objectives are now provided in international sports. The Olympic Games is one example of the potential for human democratic understanding through sports.

Educational

In the United States, in particular, sports, athletics, and physical activity are integral parts of school, university, and social agency programs. The potentials of physical activity have been found to be compatible with educational goals and with the overall purposes of educational institutions— preparation for citizenship in all its aspects.

The relationship between the goals of education in the United States and the potentials of physical activity are well noted and supported. Physical activity, properly organized and presented, can contribute to all goals of education in varying degrees. In establishing good health, physical activity makes a large and unique contribution. In democratic human understanding and self-government, it makes a large common contribution along with other school subjects. In the development of the individual as a desirable social being, it adds significantly to other school experiences.

Physical activity is a large educational force in all cultures—national and international. To achieve the potentials, however, requires leadership, as in the case of all school programs, that fully understands all educational goals and the process needed for their achievement.

Cultural

The culture of a nation is determined by the people and their social institutions. The culture is the sum total of all components of a society. Sport and all forms of physical activity are important aspects of the social world and the cultural components of social groups.

The role of sports and athletics in a culture is highly related to the leisure of man, which has increased and is increasing. Thus, sports and athletics are becoming a way of life for many people; hunting, fishing, golf, tennis, and all forms of physical activity are large parts of social institutions and of the culture. They provide a change from professional and vocational routines; they provide a challenge to man; they provide refreshment; they provide ways for social communications that are relaxing and fun; they provide ways for positive development of the human organism for protection against the stresses and the strains of modern life. Without question the role of physical activity in the world of nations is well-established. The structure provides a way for the human understanding of man that goes beyond the borders of nations.

BIBLIOGRAPHY

Boyle, R. H.: *Sport Mirror of American Life*. Boston, Little, Brown and Company, 1963.

Brailsford, D.: *Sport and Society*. Toronto, University of Toronto Press, 1969.

Brightbill, C. K.: *Man and Leisure—A Philosophy of Recreation*. Englewood Cliffs, N.J., Prentice-Hall, 1962.

Brightbill, C. K.: *The Challenge of Leisure*. Englewood Cliffs, N.J., Prentice-Hall, 1963.

Brown, R. C., and B. J. Cratty (eds.): *New Perspectives of Man in Action*. Englewood Cliffs, N.J., 1969.

Carlson, R. E., T. R. Deppe, and J. R. MacLean: *Recreation in American Life*. Belmont, Calif., Wadsworth Publishing Company, 1963.

Clark, K. A.: *Preventive Medicine in Medical Schools*. Washington, D.C., Association of American Medical Colleges, 1953.

Cozens, F. W., and F. S. Stumpf: *Sports in American Life*. Chicago, The University of Chicago Press, 1953.

Godfrey, B. B., and N. C. Kephart: *Movement Patterns and Motor Education*. New York, Appleton-Century-Crofts, 1969.

Jokl, E.: *The Scope of Exercise in Rehabilitation*. Springfield, Ill., Charles C Thomas, 1964.

Kenyon, G. S. (ed.): *Contemporary Psychology of Sport*. Chicago, The Athletic Institute, 1970.

Larson, L. A.: *Curriculum Foundations and Standards for Physical Education*. New York, Prentice-Hall, 1970.

Larson, L. A. (ed.): *Encyclopedia of Sport Sciences and Medicine*. New York, The Macmillan Company, 1971.

Loy, J. W., Jr., and G. S. Kenyon: *Sport Culture and Society*. New York, The Macmillan Company, 1969.

McIntosh, P. C.: *Sport in Society*. London, C. Watts & Co. Ltd., 1963.

Nash, J. B.: *Philosophy of Recreation and Leisure*. St. Louis, The C. V. Mosby Company, 1953.

O'Shea, J. P.: *Scientific Principles and Methods of Strength Fitness*. Menlo Park, Calif., Addison-Wesley, Publishing Company, 1969.

Pascal, A. H., and L. A. Rappina: Racial discrimination in organized baseball. Unpublished paper, proposed study to appear in forthcoming book *The American Economy in Black and White* (Tentative Title), 1970.

Shea, E. J., and E. E. Wieman: *Administrative Policies for Intercollegiate Athletics*. Springfield, Ill., Charles C Thomas, 1967.

Smith, L. E.: *Psychology of Motor Learning*. Chicago, The Athletic Institute, 1970.

Steitz, E. S. (ed.): *Administration of Athletics in Colleges and Universities*. Washington, D.C., American Association for Health, Physical Education and Recreation, 1971.

Wolfenden Committee Report: *Sport and the Community*. London, The Central Council of Physical Recreation, 1960.

Work and Activity Classifications

2

M. J. KARVONEN
Institute of Occupational Health
Helsinki, Finland

Phenomenon of Movement

Activity expresses itself in movement. The human body moves in space and time; the act of movement may be observed, recorded, analyzed, and classified. Our *motor acts* range from seemingly simple ones to the highest degrees of complexity. Painters, sculptors, dancers, and musicians use motor acts to create and carry the ideals of man and communicate the depths of his soul. The central nervous system composes the motor act in all its rich variability from contractions of bundles of muscle cells, the motor units. Muscle contraction also involves *metabolic* processes, the ultimate outcome of which is the conversion of the chemical energy of food into mechanical work and heat. The metabolic processes are measurable and may be used for scaling the intensity of physical activity in terms of energy, food, oxygen, or waste products.

When the human organism shifts from rest to activity, the increased metabolic rate recruits the support of a number of *autonomous mechanisms*. Increased ventilation brings more oxygen to the organism; the heart sends more blood to the working muscles; the sweat glands start to secrete in order to effect a loss of extra heat; and so on. In principle, each autonomously regulated body function that accompanies physical activity might be used as a measure of the intensity of exercise. Some functions are easily observable, such as the heart rate at any given moment or the rate of perspiration over a period of several hours, and have thus been widely used for the measurement of the intensity of activity.

The motor act is always the result of complex excitatory and inhibitory processes in the central nervous system and these again are influenced by the inflow of stimuli from a multitude of sensory receptors. Subjectively, man relates this process to his will. A movement may be *volitional* or *reflex*, a conditioned reflex or a combination of elements of different kinds.

The subjective experience of activity also has another side, the *perception of exercise*. Scales of the degree of subjective strain have been used to indicate the relation of activity to man. Such scales are, of course, not necessarily strictly parallel with the scaling of metabolic activities.

Purpose of Movement

Movement as Expression

Man, like other animals, expresses himself through movement. He does it when alone, and when in company; he communicates through motor acts. Even in our culture, with its rich use of verbal communication, nonverbal communication through movement still plays a large role in overcoming language barriers. Dance in its many forms is systematic expression through movement. Dance is, indeed, a language of movement. Even a system of notations has been developed for dance (Laban and Lawrence, 1947) which makes it possible to codify the choreographer's work.

Movement for Achieving Aims

Many of our motor acts are made in order to achieve aims, immediate or future. Simple reflexes are directed toward gaining something rather immediate, whereas the goals of complex volitional acts may sometimes be rather difficult to elucidate. The driving force of these goals may be predominantly turned to material benefits for the individual or his society; this we call work. On the other hand, the aims may be more on a spiritual level; here we are referring to play, games, sport, and art. The borderline between work and play is by no means sharp. The same sport may be practiced by an amateur and a professional. Expressive movement finds its place easily in work and is an integral part of play and art.

Physical Activity as Related to the Life Pattern

Work

The work of past generations has always been physical work. In modern society, however, an increasingly large proportion of working people are employed in sedentary occupations, where a minimum of physical work is involved. Work is commonly classified as very heavy, heavy, moderate, light, or very light. The assessment may be based either upon a subjective scaling or on various physiological parameters. More detailed classifications aim at listing either the occupation or the actual work done at any moment in the language of the "factory floor." The user of such a classification must be acquainted with the operations; otherwise, a description of work by occupation or by the name of the work process may easily become grossly misleading.

Sport

Professional Sport. Sport as a profession brings economic rewards like any other occupation. Nevertheless, the sportsman earns his income from maximum or near-maximum physical performances. His training program and working hours make his life quite different from that of other professions. In fact, the phenomena associated with physical activity and training are often to be observed in their most extreme form in the professional athlete.

Amateur Sport. Amateur sport is a wide concept and covers anything from sailing to running a marathon race. To use "sport" and "sportsmen" for classifying phenomena of physical activity is an inexcusable oversimplification. The sports event, the results achieved, the years of a sports career, the hours of practice per day or per week and its intensity are all needed to characterize a sportsman. The physiological literature contains too many examples where this essential information is lacking. The innate variation in structure found in people makes them individually suited for different sports, and the training required further develops quite different abilities.

Physical Education

Physical education is a program of activities that includes games, gymnastics, and sports. Its essential feature is the motivational framework. To use "physical education" as a description of physical activity thus gives very limited information. Again, the detailed program, duration, and some measure of the intensity of effort should be included in the description.

Recreation

Recreational physical activity fills a large part of the child's day. Primitive man practices it and has brought recreational activities to many cultures; dance and games are integral parts of the life pattern. However, in some cultures recreational traditions have become disrupted.

In western civilization, efforts are now being made to introduce recreational physical activity. Up to now, the success has been limited. To describe man's physical activity, some information on the nature of his recreation is essential. This becomes imperative when transcultural comparisons are made.

Fight and Flight—Emergency Situations

An animal in its natural habitat must be fit to meet enemies and other dangers. A large part of the spontaneous behavior of animals is believed to serve the purpose of keeping fit.

For human beings the dangers range from natural catastrophes and wars to myocardial infarction, from escaping an oncoming automobile to enduring the mental stresses of overwork, urban life, and interpersonal friction. Man might derive crucial benefit from physical activity if this would make him more fit to stand such stresses. Opportunities for studying this problem should be utilized to the fullest extent. Much of this study must be done on man in his normal ecological situation. Laboratory studies, even at their best, can only be supportive.

Conceptual Elements of Physical Activity

Our thinking uses concepts as its building blocks. These are, as a rule, derived from the observation of the physical world. This applies also to the conceptual structure of physical activity. Our thought processes have dissected physical activity into a number of parts that are considered largely independent of each other.

Skills

Skill is an ability to perform accurately coordinated, purposeful movements. Skills are specific to a large extent, although some skills may also have common underlying perceptual and motor factors. A skill, be it performing on gymnastics apparatus or playing the flute, may be graded by the consensus of experienced judges. The principles of grading may also be analyzed and given a verbal description. In the division of labor between academic disciplines, skills are generally handed over to the psychologist for analysis and measurement.

Strength

The unit of strength is kilogram-force (kgf). A defined scale thus exists for measuring muscle strength. In actual measurement, the conditions must be meticulously specified in order to obtain reliable results.

Speed

The speed of human movement depends on the speed of the muscle contractions as well as on the internal and external loads to be overcome. Internal loads exist, for example, in the contractions of the antagonist muscles. With heavy loads, the strength of the muscles becomes an essential determinant of the speed of contraction. In complicated movements, the skill element additionally enters the picture. Again, when the speed of human movement is being measured, the conditions of testing must be carefully standardized.

Power

Power is the concept denoting work per unit of time. The maximum power of the human machine depends essentially on the duration of the performance; maximum power is much greater in the high jump than in the marathon race. Power must always be related to the task. Work that involves large muscle groups releases more power than can be mobilized from smaller ones.

Endurance

The endurance of the organism has no place in the terminology of physics. As a physiological concept it also is heterogeneous. Static endurance, that is, the ability to keep a muscle contracted against a load, is something very different from the endurance manifested in long-distance races. In some situations, endurance in performance may indeed be a measure of a single physiological parameter, such as muscle glycogen. In other more complex situations, endurance reflects the ability of the organism to preserve its functional integrity against several interacting internal and external stresses.

Man Against Environment

Quite specific physical requirements are imposed on man in certain environments. These may be new to him, such as high altitude to a lowlander. On the other hand, he may have the background of numerous generations of adaptation to the habitat, like the pygmy to the tropical rain forest and the Eskimo to the Arctic.

Altitude and Space. The salient physiological feature of high altitude is the low partial pressure of oxygen in the air. For the climbers of high mountains and for the aviators of the recent past, the ability to endure hypoxia has been a crucial requirement. Even in spacecraft, oxygen is not supplied at its full sea level pressure. Physiological adaptation to life at high altitudes is a slow process.

Testing human performance at an altitude, natural or simulated, introduces the factor of tolerance of hypoxia. For populations living permanently at high altitudes, adaptation to the sea level conditions may also involve difficulties. Comparisons of the physical capacity of sea level and of high altitude populations are thus complex.

Diving. In diving, man exposes himself to high pressures and rapid pressure changes. The diving man shows physiological adaptations similar to those of the habitually diving mammals. Both adaptation to the environment and the degree of susceptibility to its hazards may show individual variation. High physical capacity has been considered beneficial for the diver. Whether it improves his adaptation or affords him protection against the unspecific risks of a foreign environment is not well known.

Thermal Challenges. In cold weather, the unprotected man's survival depends on his ability to produce heat by physical activity. Some minor additional mechanisms may improve adaptation. In a hot climate, other mechanisms are involved. The capacity to secrete sweat, to retain the stability of the fluid and electrolyte balance, and to keep up the orthostatic control of circulation are some of the physiological conditions that are taxed in a hot environment. In the long-term adaptation of the human species to a hot climate, humidity may play a larger role than the temperature (Hiernaux, 1968).

No simple test of physical performance capacity in a neutral sea level environment may be expected to indicate how the human body will be able to perform in widely differing environments.

Human Form and Function in Physical Activity

Physical activity may also be examined from the point of view of the human machine, of its parts and their functions. Anatomy, physiology, and biochemistry thus form the frame of reference into which the phenomena of activity are to be fitted.

Sensory and Motor Nervous System

Nerve impulses, both sensory and motor, are an essential part of every movement. Although the nervous system has a wide range of adaptability, in many situations it may become the limiting factor. Fast movements against small loads, complex movements, and repetitive work where sensory or motor fatigue may ensue are forms of activity where performance essentially depends on the performance of the nervous system.

Muscle

Muscle Strength. Muscle strength is a predominant element in many performances. It may be displayed in different ways. *Static* muscle strength is manifested by muscles that contract isometrically. Its opposite, *dynamic* strength, is connected with all muscle contractions in which the length of the muscle changes. A muscle that shortens during the contraction does *positive work* (*concentric contraction*). If, on the other hand, the load imposed on the muscle makes it longer, *negative work* (*eccentric contraction*) is said to occur. In terms of the strength of the muscle, these three types of work—isometric, concentric, or eccentric—are far from equivalent. The greatest strength may be displayed in negative work and the smallest in positive work.

Speed of Contraction. Each muscle has a maximum speed of contraction. Most rapid are the outer eye muscles, slowest are the big muscles of the trunk and legs. In sprinting, the limiting factor appears to be the speed of the contraction of the leg muscles.

Endurance of Muscle. In repetitive work, the same muscles are required to contract time after time against the same load. If the muscle group in action is relatively small, the factors limiting the performance remain local. The development of fatigue in such a situation has been much studied by physiologists but is still not completely understood.

Pacing of Work. In the contraction and relaxation of the muscle, metabolic load and recovery alternate. Not only the overall rate of the work but also the introduction of pauses at short intervals has been shown to have a major effect on the ability to perform protracted work at rates where anaerobic metabolites may accumulate (Astrand et al., 1960).

For each work cycle, a range of optimum rates exists at which the energy expenditure is lowest per cycle. However, the energy expenditure may also depend on the way the pace is imposed on the worker. In some types of work, substantially less energy is expended for work at a freely selected rate than at the same rate when observing outside pacing (Rönnholm et al., 1962; Karvonen and Rönnholm, 1964).

Supply of Energy

The contracting muscles receive their energy, through a series of enzymatic reactions involving phosphorylation and other reactions, from the chemical energy of carbohydrate and fat. The higher the intensity of the work carried out by the muscle, the larger the proportion of energy derived from carbohydrate. Body stores of fat do not become the limiting factor for exercise except in protracted starvation. However, the stores of carbohydrate in the form of muscle and liver glycogen are much smaller, and the maximum rate of carbohydrate formation from fat and protein is slow. In protracted heavy exercise, the exhaustion of the muscle glycogen stores thus determines the limit of endurance.

Although substrate is available in the muscle *in situ*, oxygen must be currently transported to it; there is practically no oxygen storage. If the supply of oxygen is not sufficient, a portion of the energy is derived from the partial breakdown of muscle glycogen into lactic acid. Aerobic and anaerobic work hence contribute a variable portion of the total energy output, depending on the intensity of the demand made by muscle contraction on the local circulatory supply and, in work involving large muscle masses, on the capacity of the heart to increase its output.

The exhaustion of carbohydrate stores may be prevented by ingesting carbohydrates during work. The supply of substrate is critical in protracted heavy exercise, such as long-distance cycling races or cross-country skiing, and in performances involving bursts of anaerobic work with its wasteful use of the muscle glycogen. When food is ingested during work, the function of the gastrointestinal tract may thus also become a critical factor in determining the maximum total performance capacity.

Internal Milieu

Heat Balance. In exercise, the larger part of the energy released is transformed to heat, which means that only a smaller part can be used for mechanical work. The extra heat is stored to some extent, but most of it must be transferred to the environment. In man, this occurs through an increase in skin temperature and through the evaporation of sweat from the skin. The capacity to sweat may thus become the limiting factor for work in a hot environment.

Water and Electrolytes. Through sweating, man loses water and electrolytes. Shifts of water and electrolytes occur also between muscles and the extracellular space. Dehydration tends to reduce the effectiveness of the orthostatic control of circulation. Increased blood viscosity slows down blood flow and thus reduces oxygen supply. Disturbances of the water and electrolyte balance may impose essential limitations on the work capacity, particularly among subjects unadapted to work in a hot climate.

Regulation of the Internal Milieu. Constancy of the internal milieu is secured through many regulatory mechanisms. Some of these are neural, some neurohumoral, some chemoneurohumoral, and so on. Several of these mechanisms use hormones as their effectors. Training the motor apparatus for higher performance also involves these mechanisms. When their functions are adapted to those of the motor act, the automatisms work smoothly. Only occasionally does an unexpected breakdown or exhaustion draw attention to their existence.

Factor Analysis of Physical Performances

Classification of work and activity is in principle also possible without recourse to any preexisting frame of reference, but purely through a formalistic approach. Factor analysis is a method that has been designed for just this type of task. It starts from a set of multiple data describing individuals, calculates a matrix of intercorrelations, and extracts the common factors from the matrix. In an ideal situation the approach is quite "blind," being unaffected by any preconceived ideas of the investigator.

In practice, however, the outcome is not completely unbiased. It is only too easy to introduce artificial factors into a factor analysis by using entries that are spuriously correlated with each other. This has been a weakness of some factor analyses in which physiological parameters have been introduced. A further limitation has been the use of data on untrained subjects at a low level of performance. Random variation of such primary data is large, dilutes the correlations of the matrix, and reduces the clarity of the outcome of the analysis.

The last part of a factor analysis consists of the rotation of the reference multidimensional space in such a way that the results can be given an understandable verbal description. The rotation may be done "blindly" or by using arbitrary guides. The interpretation of the results is quite often difficult and does not always fit preconceived ideas.

Several factor analyses of physical performances have been carried out. For example, the set of performances in the decathlon can be listed in the order of increasing uniqueness as follows (Karvonen and Niemi, 1953):

Event	Uniqueness
Shot put	0.24
100-meter (m) dash	0.27
400-m run	0.28
110-m hurdles	0.34
Broad jump	0.35
Discus	0.36
Javelin	0.47
High jump	0.57
Pole vault	0.61
1500-m run	0.77

The factor analysis revealed five factors, of which the first was called "general athletic ability." The second factor favored the jump events. The third factor remained difficult to explain; it showed negative loadings for the 110-meter (m) hurdles and the discus as opposed to a positive loading for the broad jump. The fourth factor was interpreted as "dead weight" with positive loadings in the shot put and the discus and negative ones in the 400-m run, pole vault, and 1500-m run. The fifth factor was associated with speed events but also showed positive loadings for the javelin throw and the pole vault.

Subjective Experience of Physical Activity and Work

Man judges the intensity of his work according to a subjective scale of effort. Certain work may be heavy for an old and weak man but light for a young and strong one. The perception of exercise is subject to measurement, hence, also to scientific analysis, just like other phenomena associated with work (Barry, 1967; Borg, 1971).

Also the anticipation of work situations may become associated with emotional attitudes. Genuine aversion to work may occur. An addiction to exercise may, on the other hand, develop easily. Symptoms of abstinence following an abrupt discontinuation of exercise habits have been reported.

Physical Activities of Men and Women

In each culture, there is a traditional division of men's and women's activities. This applies to both work and leisure. However, the division shows large differences among various cultures. The body build and physiological functions of men and women are different. A well-trained man performs, therefore, better in most activities than a well-trained woman. However, the best women in international sports are far superior to the great majority of the world's men (Jokl et al., 1956). Men's events and women's events in sports are distinguished more by cultural factors than by differences in ability structure.

Age Spectra of Physical Activities

The age spectra of the different forms of physical activity may be dictated by the economic necessity to work for a living or may be due to free selection of leisure-time activities. Physiological functions change with age. However, different performances do not change uniformly. In the Helsinki Olympic Games in 1952, the average age of male swimmers, cyclists, boxers, short and middle distance (100–1500 m) runners, hurdlers, and jumpers was below 25 years but was over 30 years among participants in shooting events, horse riders, fencers, walkers, and marathon runners. In swimming, the age range of the participants was from 13 to 35 years for men and from 14 to 36 years for women; in the track and field events it was from 15 to 42 for men and from 18 to 38 years for women (Jokl et al., 1956). Endurance events seem to favor older participants, at least in the running events. Altogether, age affects the physical top-performance capacity in a complex way.

The choice of recreational activities does not necessarily reflect the age spectrum of top performances. A good example is swimming; although the world elite is nowadays quite young, swimming is gaining great popularity as recreation among all ages.

Measurement of the Workload

Physiological Load

The work done by the organism may be translated into physical units using either of two approaches: one may measure the amount of mechanical work done in a standard situation, for example, using a bicycle ergometer, or one may measure the energy expended in any situation, generally from oxygen uptake. Table 2-1 shows a classification of work based on the rate of energy expenditure.

Work at the same power places a heavier load on a small machine than on a large one. In comparing the physiological load, a correction for differences in body size should be applied. Theoretically, most types of activity can be looked upon as consisting either of work done against gravity, and hence proportional to the weight of the body or of its parts, or of work independent of body weight. However, for practical purposes it is quite sufficient to effect the correction by dividing the total energy expenditure by the body weight.

A practical way of standardizing for differences in body size is to divide the energy expenditure during an activity by the energy expenditure at complete rest. The multiples of the metabolic rate at rest—or Mets—of several types of work are listed in Table 2-2 and those of leisure activities in Table 2-3.

Table 2-1 Classification of Occupational Work
(The rates of energy expenditure refer to actual work, excluding pauses.)

	Energy Expenditure, kcal/min	Heart Rate	Body Temperature, °C
Too heavy			
	12.5	175	39.0
Very heavy			
	10.0	150	38.5
Heavy			
	7.5	125	38.0
Medium			
	5.0	100	37.5
Light			
	2.5	75	37.0
Very light			

SOURCE: E. H. Christensen: Physiological evaluation of work in the Nykroppa iron works, *Symposium on Fatigue*, G. W. F. Floyd and A. T. Welford (eds.). London, H. K. Lewis, 1953.

The physiological load may also be gauged by measuring alterations in any physiological function that changes with exercise. Several possibilities offer themselves: frequency of breathing, rate of sweating, cardiac output, and so on. Heart rate is very easily observed and has been most widely used as an indicator of the physiological load. It reflects the sum total of several influences: energy expenditure, static work, rate of emotional tension, ambient heat load, and so on. On an average, the response to increasing workload is linear, but both the level and the slope show marked individual variation. Changes in the heart rate response to work reflect changes in the maximum aerobic power and are therefore being used a great deal as a training control with athletes.

Body temperature also rises during exercise. Whereas heart rate reflects all transient changes in the physiological load, body temperature tends to give an integrated measure of the load over a longer period. Table 2-1 indicates the use of body temperature for the classification of work.

Mental Load

Mental load is an elusive concept to measure. However, some methods for rough assessment are available. One of them, the simultaneous performance of multiple tasks, also lends itself easily to the study of combinations of physical and mental loads. One of the tasks has to be performed at a predetermined rate, and the rate and errors in performing a standard subsidiary task are used as indirect indicators of the variation in the mental load involved in the first task.

Hierarchy of Sports

When the best results achieved during one year by the best hundred athletes in a track and field event are plotted cumulatively on a probability

Table 2-2 Metabolic Cost of Occupational Activities

Activity	Work Metabolic Rate Divided by Basal Metabolic Rate, per min
SITTING: LIGHT OR MODERATE WORK	
a. Sitting at desk, writing, calculating, etc.	1.5
b. Driving a car	1.5
c. Using hand tools, light assembly work, radio repair, etc.	1.8
d. Just driving a truck	1.8
e. Working heavy levers, dredge, etc.	2.0
f. Riding mower, etc., as in individual work	2.5
g. Sitting for crane operator	2.5
h. Driving heavy truck or trailer rig (must include getting on and off frequently and doing some arm work)	3.0
STANDING: MODERATE WORK	
a. Standing quietly, assembling light or medium machine parts where speed is not a factor; working at own pace or a moderate rate. Can be using light hand tools	2.5
b. Just standing or just bartending	2.5
c. Using hand tools (gas station operator, other jobs where these are used other than assembly work all day)	2.7
d. Scrubbing, waxing, polishing (floors, walls, cars, windows)	2.7
e. Assembling or repairing heavy machine parts such as farm machinery, plumbing, airplane motors, etc.	3.0
f. Light welding	3.0
g. Stocking shelves, packing or unpacking small or medium objects, stocking grocery store shelves	3.0
h. Sanding floors with a power sander	3.0
i. Assembling light or medium machine parts on assembly line or working with tool or tools on line when objects appear at an approximate rate of 500 times a day or more	3.5
j. Working on assembly line when parts require lifting at about every 5 min or so, lifting involves only a few seconds at a time, parts weigh 45 lb or less	3.5
k. Same as above, parts weigh over 45 lb	4.0
l. Cranking up dollies, hitching trailers, operating large levers, jacks, etc.	3.5
m. Pulling on wires, twisting cables, jerking on ropes, cables, etc., such as rewiring houses	3.5
n. Masonry, painting, paperhanging	4.0
WALKING: MODERATE WORK	
a. Walking	4.0
b. Carrying trays, dishes, etc.	4.2
c. Walking involved in gas station mechanic work (changing tires, wrecker work, etc.)	4.5
STANDING AND/OR WALKING: HEAVY ARM WORK	
a. Lifting and carrying objects	
1. 20–44 lb (9–20 kg)	4.5
2. 45–64 lb (20–29 kg)	6.0

Table 2–2 *(continued)*

Activity	Work Metabolic Rate Divided by Basal Metabolic Rate, per min
3. 65–84 lb (30–38 kg)	7.5
4. 85–100 lb (39–45 kg)	8.5
b. Heavy tools	
1. Pneumatic tools (jackhammers, drills, spades, tampers)	6.0
2. Shovel, pick, tunnel bar	8.0
c. Moving, pushing heavy objects, 75 lb or more	
1. These can be desks, file cabinets, heavy stock furniture, such as moving van work. Also include here pushing against heavy spring tension as in boiler room, etc.	8.0
d. Other responses	
1. Laying railroad track	7.0
2. Cutting trees, chopping wood	
a. Automatically	3.0
b. Hand axe or saw	5.5
e. Carpentry	
1. Hammering, sawing, planing	6.0
f. General heavy industrial labor	
1. Handyman work, some moving, some heavy work as shoveling, carpentry, etc.; sporadic, not every day	5.0

SOURCE: G. G. Reif, H. J. Montoye, R. D. Remington, J. A. Napier, H. L. Metzner, and H. H. Epstein: Assessment of physical activity by questionnaire and interview. In M. J. Karvonen and A. J. Barry (eds.): *Physical Activity and the Heart.* Springfield, Ill., Thomas, 1967.

chart, an approximately straight line is generally obtained (Kihlberg and Karvonen, 1957, 1960). The slope, however, differs from event to event. The difference between the best and the hundredth performance appears to be smallest for the 100-m dash and largest for the javelin throw. The ranking of the slopes of the different events is given in Table 2-4.

In essentially intellectual performances, such as accumulating wealth, publishing scientific papers, or playing billiards, the slope of the best performances is uniformly about −1.5. Among sports, those that are commonly considered to require much skill come closer to the intellectual performances, whereas an event such as the 100-m dash evidently depends largely on relatively simple innate characteristics. In the running events, the requirement of endurance is associated with a decrease of the regression coefficient b from 116 for the 100-m dash to 52 for the 10,000-m run. It has been proposed that the scatter of the best performances is a measure of the multiplicity of the determinants of the event. A steep slope signifies few determinants, a gradual one many. These determinants may be physiological in the sense of a coincidence of several favorable characteristics; they may be elements in the

Table 2-3 Metabolic Cost of Leisure-Time Activities

Activity	Work Metabolic Rate Divided by Basal Metabolic Rate, per min
Flying [1]	1.5
Power boating [1]	2.5
Mowing lawn (riding mower)	
Pistol shooting [1]	
Fishing (from boat, bank, or ice) [3]	3.0
Bowling [1]	
Wood cutting (power equipment)	
Horseshoe pitching [1]	
Canoeing, rowing (for pleasure) [1]	3.5
Horseback riding [1]	
Sailing [1]	
Horseshoes [1]	
Golf (using power cart, 9 holes = 1½ hr, 18 holes = 3 hr)	
Archery [1]	4.0
Swimming (nonswimmer)	
Volleyball [1]	
Table tennis [1]	
Cycling (12 mph)	
Walking (10 blocks to the mile; 3 mph)	
Mowing lawn, power mower (not riding)	4.5
Conditioning exercise	
Military marching [1]	
Lawn work, raking, digging, filling	5.0
Gardening, weeding, hoeing, digging, spading	
Social dancing [1]	
Softball (nongame play) [1]	
Golf (9 holes = 1½ hr, 18 holes = 3 hr)	
Baseball officiating [2]	
Mowing lawn, push mower	6.0
Square dancing [1]	
Weight lifting [1]	
Cross-country hiking [3]	
Hunting (also hunter archer) [4]	
Softball (game play) [2]	
Water skiing [1]	
Stream fishing, wading [3]	
Snow shoveling [1]	
Swimming (swimmer)	7.0
Tennis [1]	
Tobogganing and sledding [1]	
Badminton [1]	
Scuba diving [1]	
Ice or roller skating	
Basketball (nongame) [1]	8.0

Table 2–3 *(continued)*

Activity	Work Metabolic Rate Divided by Basal Metabolic Rate, per min
Basketball officiating[1]	
Touch football[1]	
Mountain climbing[4]	
Snow skiing[1]	
Fencing[1]	10.0
Gymnastics[1]	
Football (competition)[1]	
Handball[1]	12.0
Squash[1]	
Basketball (game play)[1]	
Hockey[1]	
Soccer[1]	
Trampolining[1]	
Wrestling or judo[1]	
Canoeing or rowing (in competition)[1]	
Carpentry and other activities involved in interior repair, remodeling, finishing (laying of tile, painting, and so on)	4.0
Construction work involved in building and finishing cottage interior	5.0
Exterior remodeling or construction as garage, breezeway	6.0

[1] For calculation purposes, each exposure to activity is considered to last 1 hr.
[2] For calculation purposes, each exposure to activity is considered to last 2 hr.
[3] For calculation purposes, each exposure to activity is considered to last 3 hr.
[4] For calculation purposes, each exposure to activity is considered to last 4 hr.

SOURCE: G. G. Reif, H. J. Montoye, R. D. Remington, J. A. Napier, H. L. Metzner, and H. H. Epstein: Assessment of physical activity by questionnaire and interview. In M. J. Karvonen and A. J. Barry (eds.): *Physical Activity and the Heart.* Springfield, Ill., Thomas, 1967.

Table 2-4 Ranking of Sports According to the Relative Distance of the Best and the Hundredth Best Performance*

Sports Event	b	Sports Event	b
100-m dash	125	10,000-m run	61
200-m dash	90	Hop, step, and jump	−51
5000-m run	81	3000-m steeplechase	46
1500-m run	80	Broad jump	−43
800-m run	78	Pole vault	−33
High jump	−73	Shot put	−25
400-m run	72	Hammer	−25
110-m hurdles	71	Discus	−25
400-m hurdles	62	Javelin	−20

* In the equation log $N_x = a + b \log x$, N_x = number of people reaching the sports results x or better during one year; x = sports result; a and b = coefficients. The coefficients b for the 1955 results are listed.

SOURCE: J. Kihlberg and M. J. Karvonen: Comparison on statistical basis of achievement in track and field events. *Res. Quart.,* **28**:244–256 (1957).

control of the required series of movements; but they may also reflect the numbers of hours to be spent in training.

Summary

Every movement is a *motor act* that requires energy from *metabolic processes*. The organism recruits a series of *autonomous mechanisms* to support the motor act. The act may be *volitional* or *reflex*, and it is simultaneously *perceived* by the subject. Each of these aspects of human movement opens approaches to an intrinsic classification of work and activity.

Movement may be purely *expressive* or *serve aims*. It is integrated in the life pattern either as *work*, as *sport* (amateur or professional), as *physical education*, or as *recreation*. It may also be the means for dealing with emergencies, that is, *fight or flight*.

In dealing with the complex phenomenon of physical activity, our conventional analytical thought operates with the concepts of *skill, strength, speed, power*, and *endurance*. At *high altitudes, under water*, and under adverse *thermal loads*, man's performance is additionally determined by the ability of his organism to deal with the specific challenges of the environment.

The conceptual framework of anatomy, physiology, and biochemistry offers another approach for analyzing work and activity. Observations and experiments on the *sensorimotor nervous system*, on *muscle*, on the *energy supply*, and on the *al milieu* in exercise make up a body of information that is systematized in handbooks and taught in schools and at universities. However, a "blind" approach to elucidating the elements of physical activities through *factor analysis* sometimes gives answers that are difficult to fit into such an anticipated conceptual framework.

Some activities are conventionally considered as belonging to *men* and others to *women*. In some sports, only the *young* excel, whereas in others the *middle aged* may stand an equal chance.

For practical purposes, it is useful to indicate the relative load of various activities. For comparing the *physiological load*, lists of the power—the rate of energy expenditure—are convenient. *Mental loads* have not yet been systematized to the same extent.

The scatter of the world's best results may be used as a basis for an intrinsic *hierarchy of sports* events, interpreted as indicating the multiplicity of the determinants of the performance.

Thus, the classification of work and activity may be approached from many angles, either by choosing criteria from the intrinsic characteristics of human performance or by applying conceptual frameworks derived from the study of the human form and function.

REFERENCES

Astrand, I., P.-O. Astrand, E. H. Christensen, and R. Hedman: Intermittent muscular work. *Acta Physiol. Scand.*, **48**:448–453 (1960).

Barry, A. J.: Physical activity and psychic stress strain. *Can. Med. Ass. J.*, **96**:848–885 (1967).

Borg, G.: Psychological and physiological studies of physical work. In W. T. Singleton, J. G. Fox, and D. Whitfield (eds.): *Measurement of Man at Work*. London, Taylor and Francis, pp. 121–128, 1971.

Christensen, E. H.: Physiological evaluation of work in the Nykroppa iron works. In G. W. F. Floyd and A. T. Welford (eds.): *Symposium on Fatigue*. London, H. K. Lewis, 1953.

Christensen, E. H., R. Hedman, and I. Holmdahl: The influence of rest pauses on mechanical efficiency. *Acta Physiol. Scand.*, **48**:443–447 (1960).

Hiernaux, J.: La diversité humaine en Afrique subsaharienne. *Recherches Biologiques. Etudes Ethnologiques*. Bruxelles, Institut de Sociologie, Un. Libre Bruxelles, 1968.

Jokl, E., M. J. Karvonen, J. Kihlberg, A. Koskela, and L. Noro: *Sports in the Cultural Pattern of the World: A Study of the Olympic Games 1952 at Helsinki*. Helsinki, Institute of Occupational Health, 1956.

Karvonen, M. J., and M. Niemi: Factor analysis of performance in track and field events. *Arbeitsphysiologie* **15**:127–233 (1953).

Karvonen, M. J., and N. Rönnholm: Electromyographic and energy expenditure studies of rhythmic and paced lifting work. *Ann. Acad. Sci. Fenn.*, Ser. A-V, **106**, No. 19:1–11 (1964).

Kihlberg, J., and M. J. Karvonen: Comparison on statistical basis of achievement in track and field events. *Res. Quart. Amer. Ass. Health Phys. Educ.*, **28**:244–256 (1957).

Kihlberg, J., and M. J. Karvonen: Statistical distribution and predictability of top class achievement in track and field sporting events. *Wychowanie Fizyczne i Sport* **4**:145–156 (1960).

Laban, R., and F. C. Lawrence: *Effort*. London, McDonald Evans, 1947 (repr. 1965).

Reif, G. G., H. J. Montoye, R. D. Remington, J. A. Napier, H. L. Metzner, and H. H. Epstein: Assessment of physical activity by questionnaire and interview. In M. J. Karvonen and A. J. Barry (eds.): *Physical Activity and the Heart*. Springfield, Ill., Charles C Thomas, pp. 336–371, 1967.

Rönnholm, N., M. J. Karvonen, and V. O. Lapinleimu: Mechanical efficiency of rhythmic and paced work of lifting. *J. Appl. Physiol.*, **17**:768–770 (1962).

General Articles

Durnin, J. V. G. A., and R. Passmore: *Energy, Work and Leisure*. London, Heinemann, 1967.

Katsuki, S.: *Relative Metabolic Rate of Industrial Work in Japan*. Tokyo, 1960.

Passmore, R., and J. V. G. A. Durnin: Human energy expenditure. *Physiol. Rev.*, **35**:801–840 (1955).

Singleton, W. T., J. G. Fox, and D. Whitfield (eds.): *Measurement of Man at Work*. London, Taylor and Francis, 1971.

The Organism and Muscular Work

3

T. Ishiko
Juntendo University
Chiba, Japan

Skeletal Muscle

Muscle as the Origin of Human Movement

Man, like other animals, is capable of physical movement. Such movement, whether it involves only a part of the body or the body as a whole, is associated either with an external motion, such as throwing an object, or with no motion, such as maintaining posture against the force of gravity, and is an outcome of muscular contraction. Therefore, it is essential to understand the construction and function of the muscles before one can delve into the scientific investigation of physical activities.

The physical activities with which we are concerned are performed by the contraction of skeletal muscle which, in its typical form, is attached to the bones at both ends. As the muscle contracts, the bone rotates at the intervening joint. Since skeletal muscle can be activated into motion by individual volition, it is also referred to as voluntary muscle. Distinguished from these voluntary muscles are the involuntary muscles which are responsible for the movements of the heart and gastrointestinal organs, for the regulation of the blood vessels that run throughout the body, and for the control of the secretory activities of the glands. The difference between the voluntary and involuntary muscles exists in their nervous control. The former are under the control of the motor nervous system, whereas the latter are governed by the autonomic nervous system.

Voluntary muscle contracts when it receives nerve impulses that originate in the motor area of the cerebral cortex and are transmitted by the pyramidal tract and the motor nerve. These muscle contractions result in the voluntary movement of the body. This movement, although it appears quite simple, involves a large number of muscle groups that are activated by the vast concatenation of the temporal and spatial arrangements of the nerve impulses and are coordinated into an integrated movement.

Muscle Fiber

A skeletal muscle is composed of many thousands of cells, 10–100 microns (μ) in diameter and from 1 mm to 30 cm in length, called muscle fibers. The muscle fibers run side by side; a dozen or more are wrapped together by connective tissue called endomysium and form a muscle bundle. Each muscle bundle is again separately wrapped in a sheath of connective tissue called epimysium. The whole muscle, in turn, is enclosed by a membranous layer of connective tissue called perimysium. Such elaborate construction is necessary to keep these muscle fibers in place during impetuous mechanical movements that result in intensified friction within the muscle.

The skeletal muscles as a whole account for approximately 40% of the total body weight. The figure may even reach about 50% for athletes. Thus, the body is capable of very strenuous as well as delicate movements, such as those involved in sport activities.

At any given movement, one or more muscles play a leading role and will be called prime mover(s). The prime movers are assisted by synergists which work with them. The muscles that stop action or work against the movements of the prime movers and synergists are known as antagonists.

Each muscle fiber is wrapped in a thin, homogeneous cell wall called sarcolemma and has many nuclei. A majority of these nuclei are scattered close under the sarcolemma, whereas the predominant portion of the inside of the muscle fiber is occupied by several hundred to several thousand minutely thin fibrils that lie parallel to each other. The rest of the fiber is filled with a fluid substance called sarcoplasma.

Myofibril

A microscopic inspection of skeletal muscle reveals the beautifully striated pattern of the myofibrils. Skeletal muscles, therefore, are sometimes called striated muscles. Each myofibril is made up of light and dark parts alternating at regular intervals. The light and dark parts of the adjacent fibrils are lined up with each other, resulting in a cross-striations effect. The effect is due to differences in the optical properties of these parts. The light part has a single refractive property and is called the isotropic band or I band. The dark part has a double reflection property and is known as the anisotropic band or A band.

When examined under an electron microscope, the fibril is revealed to be made up of a large number of tiny filaments. These filaments have two sizes: the thinner ones are 40 Ångstroms (Å) and the thicker ones are 110 Å in their diameters. In the biochemical process of discriminatory extraction of actin and myosin, the thin and thick filaments are observed to be extracted, respectively. Therefore, the thinner filament with 40 Å diameter is considered to be the actin, and the thicker one with 110 Å diameter is regarded to be the myosin.

The schematic construction of the skeletal muscles is shown in Figure 3-1. Actin and myosin lie parallel with each other. The part on which these two kinds of filaments overlap appears dark and coincides with the A band. The I band is the light part and corresponds to an area where only one layer of actin filament exists. At the center of the A band, there is a lighter part known as the H zone (Hansen's zone). It is speculated that the actin filaments do not reach the middle of the A band, and their absence forms the H zone. The Z line, at the middle of the I band, appears the darkest. This line is considered to be a cross-sectional fixation of the actin filaments.

Huxley and Hanson (1954) proposed the "sliding theory" of muscle contraction. According to this theory, muscle contraction occurs when actin filaments slide toward myosin filaments using the chemical energy of ATP (adenosine triphosphate). The following observations provided the basis for this theory: The actomyosin filament, made up by adding actin and myosin, demonstrated *in vitro* a shortening in length when ATP was added; the space of the I band was widened when a muscle was stretched under the microscope; and the I band was narrowed as a muscle fiber contracted. (In the sarcoplasma, there are many mitochondria, which exist mainly around the area of I band and are related to the oxygen utilization of muscular contraction.)

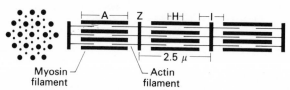

Figure 3–1. Schematic diagram of the myofibril. The thick and thin filaments consist of myosin and actin, respectively.

Muscle Innervation

The motor nerves controlling the muscles divide into branches as they descend down to the periphery before finally becoming a single nerve fiber. The axon of this nerve fiber further spreads into branches, with each of these branches reaching a muscle fiber. One nerve fiber and the muscle fibers that it controls work as a unit called a neuromuscular or motor unit. The point of connection between the nerve and muscle fiber is known as the motor end plate. When the impulses through the motor nerve reach this point, the chemical transmitter, acetylcholine, is secreted.

Within the muscle, there are muscle spindles that function as receptors of deep sensation. At the spindle, the sensory nerves originate from the bundle of intrafusal muscle fibers and are ready to sense any tension applied to these fibers. The detected changes in tension are transmitted to the central nervous system. These intrafusal muscle fibers are also supplied with a branch of efferent nerves known as gamma fibers. In the tendons, there are sensory terminal devices known as the Golgi tendon organs, which function in a manner similar to that of the muscle spindle. These devices, however, lack any connection with gamma fibers.

Thus, the muscle spindles and Golgi tendon organs detect information through tensions within the muscle and enable a person to know the posture and movements of his body and, in some cases, the impetus and weight of an object.

Muscular Contraction

When an isolated muscle is stimulated electrically, it responds with a contraction. A contraction caused by a single stimulus is called a twitch. On any mechanical recording of a twitch, a few milliseconds elapse after the onset of the stimulus before the muscle starts to contract. This time lag constitutes the latent period. After this brief interval has elapsed, the muscle develops tension and the contraction occurs. Following the periods of shortening and relaxation, the twitch is completed.

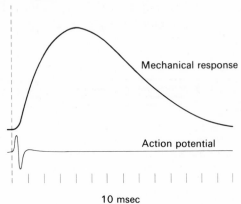

Mechanical response

Action potential

10 msec

Figure 3-2. Mechanical response and action potential during a twitch of the skeletal muscle.

If, instead of a single stimulus, a series of stimuli is applied in a short interval, the contraction becomes larger than a twitch and causes the muscle to maintain a contracted state. This state is known as the tetanus. Whenever a muscle contracts, it generates action potential, which is called spike potential due to its short duration (see Figure 3-2). In the case of repetitive stimulation, an action potential is generated that corresponds to each stimulus. Therefore, the action potentials for a tetanus are recorded separately for each individual stimulus. The voluntary movement of the human body, no matter how quickly executed, is always a tetanus; it can never be a twitch. This is evidenced by the repeated appearance of action potentials.

The contraction of a muscle may be classified in relation to the length of the muscle as follows: (1) concentric contraction, where the length of the muscle shortens as it contracts, also referred to as dynamic or isotonic contraction; (2) isometric or static contraction, where the length of the muscle stays unchanged despite the changes in its tension; and (3) eccentric contraction, where the muscle is stretched as it contracts against an external force which is greater than the maximum contractile force of the muscle.

The energy source of muscular contraction, energy-rich phosphoric acid, is liberated by the hydrolysis of ATP. Adenosine diphosphate (ADP) is the result of this process, and ATP may be resynthesized from ADP by the breakdown of either of the following two substances: (1) phosphocreatine, which breaks down to creatine and phosphoric acid, the latter also being energy rich; and (2) glycogen or glucose, which breaks down completely into carbon dioxide and water through the Krebs tricarboxylic acid (TCA) cycle. The energy of 1 mole glucose thus consumed is capable of resynthesizing 38 moles ATP. If the supply of oxygen becomes insufficient in this process, aerobic glycolysis is suspended and lactic acid is produced anaerobically, which is capable of resynthesizing only 2 moles ATP.

Muscular Strength

Normal Values

The tension produced by a muscle is called muscular strength. However, in voluntary movements, various degrees of muscle tension may be developed in accordance with the purpose of the movement. The maximum level of tension, therefore, is recorded isometrically and is termed muscular strength.

The strength of a muscle is roughly proportional to its cross-sectional dimension. The girth of the arm includes, in addition to the muscles, the bone as well as subcutaneous adipose tissue. The size of the arm girth, therefore, is not necessarily in proportion to its strength. For athletes, however, whose variance in subcutaneous fat is known to be much smaller, higher correlations are expected between muscular strength and arm girth. Ishiko (1962), for example, measured the forearm girth and the grip strength of oarsmen in regatta crews and found a close relationship between these two variables (see Figure 3-3).

According to Hettinger (1961), the muscular strength per unit dimension of muscle cross section is 4 kilograms per square centimeter (kg/cm²). In this value, males and females are quite comparable, despite the fact that females are known generally to have much weaker muscular strength than males. Ikai and Fukunaga (1968) measured the cross-sectional dimension of muscles by a method utilizing supersonic waves and obtained an average value of 6.3 kg/cm² in 245 healthy male and female subjects. There was no sexual difference.

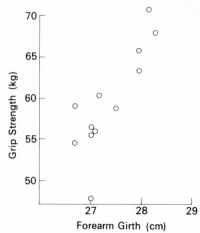

Figure 3-3. Relationship between forearm girth and grip strength of oarsmen. One circle means the average of eight oarsmen of a crew.

The measured value of muscular strength varies in accordance with differences in the technique of measurement, which involves such variation as the posture of the subjects, point of application of the dynamometer, and so on. The values of muscular strength as reported by Hettinger (1961) are listed in Table 3-1. From Table 3-1, one can see that the strength of knee extensors, which act as antigravity muscles, is four times as great as that of knee flexors.

Table 3-1 Various Muscular Strengths in Male Adults*

Posture	Movement	Application of Dynamometer	Strength, kg
Standing	Elbow flexion	Wrist	20
	Elbow extension	Wrist	30
Sitting	Trunk flexion	Chest	50
	Trunk extension	Chest	54
	Knee flexion	Chest	15
	Knee extension	Chest	60
Standing	Ankle extension	Hand	80
	Thigh abduction	Ankle	50
	Thigh adduction	Ankle	50
	Thigh flexion	Ankle	56
	Thigh extension	Ankle	52

* Rearranged by Ishiko from Hettinger.

Among the measured values of muscular strength, the most common of all may be that of grip strength. The mean values of grip strength obtained in Japan on a large number of subjects covering ages from 10 to 59 years are tabulated in Table 3-2.

Table 3-2 Grip Strength (kg) of Japanese Normal Subjects Ranging from 10 to 59 Years

Male				Female			
Age	Number	Average	SD*	Age	Number	Average	SD
10	2060	17.7	4.09	10	2055	16.3	4.14
11	2182	20.5	4.77	11	2123	19.3	4.56
12	1941	24.5	6.35	12	1945	22.5	4.63
13	2085	30.5	7.33	13	2061	25.1	4.91
14	2178	36.7	7.73	14	2192	27.0	4.94
15	3645	40.7	7.10	15	3622	27.7	5.02
16	3432	43.3	7.34	16	3526	28.4	5.24
17	3288	45.5	7.37	17	3518	28.9	5.33
18	4903	45.5	6.74	18	4429	29.4	4.82
19	3968	45.6	6.48	19	2923	29.7	4.72
20	2240	45.9	6.88	20	1710	29.1	4.80
21	605	46.8	7.10	21	455	29.3	5.29
22	616	46.9	7.41	22	351	29.0	5.39
23	503	47.9	7.00	23	227	29.3	5.55
24	320	46.6	7.96	24	192	28.3	6.47
25	300	46.5	8.00	25	201	29.7	5.47
26	285	45.8	7.92	26	199	29.3	4.82
27	234	46.3	7.19	27	164	29.0	4.83
28	246	46.9	6.74	28	173	28.8	4.66
29	239	47.0	7.83	29	159	30.1	4.71
30	537	47.7	6.69	30	436	30.7	4.63
31	453	46.5	6.33	31	433	30.9	4.64
32	491	46.4	6.79	32	509	30.5	4.68
33	499	46.2	6.45	33	534	31.3	4.83
34	567	46.2	6.36	34	610	30.3	5.00
35	585	45.9	6.46	35	608	30.5	4.53
36	555	45.7	6.70	36	592	30.3	4.74
37	593	46.0	6.64	37	560	29.9	4.55
38	531	45.7	6.40	38	556	30.1	4.57
39	553	45.4	6.39	39	561	29.7	4.75
40	543	45.0	6.45	40	516	29.9	4.74
41	622	44.3	6.51	41	462	29.7	4.64
42	628	45.6	6.06	42	444	29.6	4.64
43	540	44.8	6.21	43	386	29.7	4.84
44	492	44.8	6.49	44	347	29.3	4.64
45	518	43.8	6.48	45	386	28.7	4.14
46	431	44.8	6.51	46	316	29.5	5.14
47	408	44.2	6.38	47	291	28.7	4.59
48	384	43.7	6.69	48	260	28.9	4.86
49	352	42.9	6.12	49	227	28.2	4.17
50	332	43.5	6.57	50	219	28.0	4.29
51	314	42.6	6.30	51	205	27.8	4.24
52	311	42.5	6.38	52	197	28.4	4.92
53	300	42.4	6.44	53	179	27.2	4.63
54	322	41.4	6.28	54	171	26.9	5.01
55	316	41.7	6.24	55	154	26.9	4.20
56	275	41.1	5.91	56	147	27.3	5.01
57	234	41.6	6.30	57	135	27.3	4.79
58	205	41.4	5.65	58	129	27.3	4.47
59	312	39.4	5.72	59	158	26.2	4.08

* SD = standard deviation.

The following observations may be drawn from Table 3-2.

1. The grip strength of adult females is approximately two thirds that of males.
2. The grip strength of 10-year-old males and females amounted respectively to 38.6% and 56.3% of the value recorded for the 20-year-olds. The mean grip strength of 15-year-old males and females amounted respectively to 88.7% and 95.2% of the strength of the 20-year-olds.
3. In all age groups, the mean grip strength of the females never came up to that of the males.
4. Grip strength does not decrease as much as one might expect at middle age and older.

Muscular Strength in Athletes

Muscular strength increases through training. It is only natural that athletes demonstrate greater muscular strength than untrained persons. In addition to their originally favorable physique of mesomorphy dominance, athletes go through intensified muscular training. Table 3-3 shows the back strength and grip strength (average of left and right measurements) of Japanese athletes who trained for the 1964 Olympic Games held in Tokyo. The athletes who participated in throwing events, weight lifting, rowing, and judo registered a mean back strength exceeding 200 kg, whereas the back strength of college students 20 years old averaged only 149.5 kg. These athletes, therefore, may be said to have approximately 1.5 times the back strength of the general population. In grip strength, the same athletes showed an average exceeding 65 kg, whereas the control group recorded only 45.5 kg. Here again, the grip strength of these athletes approximated 1.5 times that of

Table 3-3 Grip and Back Strengths in Japanese Male Athletes

Activity	Back Strength, kg	Grip Strength, kg
Throwing	229.6	71.2
Weight lifting (middle)	220.0	68.8
Rowing	215.6	67.7
Judo (heavy)	205.0	65.1
Jumping	179.6	56.5
Volleyball	175.4	55.5
Basketball	174.5	55.3
Short- and middle-distance running	160.2	53.1
Soccer	148.8	52.9
Gymnastics	147.1	48.5
Swimming	142.8	48.0
Fencing	136.0	48.0
Long-distance running	124.7	43.8
General population (20 years old)	149.5	45.5

the control group. There was a very high correlation between back and grip strength with respect to the results listed in Table 3-3.

Athletes specializing in certain sport events, however, demonstrated muscular strength not appreciably superior to that of the untrained. Among these sport events, long-distance running actually does not require any exceptional muscular strength. However, the other events mentioned above do require extra strength, and the athletes in these particular sport events need further intensified training to improve their performance.

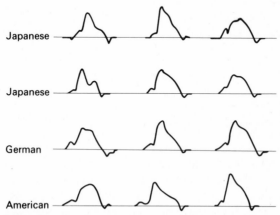

Figure 3-4. Some examples of force-time curves measured at the oar in Japanese, German, and American oarsmen.

Muscular strength usually is measured in a static condition when muscles develop tension against a resistance, such as a spring or something similar. However, by utilizing an electric device, muscular strength may be measured in dynamic motion. Figure 3-4 shows the dynamic muscular strength recorded by Ishiko utilizing subjects engaged in rowing movements. A strain gauge was attached to the oar, and the strain on the oar was recorded by a telemetering system. Then the weight was applied to the grip of the oar, and its strain was calibrated into force. The peak force during the rowing motion thus obtained was 80–100 kg.

Factors Modifying Muscular Strength

Voluntary movement is controlled by the central nervous system. Even at maximum effort, neither all of the motor units nor their maximal frequencies of discharge are mobilized. Therefore, greater muscular strength may be exerted when the muscle is artificially activated by electric stimuli. Ikai, Yabe, and Ishii (1967) compared the muscular strength developed by the thumb adductor when contracted by electric stimuli with the maximum contraction resulting from the volition of the subjects. They reported that the former produced 30% greater strength than the latter.

Thus, muscular strength is influenced by the volition of the subject or by some psychological factor. Ikai and Steinhaus (1961) reported that strength in the flexors of the upper arm improved during a hypnotized state and that the improved condition persisted for a short period after awakening. The same investigators also observed that firing a pistol immediately prior to the measurement of muscular strength resulted in significantly increased strength, which was maintained for approximately 4 sec after the firing. Muscular strength may be improved also by shouting and cheering. This phenomenon may be attributed partially to the excitation of the central nervous system, which in turn dampens its inhibitory impulses. However, the effect may also be due partially to the secretion of epinephrine, which has been elicited by these stimuli.

Muscular Work

Measuring Devices for Muscular Work

In order to observe and record the amount of work done and the corresponding changes in various physiological parameters, it is necessary to establish an experimental condition in which the subjects perform certain controllable muscular work. The bicycle ergometer and the treadmill are representative devices that have been utilized for this purpose.

Bicycle Ergometer. A bicycle ergometer is a stationary bicycle that permits a subject to pedal so as to move a flywheel. The workload can be determined by the friction resistance applied to the flywheel, utilizing a magnet, spring, or weight. The amount of work done may be computed as follows:

$$\text{Amount of work done} = \text{Resistance applied} \times \text{Circumference of the wheel} \times \text{Number of revolutions of the wheel}$$

The basic characteristics of the bicycle ergometer are described as follows:

1. The amount of work done in a given period of time as well as the total work for the entire period can be measured.
2. It is safe and easy to operate for any individual.
3. It keeps the upper limbs stationary during work so that the measurements of blood pressure and pulse rate are made easy.
4. Its purchase and running costs are low.
5. It can easily be transported to different testing places.

Motor-Driven Treadmill. The treadmill consists of a movable platform that is driven backward by a motor on which a subject runs or walks. The intensity of the work performed may be controlled by changing either the speed or the gradient of the platform. The amount of the work done may be computed as follows:

Amount of work done = Body weight of the subject × Speed of the treadmill
× Duration of the work × sin θ

where θ = gradient.

The following are the basic characteristics of the motor-driven treadmill:

1. It enables an individual to perform experimentally the basic human locomotive movements, such as walking and running.
2. It mobilizes the muscles of the entire body. Therefore, the maximum oxygen intake obtained on the treadmill is larger than that obtained on the bicycle ergometer, stepping ergometer, and so on.

Workload and Total Amount of Work Done

The amount of work performed by a subject before he comes to the state of exhaustion varies with the intensity of the work or the workload. When the workload exceeds the capacity of the subject, no work can be performed. Examples are cases where the drive speed of the treadmill is too fast for the subject to run on or the resistance applied to the wheel of the bicycle ergometer is too heavy for him to pedal.

In the case of the work of a local muscle group, the heaviest workload a subject is able to execute for just one bout of work equals his maximum muscular strength. As the workload becomes smaller, the corresponding amount of work done before reaching exhaustion becomes greater. Below a certain level of workload, a steady state is reached where the work can apparently be carried on for an indefinite period of time.

These relationships between the workload and the amount of work done may be plotted on a graph. Figure 3-5 shows such a graph obtained by Ishiko (1952) with six subjects engaged in the work of elbow flexion. The curve simulates a hyperbola, and when plotted on the logarithmic scale linearity is approximated. Thus, this relationship may be expressed mathematically as follows:

$$\log t = a \log N + b$$

where t = time of work (endurance); N = workload; and a and b are constants.

From the graph, Ishiko obtained the values for a and b, respectively, of $-2.3 \sim -3.4$ and $3.9 \sim 5.0$. Grosse-Lordemann and Müller (1936) reported a and b values of $-2.6 \sim -7.8$ and $4.0 \sim 11.0$, respectively, for their six subjects who worked on a bicycle ergometer. As the absolute value of a becomes greater, the gradient of the curve becomes steeper. Therefore, the value of *a* may be considered as an indication of muscular endurance. These processes, however, involve rather complicated manipulation and computation. Therefore, in actual practice, the muscular endurance is frequently expressed by the time or amount of work done until exhaustion applying the workload which corresponds to one quarter to one third of the maximum muscular strength.

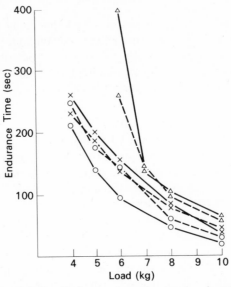

Figure 3-5. Relationship between workload and endurance time.

Dynamic Work and Static Work

Muscular contraction when accompanied by external movement is manifested as a form of dynamic work, whereas, in the case of isometric contraction where no external movement is displayed, the contraction is manifested as a form of static work. In most sport activities requiring speed and power, the work performed is dynamic in form. On the other hand, the sport of marksmanship involves predominantly static work in order to stabilize the weapon.

Dynamic work, as a rule, demands greater energy consumption than does static work of comparable nature. Ishiko (1952), utilizing an elbow flexion ergometer, compared the oxygen consumption involved in dynamic and static work tasks. For the dynamic task, the subjects flexed their arms at the elbow while holding a load. The apparatus was so arranged that no load was applied when the elbow was extended in order to remove the effect of eccentric contraction. For the static task, the subjects held the load keeping the elbow at a right angle (see Table 3-4).

Table 3-4 Comparison of Energy Requirement at Elbow Flexion Between Dynamic and Static Movements

Load, kg	O_2 Requirement, liter/min		Dynamic/Static
	Dynamic Work	Static Work	
10	1.21	0.68	1.8
8	0.66	0.40	1.6
6	0.45	0.26	1.6
4	0.38	0.15	2.8

From Table 3-4, it is apparent that dynamic work consumed approximately twice as much energy as did static work. Although the dynamic work was executed according to the cadence of one contraction every 3 sec, the actual time of contraction for each cadence was approximately 0.5 sec. When this is compared with the time factor of the static work, in which the muscles were kept contracted for the entire period, it may be said that the dynamic work consumed about ten times more energy than did the static work.

In dynamic work tasks, concentric contraction tends to pump the blood out of the muscle (milking action) and thus facilitates circulation. Such action is not associated with static work. Rather, in the case of static work, the elevated and sustained inner tension of the muscles tends to interfere with circulation and, therefore, to elicit an early fatigue.

Mechanical Efficiency of Work

The mechanical efficiency of muscular work is expressed as follows:

$$\text{Efficiency} = \frac{\text{Mechanical work done}}{\text{Energy used for the work}}$$

An accurate measure of the amount of work done can be made on a bicycle ergometer by keeping the load and the speed of revolution constant. The efficiency computed by Grosse-Lordemann and Müller (1936) appears in Table 3-5. Here the workload was held constant at 10 kgm/sec (kilogrammeters per second), while the revolution rate varied from 20 to 100 rpm (revolutions per minute). This table shows that mechanical efficiency is best

Table 3-5 Mechanical Efficiency of Bicycling Work
(Work rate 10 kgm/sec)

Pedalling, rpm	Energy Demand, cal/kgm	Efficiency, %
20	19.6	11.9
30	14.0	16.7
40	12.7	18.5
50	12.9	18.2
60	12.4	18.9
80	13.7	17.1
100	14.3	16.4

when the subject pedals at the rate of 40–60 rpm, and that the efficiency declines at rates both higher and lower than this level.

As observed above, an optimum speed is known to exist for muscular work performed by the human body. Hill (1927) explained this phenomenon as follows: At higher speeds, the innate resistance within the muscles becomes greater and thus depreciates the total efficiency; at slower rates, a large portion of the total energy is consumed by static work required in the maintenance of posture. In static work, of course, the mechanical efficiency is zero.

Differences in mechanical efficiency are not appreciable in commonplace movements, such as walking and running, in which every individual has a high degree of skill acquired through a lifetime of practice. However, in more physically demanding movements, such as swimming and skiing, in which specific experiences are indispensable for motor learning, a distinct difference is observed in the mechanical efficiencies of the skilled and unskilled performers. Ishiko and his associates (1956) measured the energy consumption in walking on snow using skis. The results are shown in Table 3-6.

Table 3-6 Energy Metabolism of Walking on Snow Ground

	Speed, m/sec	O₂ Consumption, ml/min
SKILLED		
Wearing ski with seal	1.00	1140
Wearing ski without seal	1.07	925
Carrying ski on the shoulder	0.96	1268
UNSKILLED		
Wearing ski with seal	0.85	1327
Wearing ski without seal	1.00	1592
Carrying ski on the shoulder	0.97	1522

Skilled and unskilled skiers of approximately comparable physique were required to walk on the snow-covered ground under three conditions: wearing skis with seal; wearing just skis; and on foot, carrying the skis on their shoulders. In all the conditions, the oxygen consumption was less for the skilled than for the unskilled skiers. An especially marked difference was found when the subjects just wore skis. Skilled skiers consumed only 60% of the energy required for the unskilled skiers. It was concluded that the skilled movements were performed more economically, avoiding wasteful motions. Therefore, better mechanical efficiency is characteristic of skilled performers.

Effects of Muscular Training

Morphological Change

Among the tissues of the human body, the muscles demonstrate the most significant response to training. Through physical training, the mass of the muscles and their work capacity are increased; at the same time, the metabolism and circulation in these muscles are improved.

Morpurgo (1897) had dogs and rats undergo a muscular workout and compared anatomically the cross sections of their muscles before and after the workout. He also counted the number of muscle fibers. The result showed a 20–50% increase in the muscle cross-section as a result of training. This increase was not caused by an increase in the number of muscle fibers, but rather was attributed to the hypertrophy of the fibers, the number of which remained unchanged. It was also found that the variance in the diameter of these fibers became smaller, which indicated that the thinner fibers achieved the greater degree of hypertrophy.

Hettinger and Müller (1953) studied muscle cross section and muscular strength in men before and after static training. A significant increase was found in both variables. However, the ratio of these two variables remained unchanged even after training (see Table 3-7). Therefore, it was concluded

Table 3-7 Change in Muscular Strength by Training

Subject	Status	Muscular Strength, kg	
		Raw Score	Per Unit Cross Section
1	Before training	180	6.4
	After training	228	6.5
2	Before training	192	6.6
	After training	336	6.7
3	Before training	194	6.7
	After training	288	6.6

SOURCE: T. Hettinger and E. A. Müller: Muskelleistung und Muskeltraining. *Arbeitsphysiol.*, **15**:111–126 (1953).

that the increase in muscular strength is due to the increase in the cross section of the muscle. This finding was also confirmed by Ikai and Fukunaga (1968). The basis for such hypertrophy, however, has not been established.

Petren and his coworkers (1936), who had mice run for a certain period of time, failed to observe an increase in the size of muscle fibers. However, they found 40–45% more capillaries in the muscles of the heart and the gastrocnemius of these mice than those of the untrained animals. Vannotti and Pfister (1934) also observed that training produced a large number of anastomoses among capillaries enabling them to transport more blood to the active muscles. Increased blood flow through the muscle is, of course, closely associated with an increase in the endurance of the muscle.

Gollnick and King (1969) trained male albino rats on motor-driven work wheels and observed, with an electron microscope, that the mitochondria were more numerous and larger in the trained gastrocnemius muscle than in the untrained muscle. Moreover, cristae were more densely packed in the mitochondria of the trained muscle. Holloszy (1967) reported that a training program of strenuous running increased the oxidative capacity, total protein, and enzymatic activity of the mitochondrial fraction of rat skeletal muscle.

Chemical Change

Myoglobin is considered to play an important role in supplying oxygen to muscular tissue. According to Millikan (1936), myoglobin has a greater affinity for oxygen than hemoglobin. He found that, when a tetanus was induced in the soleus muscle of a cat, 20% of the oxygen bound with myoglobin was utilized by the muscle in 1 sec, and within 4 sec more than 50% was utilized. According to Wipple (1926), a sedentary house dog contained 400 mg of myoglobin per 100 g of muscle tissue, whereas an active hunting dog would receive a greater oxygen supply to its muscles.

An increase in the glycogen content of muscle tissue as a response to training has been confirmed by Embden and Habs (1926). They trained one leg of a rabbit by inducing tetanus with electric stimuli, while the other leg was kept stationary. After several weeks, the glycogen content of the trained leg was two to three times greater than that of the untrained leg.

Bergström and Hultman (1966), utilizing a modern technique of biopsy in the human quadriceps femoris muscle, demonstrated an increase of glycogen in the trained muscle. They trained one leg of two subjects with exhaustive work on a bicycle ergometer, whereas the other leg was kept untrained. After the training, a high carbohydrate diet was supplied. After 1 day the glycogen content in the exercised leg rose from practically zero at the termination of training to higher values than that in the untrained leg. The glycogen content continued to rise during the following 2 days until it reached about twice that in the untrained leg.

Palladin and Ferdmann (1928) found that the phosphocreatine content in the muscles of rabbits increased after 5 days of training, and this increased state was maintained for 6 days after the cessation of training.

The behavior of the potassium content of muscles accompanying training has also drawn attention. Brumann and Jenny (1936) reported a 6–20% increase in potassium content associated with the hypertrophy of the muscle after 2 months' training involving rabbits. Fomin (1930) reported that the level of increase in potassium content varied in accordance with the time elapsed between the termination of training and the measurement. The value decreased slightly 20–48 hr after the end of training, but increased remarkably after 3–4 days; after 6 days it increased moderately. According to Nocker et al. (1958), training caused an increase in the potassium content of skeletal muscle; however, the potassium level of trained muscle decreased more than that of untrained muscle during exhaustive work.

As discussed in the foregoing, vast changes take place in muscles in association with training. The outcome of these changes is an increase in muscular strength and endurance. This increase is a manifestation of the adaptation mechanism possessed by muscles caused by frequent and intense use. The reverse is also true, since definite atrophy and deterioration are known to be exhibited by muscles not used or immobilized in a plaster cast for a prolonged period of time.

REFERENCES

Bergström, J., and E. Hultman: Muscle glycogen syntheses after exercise: An enhancing factor localized to the muscle cells in man. *Nature*, **210**:309–310 (1966).

Brumann, F., and F. Jenny: Untersuchungen zum Studium des Trainiertseins. VIII. Miteilung. Trainingszustand und Kaliumgehalt der Muskulatur. *Arbeitsphysiol.*, **9**:147–151 (1936).

Embden, G., and H. Habs: Beitrag zur Lehre von Muskel-training. *Scand. Arch. Physiol.*, **49**:122–123 (1926).

Fomin, S. W.: Uber den Einfluss des Trainiertens auf die mineralischen Substanzen der Muskeln. *Biochem. Z.*, **217**:423–429 (1930).

Gollnick, P. D., and D. W. King: Effect of exercise and training on mitochondria of rat skeletal muscle. *Amer. J. Physiol.*, **216**:1502–1509 (1969).

Grosse-Lordemann, H., and E. A. Müller: Der Einfluss der Leistung und der Arbeitsgeschwindigkeit auf das Arbeitsmaximum und den Wirkungsgrad bein Radfahren. *Arbeitsphysiol.*, **9**:454–475 (1936).

Hettinger, T.: *Physiology of Strength.* Springfield, Ill., Charles C Thomas, 1961.

Hettinger, T., and E. A. Müller: Muskelleistung und Muskeltraining. *Arbeitsphysiol.*, **15**:111–126 (1953).

Hill, A. V.: *Muscular Movement in Man.* New York, McGraw-Hill (1927).

Holloszy, J. O.: The effects of exercise on mitochondrial oxygen uptake and respiratory activity in skeletal muscle. *J. Biol. Chem.*, **242**:2278–2282 (1967).

Huxley, H. E., and J. Hanson: Changes in the cross-striations of muscle during contraction and stretch and their structural interpretation. *Nature*, **173**:973–976 (1954).

Ikai, M., and A. Steinhaus: Some factors modifying the expression of human strength. *J. Appl. Physiol.*, **16**:157–163 (1961).

Ikai, M., and T. Fukunaga: Calculation of muscle strength per unit cross-sectional area of human muscle by means of ultrasonic measurement. *Int. Z. Angew. Physiol.*, **26**:26–32 (1968).

Ikai, M., K. Yabe, and K. Ishii: Muskeldraft und muskläre Ermüdung bei willkürlicher Anspannung und elektrischer Reizung des Muskels. *Sportarzt Sportmed.*, **5**:197–204 (1967).

Ishiko, T.: Relationship between work load and endurance time. *J. Physiol. Soc. Jap.*, **14**:489–493 (1952) (in Japanese).

Ishiko, T.: Energy expenditure of elbow exflexion. *J. Physiol. Soc. Jap.*, **14**:494–497 (1952) (in Japanese).

Ishiko, T.: *Sports and Human Body.* Iwanami (1962) (in Japanese).

Ishiko, T.: Biomechanics of rowing. *Med. Sport*, **6**:249–252 (1971).

Ishiko, T., et al: Energy metabolism of skiing. *Res. J. Phys. Educ.*, **2**:130–137 (1956) (in Japanese).

Japan Sports Association: *Report of Sports Sciences for the 18th Olympic Games in Tokyo* (1965) (in Japanese).

Millikan, G. A.: The role of muscle haemoglobin. *J. Physiol.*, **87**:38P–39P (1936).

Ministry of Education in Japan: *A Report on Physical Fitness of Japanese*. 1971 (in Japanese).

Morpurgo, B.: Über Activitats-Hypertrophie der willkürlichen Muskeln. *Virchow Arch. Pathol. Anat.*, **150**:522–554 (1897).

Nocker, J., D. Lehmann, and G. Schleusing: Einfluss von Training und Belastung auf den Mineralgehalt von Herz und Skeletmuskel. *Int. Z. angew. Physiol.*, **17**:243–251 (1958).

Palladin, A., and D. Ferdmann: Über dem Einfluss des Trainings der Muskeln auf ihren Kreatingehalt. *Hoppe Seyler's Z. Physiol. Chem.*, **174**:284–294 (1928).

Petern, T., T. Sjöstrand, and B. Sylven: Der Einfluss des Trainings auf die Häufigkeit der Capillaren in Herz und Skeletmuskulatur. *Arbeitsphysiol.*, **9**:376–386 (1936).

Vannotti, A., and H. Pfister: Untersuchungen zum Studium des Trainierstseins. IV. Mitteilung: Die Blutversorgung des ruhenden Muskels am Tramierten Tiere. *Arbeitsphysiol.*, **7**:127–133 (1934).

Wipple, G. H.: The hemoglobin of striated muscle. I. Variations due to age and exercise. *Amer. J. Physiol.*, **76**:693–706 (1926).

Neuromuscular Performance

4

E. Karvinen and P. V. Komi
University of Jyväskylä
Jyväskylä, Finland

Neural Control of Muscular Activity

Motor Unit

The basic functional unit that initiates movement in muscle tissue is called the motor unit. It consists of a single alpha motor neuron, its axon, and all the muscle fibers innervated through the axonal branches. The number of muscle fibers in one motor unit varies widely. There is a general agreement that muscles controlling fine movements and adjustments have the smallest number of muscle fibers per motor unit, whereas large coarse-acting muscles have large units. Thus, it has been estimated, for example, that motor units of human extraocular muscles contain five to six muscle fibers, human laryngeal muscles two to three fibers, and the medial head of the human gastrocnemius 2000 muscle fibers per motor unit.

The individual fibers of a motor unit may be widely scattered and intermingled with fibers of other motor units.

The spike potentials of each motor unit seem to be localized in an approximately circular region, with an average diameter of 5 mm, to which the fibers of the motor unit are confined. Many overlapping motor units are found in this 5-mm area as well.

Conduction Along the Motor Neuron. Under natural conditions the contraction of a muscle fiber is initiated by the arrival of a nervous impulse. The motor neurons have a resting membrane potential of 50–80 millivolts (mv). The membrane has a neutral pump extruding sodium ions (Na^+) and taking up potassium ions (K^+), thus generating concentration gradients of these ions across the membrane. An imbalance in back diffusion of ions functions to separate the electric charge; since K^+ can penetrate more easily than Na^+, the excess K^+, diffusing outward, charges the outside of the membrane positively and thus generates the transmembrane voltage.

The nervous impulse is propagated in the form of an action potential or spike that reaches a peak of 40–50 mv, positive inside, and swings rapidly back to the resting level. An increase in Na$^+$ permeability is responsible for the rising phase of the action potential, whereas K$^+$ permeability increases as the action potential declines. The action potential leaves behind a short refractory period of 1 to a few milliseconds (msec) during which the fiber is unable to carry a second signal.

Neuromuscular Transmission. While nervous impulses travel along the axons in the form of action potentials, the transfer from nerve to muscle takes place by means of a chemical transmitter, acetylcholine (ACh). It has been shown that ACh is released from a presynaptic site and that it acts on a postsynaptic site. Schematically, neuromuscular transmission involves the following steps (Katz, 1966):

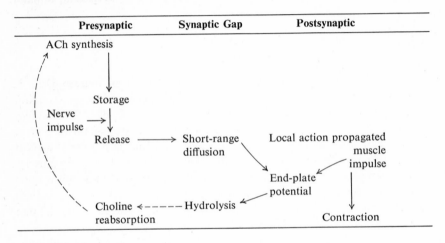

When a nervous impulse reaches the terminal branch, a small amount of ACh is set free into the synaptic gap that separates nerve and muscle. By diffusion, ACh reaches the muscle membrane and acts upon it in such a way that it suddenly becomes freely permeable to both Na$^+$ and K$^+$. The membrane loses its resting potential and an end-plate potential is produced. If the end-plate potential reaches a critical firing level, a propagated muscle action potential is produced. ACh is immediately broken down by an enzyme, cholinesterase, found in the area. Neuromuscular transmission can be blocked by curarine, which occupies the sites where ACh should act, or by anticholinesterases (for example, insecticides or nerve gases).

Conduction Along the Muscle Fiber. Conduction along the membrane of the muscle fiber is rather similar to that along the neuron. The end-plate potential gives rise to a propagated muscle action potential of an all-or-nothing type that displaces the resting membrane potential of the muscle fiber from −90 mv to a peak of +35 mv. The action potential, traveling along the membrane at a speed of about 5 m/sec, serves to produce sufficiently quick "mobilization" of the contractile apparatus of the muscle fiber. In a long muscle fiber, however, the excitation cannot reach all parts simultaneously.

The action potential gives rise to contraction by a sequence of at least two main events. First, the action potential generates a signal that is conducted inwardly by an internal membranous structure called the T system and rapidly transforms the electrical charge at the cell membrane into an equivalent charge in close proximity to the myofibrils. Second, this signal causes a release from stores within the sarcoplasmic reticulum of a chemical agent, very likely the calcium ion (Ca), which triggers an enzyme action associated with myosin (the contractile protein of the fibrils) to bring about the hydrolysis of adenosine triphosphate (ATP) with the release of energy for the contraction of the fibrils. The active shortening of the fibril is brought about by the interaction of two different kinds of protein filaments, actin and myosin.

Active State and Mechanical Reaction

After the action potential passes over the muscle fiber, there is a latent period of a few milliseconds before the contraction begins. When this latent period is over, the muscle immediately passes into an active state involving the contractile proteins; this active state is maintained for a short period of time. Mechanical tension is produced at the same time but, due to elastic elements present in series with the contractile elements, tension develops more slowly, reaching its peak while the active state is already disappearing. The duration of a single twitch contraction, which is produced in response to a single muscle action potential, is about 30 msec, but there is a wide range in duration from fast to slow muscle fibers.

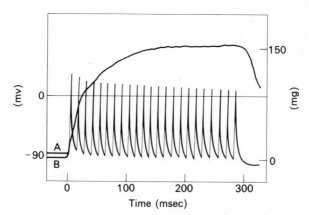

Figure 4-1. Intracellularly recorded action potentials and mechanical tension during tetanization of a single muscle fiber. *A*. Membrane potential (mv). *B*. Isometric tension (mg). [From E. Asmussen: *The Neuromuscular System and Exercise*. New York, Academic Press, 1968.]

If a new muscle action potential arrives before the twitch has completely died away, the second mechanical response becomes fused to the first. If action potentials arrive regularly at a high enough frequency, the individual responses can no longer be detected, and the muscle shows a smooth maintained contraction or tetanus (see Figure 4-1)

Proprioceptive Control of Muscular Contraction

For effective control of muscular activity by the brain and spinal cord, a constant supply of sensory information must be fed back as the movement progresses. This feedback of sensory information about movement and body position is called proprioception. There are two types of proprioceptive receptors: kinesthetic and vestibular.

Kinesthetic Proprioceptive Receptors. Three types of receptors serve the muscle sense or kinesthesis: (1) the muscle spindle, (2) the Golgi tendon organ, and (3) the joint receptors.

The Muscle Spindle. The muscle spindle is an elongated capsule lying parallel with the muscle fibers. It contains thin modified muscle fibers called intrafusal muscle fibers. Each intrafusal fiber consists of two contractile polar portions striated in the same way as normal (extrafusal) muscle fibers and a central part, the nuclear bag, which is noncontractile. The polar portion is supplied by a thin motor nerve of the gamma (γ) type. The sensory end organs within the spindle are of two types: the annulospiral primary ending in the midportion, and the flower spray secondary ending in the transitional zone between the nuclear bag and the contractile part. There are two types of afferent nerve fibers. The annulospiral ending discharges into its large type I sensory nerve (fast conducting), whereas the flower spray ending discharges into its type II sensory nerve (slow conducting).

Sensory impulses are generated in the muscle spindle when the central portion of the nuclear part between the polar regions becomes stretched (see Figure 4-2). This may happen (1) when the whole muscle is passively stretched or (2) when increased activity of the γ fibers causes the polar portions of the intrafusal fibers to contract. A contraction of the whole muscle tends to shorten the muscle spindle and, thus, stops the generation of sensory impulses in the spindle.

Adaptation of the muscle spindle occurs slowly. Its discharge into the afferent nerve continues for as long as the muscle is stretched, though the frequency of the discharge gradually declines. A stimulus that increases slowly in intensity produces a lower frequency of sensory impulses than a stimulus rising rapidly to the same level. Thus, the muscle spindle is a receptor to measure the length of the muscle, the extent of mechanical stimulation, and the rate at which the stretch is applied.

The Golgi Tendon Organ. The Golgi tendon organ (see Figure 4-2) is located at the insertion of the tendon into the muscle. Thus the tendon organ is in series with the muscle fibers. It is stimulated by tension in the tendon, either by stretching or by active contraction of the muscle. A sensory difference is found between passive stretching and muscle contraction. In active contraction, the tendon organ discharges but the muscle spindle does not because it is parallel with the extrafusal muscle fibers and is thus unloaded when the extrafusal fibers shorten. In passive stretch, the spindle discharges only because the tendon organ has a very high threshold for stimulus. At high tension, the tendon organ will fire.

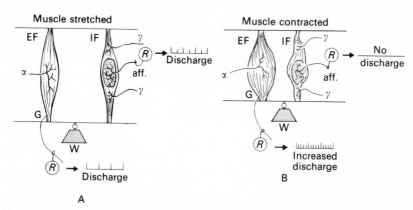

Figure 4-2. Schematic illustration of the activity in afferent fibers from muscle spindle (*aff.*) and Golgi tendon organ (*G*, lower record) when the muscle is (A) stretched and (B) contracted. *EF*. Extrafusal muscle fibers. *IF*. Intrafusal muscle fibers. *R*. Recording instrument with its record of nervous discharge. The muscle spindle is stimulated by stretch, but there is eventually a pause in its discharge during muscle contraction during which there is an accelerated rate of discharge from the tendon organ. [From *Textbook of Work Physiology* by P.-O. Astrand and K. Rodahl. Copyright 1970. Used with permission of McGraw-Hill Book Company.]

Joint Receptors. Joint receptors are located in the ligaments and the capsules of the joints. Some of these receptors are specialized to respond to movement of the joint, whereas others discharge when the joint is in a certain position but are less sensitive to movements.

The Vestibular Receptors. The vestibular receptors are located in the nonauditory labyrinths of the inner ear. There are two proprioceptive receptors in the inner ear: the crista and the otolith organ. The crista is stimulated by the movement of fluid in three small canals called semicircular canals. The cristae provide sensory information on rotational acceleration or deceleration of movement; rotational movement in itself is not recognized. The otolith organ provides information on the direction of gravity or linear acceleration. Thus we can recognize the posture of the body in space.

Spinal Reflexes. Much of the neural control of muscular activity is reflex in nature. A reflex is an involuntary motor response to a stimulus and, in a simple form, the reflex consists of a discharge from a sensory nerve ending receptor from which impulses are conducted over the sensory (afferent) nerve fiber to a synapse or junction with a motor neuron in the spinal cord. When the motor (efferent) neuron is stimulated to discharge, impulses are conducted to the effector muscle, producing the reflex response.

The Myotatic or Stretch Reflex. Myotatic or stretch reflex is a simple spinal reflex (see Figure 4-3). Its receptors are the annulospiral endings in the muscle spindle. When this part of the spindle is stretched, impulses are sent to the spinal cord where motor neurons of the same muscle are stimulated to discharge, with the result that motor units in the same muscle that contains the stretched muscle spindle will contract. When the muscle contracts, the ends of the muscle spindle come closer together and the stretch on the annulospiral ending is reduced. The stimulus to the receptor will then become less or cease entirely.

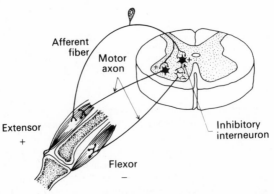

Figure 4-3. The stretch reflex. If the extensor muscles are stretched, an impulse is evoked that goes from the muscle spindles in the afferent fibers, which synapse with the motorneurons of the extensor muscles, stimulating them to contraction (+). Other branches of the afferent fibers synapse with interneurons which, however, will cause an inhibition of the motorneurons of the flexor muscles, which therefore will relax (−) (reciprocal inhibition). [From *Textbook of Work Physiology* by P.-O Astrand and K. Rodahl. Copyright 1970. Used with permission of McGraw-Hill Book Company.]

Stretch on the muscle spindle can be produced by passive stretching of the whole muscle; for example, in a routine medical examination, tapping the quadriceps tendon stretches the muscle and its muscle spindles and results in the knee reflex, a jerk of the lower leg.

The myotatic reflex is the basic reflex in postural control. The muscles antagonizing the pull of gravity are stretched and thereby the muscle spindles of these muscles are also stretched. By means of the myotatic reflex the muscles then contract so that the pull of gravity is counterbalanced or relieved.

Antimyotatic Reflex. Antimyotatic reflex is initiated from the Golgi tendon organ. The tendon organ has a much higher threshold of stimulus than the muscle spindle. Therefore, the antimyotatic reflex is elicited only by powerful tension applied to the tendon, either passively or by active contraction of the muscle. The reflex response is a reflex relaxation of the muscle connected with the tendon. The relaxation is probably caused by an inhibition of the γ neurons resulting in a decrease in the stretch applied on the annulospiral ending and thus reducing the myotatic reflex contraction of the muscle. The antimyotatic reflex serves in preventing overstretching of the tissues.

Renshaw Feedback. Alpha motor neurons have recurrent axons that synapse with internuncial neurons, called Renshaw cells, in the spinal cord (see Figure 4-4). The Renshaw cells send axons, having inhibitory synaptic connections, to the same alpha motor neuron and other motor neurons at the same segmental level of the cord. This system constitutes a feedback loop: The alpha neuron activation is fed back and used to inhibit the same and other motor units not to make the contraction too strong. This may protect against convulsive activity and overloading of the muscles.

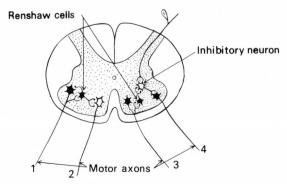

Figure 4-4. Some motorneurons give off branches before they leave the spinal cord. These branches synapse with inhibitory internuncial cells, called Renshaw cells. They synapse, in turn, with the same or other motorneurons. To the left in the figure the activated motorneuron (**1**) stimulates the Renshaw cell, which then inhibits both motorneurons (**1**) and (**2**). To the right we have an example of inhibition of inhibition: An impulse in the afferent nerve (upper right) stimulates the inhibitory neuron, and therefore, the motorneuron (**4**) will become inhibited. If the motorneuron (**3**) is now stimulated it excites, via its branches, the Renshaw cell, which in turn inhibits the inhibitory neuron and, as a consequence, the motorneuron (**4**) will be released from the inhibition and may more easily respond to excitatory impulses. [From *Textbook of Work Physiology* by P.-O. Astrand and K. Rodahl. Copyright 1970. Used with permission of McGraw-Hill Book Company.]

Internuncial Cells. Only a few sensory signals entering the spinal cord or signals from the brain terminate directly on the α motor neurons. Instead the signals are transmitted first through internuncial cells where they are appropriately processed before stimulating the motor neurons. The internuncial

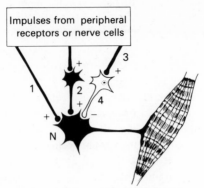

Figure 4-5. The motorneuron (*N*) in the spinal cord can be excited (+) directly (*1*) or via an internuncial cell (*2*). Thereby, an impulse is propagated in the nerve fiber and the muscle is stimulated, causing muscular activity. However, other nerve terminals can prevent the motorneuron from responding to the exciting impulse. Schematically this is illustrated as follows: Nerve ending (*3*) stimulates an inhibitory internuncial cell (*4*). This cell inhibits (−) the motorneuron to react to the stimulation by nerve *1*. [From *Textbook of Work Physiology by* P.-O. Astrand and K. Rodahl. Copyright 1970. Used with permission of McGraw-Hill Book Company.]

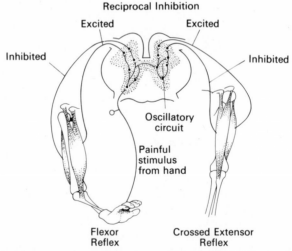

Figure 4-6. Reciprocal inhibition. A painful stimulus from the hand results in a withdrawal of the hand by the contraction of the flexor muscles (flexor reflex). Other branches of the afferent fibers from the hand, however, synapse with internuncial cells, which will cause an inhibition of the motorneurons of the extensor muscles which therefore will relax (reciprocal inhibition). Some internuncial cells connect the left and right sides of the body. Thus crossed reflexes are produced. For instance, the flexor reflex on the left side leads to an extensor reflex on the right side (crossed extensor reflex) and to an inhibition of the flexor muscles on the right side. [From A. C. Guyton: *Textbook of Medical Physiology*, 3rd ed. Philadelphia, W. B. Saunders, 1966.]

cells are therefore responsible for the convergence of motor stimulatory signals from many different sources. Thus, they are responsible for the integrative functions of the spinal cord.

For instance, excitation of one muscle often produces inhibition of another muscle via the internuncial cells (see Figure 4-5). This is the case when a stretch reflex of one muscle produces simultaneously an inhibition of the antagonistic muscle. This phenomenon is called *reciprocal inhibition* (see Figure 4-6). Likewise, internuncial cells are responsible for reciprocal relationships between the right and left sides of the body. For instance, a flexor reflex on one side leads to an extensor reflex on the opposite side as well as an inhibition of the flexor on the opposite side.

Higher Control of Muscular Activity

The motor neurons are activated or inhibited by nervous impulses which constantly travel either through descending tracts from the brain or reflexly through sensory nerves from receptors in the muscles or other organs. The excitability of the motor neurons is increased or decreased depending on the algebraic sum of the excitatory and inhibitory activity arriving at the synaptic knobs from different sources.

Pyramidal and Extrapyramidal Systems. Motor pathways descending from the brain fall into two major categories: pyramidal and extrapyramidal systems. The *pyramidal* tracts are direct paths from the motor centers in the cortex to the spinal cord where they synapse with internuncial neurons, which, in turn, synapse with the motor neurons to the muscles. The pyramidal tracts initiate discrete voluntary contractions in different muscles.

The term *extrapyramidal* is used to describe all of the influences of the brain on the lower motor neurons that are not effected through the pyramidal system. The extrapyramidal tracts also originate in subcortical centers and in the brain stem. The movements initiated through them are more massive and diffuse muscular contractions involving several muscles and joints. The reticulospinal tracts are the most common pathways by which these effects are transmitted to the motor neurons of the spinal cord. The extrapyramidal system may be either excitatory or inhibitory.

The Gamma (γ) System. There are muscular contractions that are initiated in the brain but are not elicited though direct pathways from the brain.

The reticular formation of the brain stem both receives impulses from other areas of the brain and initiates nervous impulses that are then transmitted via the reticulospinal tracts to the γ neurons innervating the intrafusal muscle fibers (see Figure 4-7). When the contractile portions of the intrafusal fibers contract, sensory impulses are generated in the muscle spindle. These impulses will then elicit a myotatic reflex and a number of extrafusal muscle fibers will contract.

Thus, a muscular contraction has been produced by means of the γ loop

(Granit, 1956) without the involvement of direct pathways from the brain to the extrafusal muscle fibers. The direct pathways are probably more important for skilled and sudden movements, whereas the γ loop may be more important for postural control and automatic movements, such as walking.

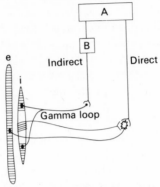

Figure 4-7. Schemes of indirect motor pathway via γ loop, and direct pathway. *A.* Higher motor centers. *B.* Centers in reticular formation. *i.* Intrafusal fibers. *e.* Extrafusal muscle fibers. [From E. Asmussen: *The Neuromuscular System and Exercises.* New York, Academic Press, 1968.]

Cerebellar Control. Information from the motor cortex concerning the stimulation of the pyramidal system is passed to the cerebellum. Thus, the cerebellum is informed of the desired force and rate of muscular contraction. During the contraction, proprioceptive impulses are also sent to the cerebellum informing it of the actual progress of the contraction. The cerebellum then compares the two sets of information and sends out corrective impulses so that the force and rate of contraction will be adjusted to the intended level. Thus, the cerebellum acts as a comparator in a servomechanism. The extrapyramidal system is controlled by the cerebellum in a similar way.

Many highly skilled movements are so rapid that there is no time to execute cerebellar control over them. Such skilled movements are controlled completely by the cerebral cortex. These movements are produced by some kind of patterned sequence of controls summoned into action on appropriate command.

Coordination of Muscular Activity. Normally a movement is an interplay of muscles (agonists, antagonists, synergists, and stabilizing muscles), and it results from the integrative action of the nervous system on different levels (cortical, cerebellar, subcortical, and spinal) (see Figure 4-8). Volitional movements are initiated in the cortex; the rate and force of the contraction is controlled by the cerebellum; and the stability of the limb for the execution of the movement is secured by the globus pallidus (one of the basal ganglia), which provides tonic contraction of the muscles in the proximal part of the limb. The signals from these and other nervous centers, as well as sensory impulses, finally converge on the spinal level.

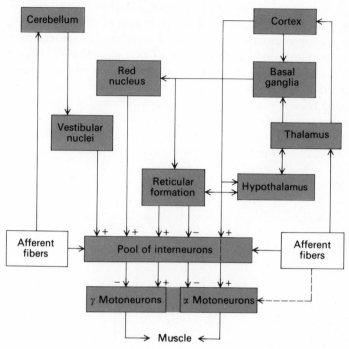

Figure 4-8. Schematic illustration of some of the connections with the central nervous system essential for coordinated muscular activity. (For simplicity most of the connections to and from the cerebellum are excluded.) The spinal motoneurons and interneurons are exposed to excitatory ($+$) as well as inhibitory ($-$) impulses from various levels of the central nervous system. The α and γ systems are, in a way, independent of each other, but are normally linked together via the interneurons. The afferent fibers come from muscle spindles, Golgi tendon organs, joint receptors, cutaneous receptors, and vestibular organs. They constitute feedback channels used in the integration of motor activity. [From *Textbook of Work Physiology* by P.-O. Astrand and K. Rodahl. Copyright 1970. Used with permission of McGraw-Hill Book Company.]

Interrelationship Among Electrical (Neural) Activity and Mechanical Responses of Muscle

Gradation of Muscular Contraction

A greater volitional input to the muscle usually brings about an increased mechanical output, that is, the muscle tension increases. This increase in tension indicates that (1) a single motor unit is discharging more frequently and/or (2) more motor units are being activated. Since the motor units are the smallest functional units of muscle tissue, it seems logical to investigate the mechanism of gradation of muscle contraction from the behavior of these motor units.

During voluntary contraction, the discharge rates of single motor units vary from 5 to 50 (or more) impulses per second when the tension is increased from light to maximum. By using the technique of electrical stimulation, it has been well demonstrated that the increase of motor unit tension is caused by a summation in individual twitches of that motor unit. The summation starts at the minimal rate of steady firing of the motor neuron. The gradation of contraction of the whole muscle proceeds in the same manner. The smooth pull on the muscle results from continuous twitches of several motor units that discharge at different frequencies. Because the tension produced by a single motor unit is relatively small (only a few grams), a strong contraction of skeletal muscle requires the contraction of many such motor units.

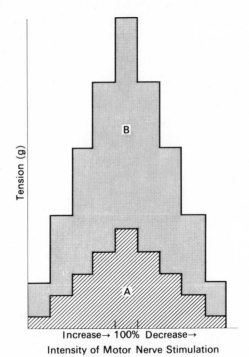

Figure 4-9. Diagram illustrating the different patterns of tension change by muscles with small (*A*) and larger (*B*) motor units. For the purposes of the diagram, it is assumed that the motor unit sizes are uniform within each hypothetical muscle. [From Barry Wyke: *Principles of General Neurology*. Amsterdam, London, New York, Elsevier Publishing Co., 1969.]

The minimum tension that a muscle can exert is the tension of its smallest motor unit. Some skeletal muscles contain mainly small motor units (those having few muscle fibers per unit), whereas other muscles may have predominantly large motor units. This means that, if more motor units are being activated in the muscle containing primarily large units, a much coarser (less smooth) gradation of tension is observed than if the motor units were smaller in size (see Figure 4-9).

In addition to the size spectrum of the constituent motor units, the smoothness of voluntary movement also depends on the degree of asynchrony among the volleys of impulses coming down the many axons. In the past, it was an accepted opinion that the asynchrony of motor unit contraction was relatively complete in the entire physiological tension range. Recent experiments with fine techniques of cross-correlation analysis (Person and Kudina, 1968) have shown, however, that the asynchronous motor unit activity in healthy subjects takes place only during very weak contractions. As Figure 4-10 suggests, the degree of synchronization seems to be related to the intensity of contraction. This existence of synchronization, to which fatigue and certain neuromuscular disturbances such as poliomyelitis and hemiparesis contribute, is probably due to some mechanism that inactivates impulses at the spinal level (Person and Kudina, 1968).

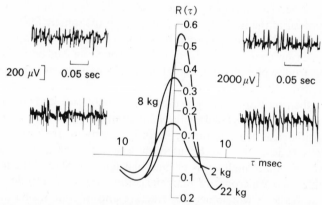

Figure 4-10. Cross-correlation (synchronization) functions of two electromyographs of m. biceps brachii in a normal subject under different loads. Surface electrodes. $R(\tau) =$ maximum value of cross correlation. [From R. S. Person and L. P. Kudina: Cross-correlation of electromyograms showing interference patterns. *Electroencephalogr. Clin. Neurophysiol.*, **25**:58–68 (1968).]

Muscular Tone

The concept of muscular tone has been widely used by neurophysiologists, physiotherapists, and physical educators. However, the real meaning of the term has been different for different people. To some it has meant mainly those nervous factors (either α or γ control) that bring the muscle into a state of activity. However, it is generally agreed among most of the investigators that resting, relaxed muscle displays electrical silence; that is, no electromyographic activity can be recorded from the muscle. Yet, a relaxed muscle possesses tone which is a result of the natural elasticity of the muscular and fibrous tissue. Thus, resting muscle tone is of mechanical origin. This can be demonstrated by the fact that a muscle will show resistance to stretch without relying on nervous control.

The report by Long (1970) suggests that at a certain threshold level reflex activity can be detected; above this level, tone is a result of both neural and mechanical factors. Apparently the quality (and quantity) of the connective tissue determines the mechanical (resting) muscle tone because it seems to be age dependent in men and always greater in men than in women.

Relationship Between Electrical Activity and Tension in the Skeletal Muscle

The motor unit is activated by a variety of nervous pathways that include impulses from the motor cortex and excitatory and inhibitory effects from various reflex sources. For this reason one should not assume that the motor unit potential, which precedes the contraction, is a result of voluntary activation alone. This motor unit potential, which is a summated waveform consisting of all of the individual potentials from the muscle fibers belonging to that motor unit, can be recorded by means of electromyography (EMG). In EMG measurements the activation of motor units can be picked up by surface electrodes placed upon the skin of the muscle, by inserted needle electrodes, or by fine wire electrodes. Needle and fine wire electrodes are very selective in their pick up and can be used in the qualitative study of motor unit activation. If one is interested in the activation of the whole muscle in the entire physiological tension range, surface electrodes are preferred. Wire inserted electrodes can also be used in kinesiological and physiological studies, which require high levels of muscular tension. Due to the fineness of the wire [25–50 μ (microns) in diameter], this type of electrode is usually painless; however, it will sometimes fracture and migrate inside the muscle (Jonsson and Bagge, 1968). The repeatability of measurements is better with surface than with wire inserted electrodes (Komi and Buskirk, 1970).

Integrated EMG versus Isometric Tension. To investigate the relationship between EMG activity and muscular tension, the EMG must be quantified by some means, for example, electronic integration. The integrated EMG (IEMG) has been shown to increase with an increase in muscle tension (see Figure 4-11). The slope of the regression line indicates that this relationship depends on (1) which muscle is being studied, (2) the condition of the muscle, and also (3) the recording technique used. There is also a fairly large interindividual variability in the amount of IEMG activity per unit of tension. This will make it necessary to avoid comparing two different individuals with regard to their electrical activity per certain amount of muscle tension. Although the IEMG value stays relatively constant for each muscle under normal conditions, it must not be regarded as an indicator of the level of muscular tension produced unless the calibration curve for the relationship between IEMG and tension is known for each individual and each muscle studied. A great variability has been observed also in the amount of IEMG among different muscles of the same subject. A relatively poor correlation

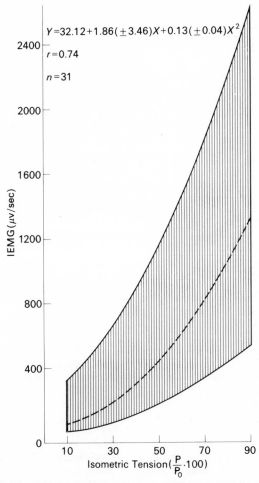

$$Y = 32.12 + 1.86(\pm 3.46)X + 0.13(\pm 0.04)X^2$$

$$r = 0.74$$

$$n = 31$$

Figure 4-11. Relationship between integrated electrical activity (IEMG) of the m. biceps brachii (surface electrodes) and the forearm flexor isometric tension. The shaded area represents the range of the regression lines of 31 male subjects. [From P. V. Komi and E. R. Buskirk: Effect of eccentric and concentric muscle conditioning on tension and electrical activity of human muscle. *Ergonomics.* **15**(4):417–434 (1972).]

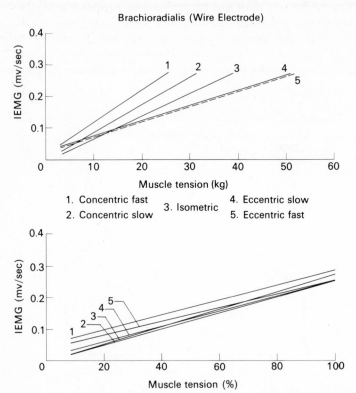

Figure 4-12. Comparison of the relationship between IEMG and tension for the brachioradialis muscle at different contraction velocities, when muscle tension is expressed in absolute values (above) and in percent of the maximum voluntary contraction of the elbow flexors (below).

Note: The contraction velocity was measured from the biceps brachii muscle of an adult man of average size. Because in the measuring dynamometer all the velocities stayed constant and reliable, the recorded value was used for all male subjects (16), and was identified as follows:

Concentric fast	+4.5 cm/sec
Concentric slow	+1.4 cm/sec
Isometric	0 cm/sec
Eccentric slow	−1.4 cm/sec
Eccentric fast	−4.5 cm/sec

[From P. V. Komi: Relationships between muscle tension, EMG, and velocity of contraction under concentric and eccentric work. In J. E. Desmedt (ed.): *New Developments in Electromyography and Clinical Neurophysiology*, Vol. 1. Basel, Karger, pp. 596–606, 1973.]

coefficient has been observed between IEMG and absolute tension in kilograms. This finding strengthens the assumption that the amount of IEMG should not be used directly to indicate how much force has been exerted.

Several factors may have an effect on the regression line of IEMG per tension. In certain pathological conditions and during fatigue the regression line becomes steeper, indicating that a greater neural input is needed to produce a certain amount of muscle tension. In a normal muscle the relationship between IEMG and muscle tension can be quadratic (see Figure 4-11) or linear. The recording technique may affect the nature of the relationship, but the nonlinear regression line could also be due to the effect of the increased role of motor unit synchronization, which comes into play in higher muscle tensions.

Electrical Activity in Isotonic Contractions. The information concerning the relationship between IEMG and muscle tension has usually been obtained under isometric conditions of muscle contraction. When other types of contraction are investigated, the IEMG will be a function of (1) tension, (2) velocity of contraction, (3) acceleration of movement, and (4) the external

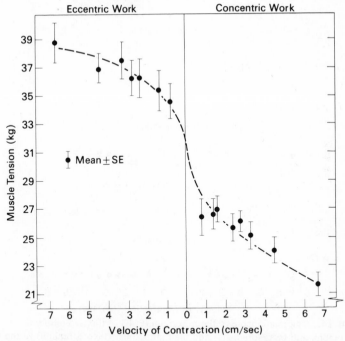

Figure 4-13. The force-velocity relationship for the elbow flexor muscles in eccentric and concentric work ($n = 16$). [From P. V. Komi: Measurement of the force-velocity by relationship in human muscle under concentric and eccentric work. *The Third International Seminar of Biomechanics,* Rome, 1971.]

mechanical work. If the velocity of muscle shortening and lengthening is held constant, which is possible only with fairly complex measurement techniques, then the regression line (IEMG/tension) is much steeper in concentric than in eccentric contraction (see Figure 4-12). This implies that for a certain level of tension one will have to use more electrical (neural) input energy to the muscle when this tension is exerted concentrically. This also means that fewer muscle fibers are needed in eccentric than in concentric work to produce the same force. Figure 4-12 also shows that the regression line becomes steeper the faster the muscle contracts concentrically. And, if the IEMG is related to the relative (percent) muscle tension, then the regression lines become superimposed, suggesting that despite the type or velocity of contraction the IEMG/muscle tension ratio stays the same.

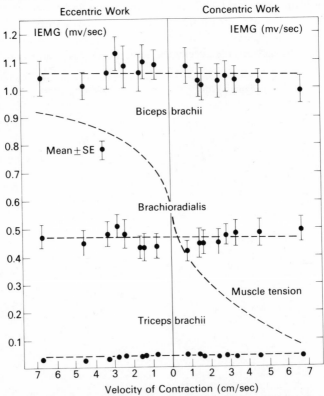

Figure 4-14. The relationship of the maximum IEMG of the two elbow flexor muscles (biceps brachii and brachioradialis) and their antagonist (triceps brachii) to the velocity of contraction in eccentric and concentric work ($n = 16$). The EMG's were recorded simultaneously with the force-velocity data of Figure 4-13. [From P. V. Komi: Measurement of the force-velocity relationship in human muscle under concentric and eccentric work. *The Third International Seminar of Biomechanics*, Rome, 1971.]

Dependence of the Maximum Electromyographic Activity on the Velocity of Contraction. The force-velocity relationship in human muscle under concentric and eccentric contractions can be measured with a special electromechanical dynamometer, which allows accurate control of both velocity and direction of movement (Komi, 1971). As the obtained force-velocity curve (see Figure 4-13) indicates, the difference in maximum tension between eccentric and concentric contraction becomes greater when higher velocities are used in shortening and lengthening. The behavior of IEMG under these conditions does not seem to follow the same pattern. The maximum IEMG is relatively the same at different contraction speeds and in all types of contraction (isometric, concentric, and eccentric) (see Figure 4-14). This suggests that the muscle's contractile component, which is the portion of muscle to receive the efferent neural command, could be activated to the same extent in any kind of maximum contraction.

Conditioning of the Neuromuscular System

Active physical conditioning also has its effects on the functional state of the neuromuscular system. In this system, both the neural (input) component and the muscle function (output) will be affected by training. Because the movement of the muscle is directed by several neural command and feedback systems, it is often difficult to assess in which of the two components the changes caused by training have been most remarkable. Furthermore, it is often impossible to differentiate the pure effects of training from those of learning. Training causes a motor act to be learned. Thus, learning involves training, either physical, mental, or both. In the following sections, focus is given to the principles that govern the relationship of conditioning to coordination and the interplay of muscles, to muscle strength, and to the force-velocity relationship of the muscle.

Coordination of Movement

The neuromuscular system has been developed to produce coordinated movements. For example, in a simple flexion-extension movement of the elbow joint the agonist-antagonist activity should be fairly well coordinated. A nontrained subject will execute this movement in a nonstereotyped fashion, which is seen by the jerky nature of the movement and continued activity of the antagonist muscles. The movement will be performed mainly because of the alternating predominance of the effort of one muscle over that of the other. After a series of training sessions, the movement will become more stereotyped, synchronized, smooth, and it will follow the classical concept of reciprocal relations in rhythmic movements.

The effect of training on the coordination of the muscles in a complex movement, such as the knee circle mount on the horizontal bar, has been

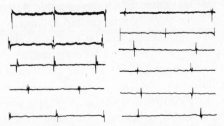

Figure 4-15. Example of a subject's ability to isolate eleven different motor units of the abductor pollicis brevis muscle. [From J. V. Basmajian, M. Baeza, and C. Fabriger: Conscious control and training of individual spinal motor neurons in normal human subjects. *J. New Drugs*, **5**:78–85 (1965).]

clearly demonstrated by Kamon and Gormley (1968). In this type of movement a pattern of muscular activity for a trained subject is manifested by (1) a decrease in total neural (EMG) activity, (2) a reduction in the amount of overlap between muscles taking part in the execution of the movement, and (3) a shorter and sharper function of each muscle involved. Thus, a skilled movement shows improved economy in the use of the muscles and good coordination in the timing of muscle interplay.

Motor Unit Training

Coordination of activity can also take place "inside" the muscle, that is, among the several hundred motor units responsible for the muscular activity. Basmajian (1963) introduced the concept of "motor unit training," which means that human subjects are consciously able to control the firing of the

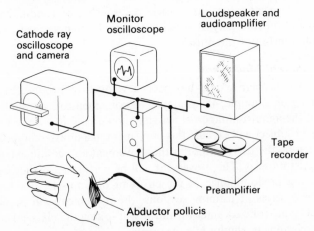

Figure 4-16. Arrangement of the recording and monitoring system for motor units training. [From J. V. Basmajian: Conscious control of single nerve cells. *New Sci.*, **20**:662–664 (1963).]

motor unit in any skeletal muscle. After a relatively short period of training almost all persons are able to isolate one motor unit from a muscle and turn it on and off in a desired manner. However, isolation of several motor units (see Figure 4-15) requires special high-order control by the subject. Motor unit training can also lead to such skills as the ability to control or deliberately change the firing rate of one spinal motor neuron. For training of these specific skills the use of both visual and auditory feedback systems is advisable (see Figure 4-16).

Effects of Training on the Relationship Between EMG and Muscle Tension

A trained person possesses the ability to produce a greater muscular force output than an untrained person, given the same amount of neural (EMG) energy (see Figure 4-17). Conditioning and training should then lead to a reduction in the EMG activity needed by a muscle to reach a certain level of muscular tension.

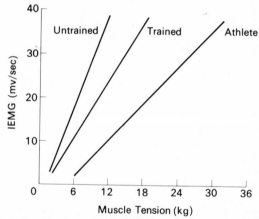

Figure 4-17. Relationship between IEMG and muscle tension during a progressively increasing isometric contraction by an untrained, normal trained, and a prominent sportsman. For an equal amount of neural energy (IEMG) the trained person is capable of exerting higher muscle tension than the untrained one. [Redrawn from A. Fischer and J. Merhautova: Electromyographic manifestations of individual stages of adapted sports technique. In *Health and Fitness in the Modern World*. Chicago, Athletic Institute, 1961, Chap. 13.]

Some authors (for example, Stoboy and Friedeboldt, 1968) suggest that conditioning of the muscle could also lead to a reduced role for the synchronously firing motor units in producing the force of the muscle. This beginning of the "desynchronization" phase depends apparently on the functional state of the muscle before the conditioning period starts. An atrophied muscle requires a longer conditioning period before the desynchronization can be triggered, whereas in a "fit" muscle this increased economical behavior can be demonstrated at a fairly early stage of training. The physiological mechanism responsible for the possible desynchronization phenomenon is unknown.

Conditioning of Muscular Strength and Speed

Overload Principle and Eccentric Training. For many decades scientists have been puzzled by the lack of information concerning the best method to increase muscle strength through training. When Hellebrandt and Houtz

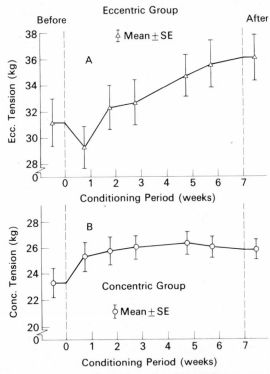

Figure 4-18. Increase of muscle strength by eccentric and concentric conditioning. *A.* Eccentric group, trained with maximum eccentric contraction of forearm flexors six times daily four times a week. Note a decrease in eccentric tension during the first conditioning week, which was due to muscle soreness. *B.* Concentric group, trained with maximum concentric contractions; the daily repetitions were the same as for the eccentric group. Despite the muscle soreness during early conditioning, the eccentric group attained a higher average tension in all contraction types (isometric, concentric, and eccentric) than did either the concentric or the control group. [From P. V. Komi and E. R. Buskirk: Effect of eccentric and concentric muscle conditioning on tension and electrical activity of human muscle. *Ergonomics,* **15**(4):417–434 (1972).]

(1956) introduced the term "overload principle," which is similar in concept to what the Germans already had discussed in the late 1800s (Roux, 1895), a considerable clarification was brought to the understanding of strength training methods. A present-day interpretation of this overload principle is that the higher the intensity of tension in conditioning, the greater would be the increase in muscular strength. In practical terms this means that if two different weights are lifted by two different persons using similar training methods, then the training effect of the heavier load on muscular strength should be greater than that of the lighter one. In looking at Figure 4-13, it is suggested that this principle will also lead to the conclusion that the greatest gains in muscular strength will be obtained by eccentric training, because the maximal muscle tension is always higher in eccentric than in any other type of muscular contraction.

Indeed, recent experiments (Komi and Buskirk, 1972) suggest the superiority of eccentric conditioning over other methods to improve muscle strength. In this study, two experimental groups, eccentric and concentric, performed at the same contraction speed several maximal contractions of the forearm flexors four times weekly for a period of 7 weeks. On the average the eccentric group gained more in muscle strength (either eccentric, isometric, or concentric) than did the concentric or control groups.

A most remarkable finding was, however, that all the subjects who trained eccentrically experienced muscle soreness in their exercised muscles during the first weeks of training. During this period, maximum tension decreased (see Figure 4-18). When the symptoms of pain disappeared an increase in tension occurred almost in a linear fashion. Although the concentric group also trained with maximum contractions, no soreness was felt by any of the subjects. In the eccentric group the pain could be localized in the tendon attachments of the muscles involved, that is, biceps brachii, brachioradialis, and brachialis. Thus, high tension eccentric work appears to give greater load to the elastic elements of the muscle (sarcolemma, connective tissue among fibers, and tendon), but its training effect will not show up until the elastic tissue has recovered from forceful stretching.

Muscle Conditioning and the Force-Velocity Curve. The force-velocity curve (see Figure 4-13) determines the basic principles concerning how and for what purpose the muscles should be conditioned or trained. If one wants mainly to train the velocity component of the muscle function, then the loads and contraction speeds should be selected from the low end (concentric work) of the curve (see Figure 4-13). To improve mainly the force component of the muscle function, high loads should be selected. Thus training with fast contractions specifically improves the speed of the muscle, whereas training stimuli of high tension have the specific effect of improving muscle strength. However, if one is interested in an overall power conditioning (power = force × velocity), then the contraction velocities for conditioning should be selected to correspond to 30–60% of the maximum isometric strength (P_o). Figure 4-19 summarizes this important work of Ikai (1970). So far this principle seems to be applicable only to concentric work because similar studies have not been reported on eccentric work.

Muscular Fatigue

Muscular fatigue means diminution of activity of a specific muscle or muscle group; that is, the mechanical output of the muscle decreases after a

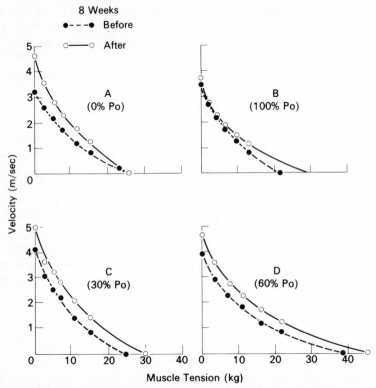

Figure 4-19. Specific effects of the different training loads and speeds on the force-velocity curve. *A*. The subject who trained his forearm flexors with maximum contraction without load (0 × P_0) showed no increase in strength but a considerable improvement in the velocity under the small load. *B*. Training with maximum load but zero velocity (1 × P_0) resulted in an increase of strength and velocity under larger loads. *C* and *D*. Training with the loads of 0.3 × P_0 (*C*) and 0.6 × P_0 (*D*) showed all-around improvement in the force-velocity relationship. The data suggest that training with maximum strength or maximum speed is effective merely to its own direction and that training by dynamic contraction with adequate load could improve both the force and velocity factors, resulting in improvement of the power. [Redrawn from M. Ikai: Training of muscle strength and power in athletes. A paper presented during FIMS Congress, Oxford, England, 1970.]

sufficiently prolonged and intense period of exercise. In isolated muscles, this is seen as a decreasing contraction or tension production in spite of constant stimulation. As the muscle fibers become fatigued their output per twitch decreases, but new units are then mobilized to compensate for the lost power.

Although fatigue is localized in the neuromuscular system, the major cause of fatigue is chemical. It can be due either to accumulation of intermediate or final end products of energy metabolism (carbon dioxide, lactic acid, pyruvic acid, acid phosphates, and so on) or to the deficiency of energy-furnishing materials. The adequacy or inadequacy of oxygen supply to the muscles during exercise determines the extent of accumulation of the intermediate or end products of metabolism and influences the resynthesis of the energy-furnishing substances. Recovery from fatigue caused by lactic acid accumulation can occur within 1 hr, but if the depletion occurs in the glycogen stores, which are important in rebuilding the energy-rich phosphates, then the replenishing of these stores may take several days (Hultman, 1967).

Electrical changes that occur in muscle tissue during sustained contraction have been studied quite extensively. Most of the researchers agree that with sustained contractions occurring in a state of fatigue there is a reduction in the amplitude and a lengthening in the duration of the muscle action potential. Considerable modifications also occur in the organization of the electrical activity recorded from the whole muscle. For example, during continuous voluntary isometric contraction of a muscle, the integrated electrical activity gradually increases as fatigue sets in despite the fact that the tension is kept constant (Edwards and Lippold, 1956). This phenomenon is assumed to be due to recruitment of motor units to compensate for the decreased force of contraction in the fatigued muscle fibers. Other electrical changes in muscle during fatigue are the synchronous firing of motor units and the appearance of large waves with a frequency of 25–30 cycle/sec (Lippold, et al., 1960).

REFERENCES

Asmussen, E.: The neuromuscular system and exercise. In H. B. Falls (ed.), *Exercise Physiology*. New York and London, Academic Press, 1968.

Astrand, P.-O., and K. Rodahl: *Textbook of Work Physiology*. New York and London, McGraw-Hill, 1970.

Basmajian, J. V.: Conscious control of single nerve cells, *New Sci.*, **20**:662–664 (1963).

Basmajian, J. V., M. Baeza, and C. Fabrigar: Conscious control and training of individual spinal motor neurons in normal human subjects. *J. New Drugs*, **5**:78–85 (1965).

Edwards, R. G., and O. C. J. Lippold: The relation between force and integrated electrical activity in fatigued muscle. *J. Physiol.*, **132**:677–681 (1956).

Fischer, A., and J. Merhautova: Electromyographic manifestations of individual stages of adapted sports technique. In L. A. Larson (ed.), *Health and Fitness in the Modern World*. Chicago, The Athletic Institute, 1961, Chap. 13.

Granit, R.: *Receptors and Sensory Perception.* New Haven, Yale Univ. Press, 1956.

Guyton, A. C.: *Textbook of Medical Physiology*, 3rd ed. Philadelphia and London, W. B. Saunders, p. 777, 1966.

Hellebrandt, F., and S. Houtz.: Mechanism of muscle training in man: experimental demonstration of the overload principle. *Phys. Ther. Rev.*, **36**(6):371–383 (1956).

Hultman, E.: Physiological role of muscle glycogen in man with special reference to exercise. *Circ. Res.*, **20, 21**:suppl. 99–112 (1967).

Ikai, M.: Training of muscle strength and power in athletes. A paper presented during the FIMS Congress, Oxford, England, 1970.

Jonsson, B., and U. E. Bagge: Displacement, deformation and fracture of wire electrodes for electromyography. *Electromyography*, **8**:329–347 (1968).

Kamon, E., and J. Gormley: Muscular activity pattern for skilled performance and during learning of a horizontal bar exercise. *Ergonomics*, **11**(4):345–357 (1968).

Katz, B.: *Nerve, Muscle, and Synapse.* New York, McGraw-Hill, 1966.

Komi, P. V.: Measurement of the force-velocity relationship in human muscle under concentric and eccentric work. *The Third International Seminar of Biomechanics*, Rome, 1971.

Komi, P. V.: Relationship between muscle tension, EMG, and velocity of contraction under concentric and eccentric work. In J. E. Desmedt (ed.), *New Developments in Electromyography and Clinical Neurophysiology*, Vol. 1. Basel, Karger, pp. 596–606 (1973).

Komi, P. V., and E. R. Buskirk: Reproducibility of electromyographic measurements with inserted wire electrodes and surface electrodes. *Electromyography*, **10**(4):357–367 (1970).

Komi, P. V., and E. R. Buskirk: Effect of eccentric and concentric muscle conditioning on tension and electrical activity of human muscle. *Ergonomics*, **15**(4):417–434 (1972).

Lippold, O. C. J., et al.: The electromyography of fatigue. *Ergonomics*, **3**:121–131 (1960).

Long, C.: Normal and abnormal motor control in the upper extremities. Final report, Social and Rehabilitation Services, Grant No RD-2377-M Ampersaad Research Group, Cleveland, 1970.

Person, R. S., and L. P. Kudina: Cross-correlation of electromyograms showing interference patterns. *Electroenceph Alogr. Clin. Neurophysiol.*, **25**:58–68 (1968).

Roux, W.: *Gesammelte Abhandlungen über Entwicklungsmechanik der Organismen*, Band I, Funktionelle Anpassung. Leipzig, 1895.

Stoboy, H., and G. Friedeboldt: Changes in muscle function in atrophied muscles due to isometric training. *Bull. N. Y. Acad. Med.*, **44**:553–559 (1968).

Wyke, B.: *Principles of General Neurology.* Amsterdam, London, New York, Elsevier Publishing Co., p. 414, 1969.

The Organism and Speed and Power

5

P. R. TRAVERS AND W. R. CAMPBELL

St. Luke's College,
Exeter, England

An organism obtains both speed and power from muscular contractions. The skeletal muscles will shorten when contracting against a submaximal load, the degree of shortening varying inversely with the magnitude of the load applied. Initially, the muscle will contract without shortening (isometrically), until it has developed a tension which is equal to the load applied; thereafter it will contract and shorten (isotonically). From this it follows that a load will eventually be reached which equals the maximum isometric tension of which the muscle is capable; in this instance no shortening can occur, and the whole contraction is isometric. Thus, maximal isometric tension of a muscle is known as the muscle strength and is measured in practice with a dynamometer. It should be noted that, since true muscle strength is a measure of the maximal isometric tension, it is important that the dynamometer used allows only the very minimum of joint movement when making the test. In measuring strength there is also the question of whether a subject can voluntarily exert the maximal isometric tension of which a muscle is capable; indeed Asmussen (1969) has postulated that, "This may mean that one has a reserve of strength that normally cannot be mobilized but which may be called up in emergencies."

It should be noted that, when a muscle contracts isometrically it will expend energy but, paradoxically, it will do no mechanical work because no joint movement occurs. In movements of the whole or part of the organism there must be joint movement and, hence, there must be shortening of the muscles (prime movers) which bring about that movement. In the movement of any mass, be it the whole body, a body part, or an object propelled by the body, power is developed. Power is defined as the rate of doing work and may be derived from the formula

$$\text{Power} = \frac{\text{Force} \times \text{Distance}}{\text{Time}}$$

From this formula two others may be derived

$$\text{Power} = \text{Force} \times \text{Velocity}$$

$$\text{Power} = \frac{\text{Work}}{\text{Time}}$$

The force in this instance is the force necessary to overcome the load against which the muscle acts. The greater the force, the greater the power-potential of the organism. Thus, although raw strength is an important factor in power output, so too is speed. An individual may possess great strength but, unless he can exert that strength quickly, he will not be powerful. This is important because we need power rather than strength in the majority of sporting activities.

The rate at which a muscle will contract varies inversely with the load against which it works. The heavier the load, the slower the rate of contraction. In 1938, Professor A. V. Hill deduced the equation:

$$V = \frac{(P_0 - P)b}{(P + a)}$$

where V is the velocity of contraction, P is the force acting, P_0 is the isometric force that the muscle can develop at its optimal length, and a and b are constants. This equation is valid only for the length of the muscle L_o at which P_o is optimal; however, it can be modified for different muscle lengths.

In the isolated muscle preparation the power output when the muscle is stimulated electrically varies with the load, reaching a maximum when the load approximates to one-third of the maximum isometric tension. In experiments with human subjects once again the power output is found to be maximal when working against submaximal loads. This can be demonstrated simply as follows.

A subject lifts a weight and the time taken to move it vertically through a given distance is measured. From these measurements the power output may be calculated. The experiment is repeated using different weights varying from the maximum that can be lifted to zero. The speed of limb movement is measured by a photoelectric timer (Figure 5-1). A graph is then drawn showing the relationship of power output to weight lifted (Figure 5-2).

When lifting heavy weights the speed of movement will be low and so will the power output. As the weight is reduced the speed of movement will increase, and, provided that the increment in speed exceeds the decrement in weight, the power output will increase. Experimentally it has been found that

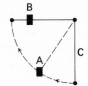

Figure 5-1.   Measurement of speed of limb movement.

the maximum power output is achieved when lifting a weight which is between one-half and two-thirds of the maximum that can be moved. This maximum weight which can be moved through the middle range of joint movement is found to be approximately three-quarters of the maximum isometric tension of the muscle group which produces the movement. Thus, we find that the maximum power output is achieved when lifting a weight which is approximately one-third of the maximum isometric tension of the muscle group involved. This correlates well with the results of the isolated muscle experiments. It should be noted that the exact fraction of the maximum weight with which the maximum power can be achieved depends upon the length of the levers involved. An individual with long limbs (levers) will produce his greatest power output with a smaller fraction of his maximum weight than someone with shorter limbs (levers). This means that body type exerts an influence upon power output.

It must be noted that even when a muscle contracts isometrically there will be some shortening of the muscle fibers as the muscle "takes up the slack." This is because a muscle must be considered as a complex system of contractile and elastic elements. Starling and Evans (1968) describe three elements (Figure 5-3): the parallel elastic component (PEC), the contractile

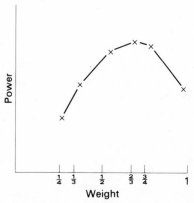

Figure 5-2.   Relationship of power output to weight lifted.

component (CC), and the series elastic component (SEC). The PEC operates only when the muscle is stretched beyond its resting length; the CC is capable of active shortening; and the SEC transmits and modifies, to some extent, the force of the CC. The SEC is found in the fibrous muscle attachments, whereas the PEC constitutes the interstitial fibrous tissue and, to some extent, the sarcolemma.

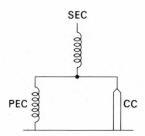

Figure 5-3.   Contractile and elastic elements in muscle.

During contractions from a position of rest the CC contracts to produce active shortening (concentric work). During eccentric work from the fully shortened position to the resting length, the CC lengthens against the load. However, when eccentric work continues beyond the resting length, that is to say in the outer range, the PEC comes into play and assists the CC as it "pays out." Similarly, the PEC assists the CC in concentric work from the outer range to the resting length.

The rate of contraction of human muscle fibers varies. Basically these fibers are divided into two groups, fast and slow firing, although it must be appreciated that the boundaries of the two groups are somewhat indefinite. The fast firing fibers have the larger cross section and are supplied by neurons of larger size and having high thresholds. Thus, they operate only at higher work intensities. The slow firing fibers are smaller in cross section and are supplied by neurons of smaller size and having lower thresholds. They, therefore, are active at all work intensities.

The fast firing fibers contain an abundance of glycolytic enzymes and are able to produce a high work output; however, the duration of their work is limited by the production of lactic acid because they work largely anaerobically. On the other hand, the slow firing fibers have many mitochondria and a higher concentration of myoglobin and other respiratory enzymes. They are therefore capable of more prolonged oxidative processes and can sustain a contraction for longer periods than can the fast firing fibers. The greater myoglobin content of the slow firing fibers has led to them being called "red" muscle fibers as opposed to the "white" fast firing fibers. This terminology is now seldom used because all muscle fibers are pink in color. Some authorities call the fast firing fibers large muscle fibers, owing to their greater cross section. Thus, we have large or fast firing fibers and small or slow firing fibers.

Each individual muscle will contain both red and white fibers, and it is evident that the function of the muscle will dictate the relative numbers of each. In addition, it must be remembered that functionally we are concerned with motor units rather than with individual muscle fibers. The motor unit is defined as a motor neuron and its associated muscle fibers. The larger the motor neuron, the larger the number of terminal axon fibrils, and hence the greater the number of muscle fibers that it supplies. Since the fast firing fibers are supplied by larger motor neurons, they will also be found in the larger motor units. Muscles which contain many fast firing fibers are therefore capable of producing great strength but, because they have an abundance of large motor units, cannot produce fine gradations of movements. Muscles of this type include the quadriceps femoris and the spinal muscles.

On the other hand the slow firing muscle fibers will be found in the smaller motor units, which means that the muscles containing predominantly these fibers will be capable of sustained action and also of very fine gradations of movement. In man these muscle fibers are found predominantly in the postural muscles, which must sustain continuous activity for long periods, in the small muscles of the hand, and in the muscles which control eye movements.

Bach (1948) showed that by changing the function of a muscle in an experimental animal it was possible to change red (slow firing) into pale (fast firing) fibers. He transplanted the tendon of soleus (red) into that of the synergist (pale) tibialis posterior. When the animals were killed 6 months later, he found that the iron and hemoglobin content of the transplanted muscle had changed toward that of the tibialis posterior. The iron content of tibialis posterior was 32.5 mg per 5 g of muscle, that of the normal (untransplanted) soleus was 53.49 mg, and that of the transplanted soleus was 34.00 mg. Additionally, he showed that the tetanic contraction of the transposed soleus when stimulated reflexly had changed and approximated that of the tibialis posterior. This experimental work suggests that, if the same changes occur in human muscles, this may be part of the mechanism by which strength is gained through strengthening exercises.

Certainly it is true that the circumference of a muscle will increase as a result of strengthening exercises. In part this increase in cross-sectional area is due to an increase in the diameter of the muscle fibers, in part to an increase in the capillary bed, and in part to an increase in the interstitial tissues. This relationship between the cross-sectional area and strength of a muscle was first investigated by Fick (1911). He compiled tables of the physiological cross section of various muscles related to their strength. The physiological cross section of a muscle is defined as a section through the muscle at its greatest diameter and at right angles to the direction of its fibers when the muscle is in its midshortened position. Thus in a fusiform muscle it is a section through the thickest part of the muscle at right angles to its longitudinal axis. The physiological cross section of other muscles is obtained by taking several sections each at right angles to the fibers so that all fibers are included (Fig. 5-4). Fick assumed that a muscle could develop a strength of 10 kgm/cm² of physiological cross section. This figure is nowadays accepted as being too high, and 3–4 kgm/cm² of cross section is recognized as being more correct.

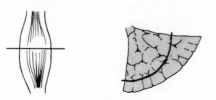

Figure 5-4.   Physiological cross section of muscle.

In many human activities the acceleration of the body as a whole or the acceleration that the body can impart to an external object is of importance. The thrust that a muscle can exert must therefore be considered. Thrust is a force, and therefore the maximum thrust that can be exerted is equal to the maximum isometric strength of a muscle. When the human body is being accelerated, the thrust of the legs is exerted against the ground and is exactly balanced by the reaction of the ground to the thrust. In the same way, the thrust exerted upon an external object is exactly balanced by the reaction of that object. Thus, if a weight is being lifted at a uniform rate, the thrust of the muscles which are being used is exactly equal to the weight lifted.

If an object is accelerated from zero velocity by a thrust which acts for a given time, the product of the thrust and the time is said to be the impulse. Consider the case of a subject making a vertical jump. He exerts a thrust against the ground, the force of which can be measured with a force platform. The thrust lasts for a finite time, until his feet leave the ground. The impulse can therefore be calculated by multiplying the thrust by the time during which it acts.

It is also apparent that when a subject makes a vertical jump he does mechanical work equivalent to the product of his body weight and the height jumped. The energy for the jump was generated while he was exerting thrust against the ground. The time during which this thrust is exerted can be measured accurately and simply by using a spring platform incorporating a microswitch that starts a timing device as soon as the subject begins to exert a force against the platform. The time clock is stopped as soon as he leaves the ground. Now, we know that all the energy generated during the thrust against the ground is dissipated by the time that he reaches the top of his jump; a measure of his power output can therefore be obtained by dividing the work done in the jump by the duration of the thrust.

$$\text{Power output} = \frac{\text{Body weight} \times \text{Height of jump}}{\text{Duration of thrust}}$$

This equation is of interest because it is often found that the height of the jump varies directly as the duration of the thrust, but this in turn means that the higher the jump the lower the power output for these subjects.

The time during which the thrust takes place is of importance in a number of sporting skills. The long last stride of the high jumper allows a long time for the operation of the thrust of his jumping leg to obtain the maximum velocity for his center of gravity. The arc of a golfer's swing and the point at which the club head strikes the ball dictates the length of the period of contact between the club head and the ball and, hence, the duration of the thrust. On the other hand, a basketball player or a soccer player who needs to exert thrust for a long time when jumping for the ball will be beaten to it by another player who, being more powerful, is able to generate the necessary impulse for his jump from a shorter ground-contact time. Serial vertical jump tests made during weight training programs at Saint Luke's College, Exeter, England, have shown that an improvement in the power output of a subject occurs not only as a result of a greater height of jump but also from a decrease in the time of thrust needed to achieve the same height.

It has been mentioned that the magnitude of the fraction of the maximum weight with which the greatest power output can be generated varies with the length of the limb. The longer the limb the smaller the fraction of the maximum weight that can be used to produce the greatest power output. Thus, it is apparent that both power and speed depend, to some extent, upon body type. The tall, asthenic ectomorph with his long levers is at a mechanical disadvantage compared to the more compact mesomorph. This disadvantage is magnified by differences in the cross section of the skeletal muscles, which are also inherent in the different body types. It has been shown that the strength of a muscle varies directly as its cross section; therefore, we find that the mesomorph is capable of producing greater strength by virtue of the greater cross section of his muscles when compared with an ectomorph or endomorph of similar body weight. It should be noted that there is also a psychological factor to be considered, since each body type tends to have a related psychological outlook toward exericse and physical activity. This different approach is admirably summed up by Karpovich (1965) as follows:

> An extreme endomorph prefers to take life easy, and usually enjoys watching vigorous activities more than participating in them. An extreme mesomorph enjoys strenuous physical activities and excels in them. An extreme ectomorph dislikes physical activities involving bodily contacts

or feats of strength, although he may enjoy such individual activities as hiking and swimming.

Although Karpovich refers to the extremes of body types, it is evident that these trends may be found to be true to a lesser degree among those of more mixed somatotype.

This relationship between the physical and psychological makeup of an individual is important when we consider the effects of training on strength and power. Not only must we consider the physical body type of each individual but we must also take note of his psychological outlook toward exercise, and particularly toward training, if we are to help him to achieve his best possible performance. Thus the approach used with an overenthusiastic mesomorph will be different from that adopted for the more introverted ectomorph.

Whenever muscles are active, they not only expend energy but also increase their rate of wear and tear. During training to increase strength and power there is an increase in the size of the muscles and in the total body weight. The increase in the size of the muscle is in part due to an increase in the diameter of the individual fibers. Muscle fibers contain 20% protein, and therefore any increase in the size of a muscle must mean that there will be an increase in the total body protein. During vigorous activity the daily intake of protein must be increased from a normal level of 69 g/day to 120 g/day. This additional protein is metabolized to allow for the increase in the total body protein and to provide for an increased rate of repair following the increased rate of breakdown of muscle tissue caused by the increased rate of work.

This need for additional protein has been recognized by sportsmen, particularly by field events athletes, but it must be emphasized that this extra protein must be taken during training; it is faulty logic to assume that a large protein meal shortly before competition is helpful or even desirable. In two recent double-blind experiments, the effects of supplementary protein in the diet of college students taking part in a strength training program were investigated. In each trial it was shown that the group taking the protein supplement increased their strength gain to a greater extent than another group taking a carbohydrate supplement and a third control group who took no supplement at all.

Protein foods are in general the most expensive available, and therefore the minimum protein requirement must be studied in some detail. It must be realized that the association of protein foods and strength extends back to the time of the Greeks. Cooper believes that the heavily meat-based diet came into vogue in Stymphalus in about 500 B.C. Unfortunately, protein is poorly metabolized and cannot be stored in any significant amounts in the body; it is therefore necessary to "top up" our protein store daily.

After metabolism, protein is excreted mainly as urea and uric acid, both of which are nitrogen-containing substances. The amount of nitrogen excreted must therefore be balanced by an equivalent amount of nitrogen taken in as protein. When this occurs the individual is said to be in nitrogen balance. However, the amount of protein required to maintain nitrogen balance depends to some extent upon the amount of fat and carbohydrate in the diet. If these are not supplied in sufficient amounts, some of the protein must be metabolized to provide energy. Indeed, in animal experiments it has been shown that animals in nitrogen balance may show evidence of nitrogen retention when the carbohydrate content of the diet is increased.

Proteins provide the necessary amino acids from which body proteins can be synthesized. The amino acid content of the protein intake must therefore be considered. Ross et al. (1955) established that eight amino acids are essential for humans. These amino acids and their minimum daily requirement are as follows:

Amino Acid	Grams per Day
L-Lysine	0.80
L-Trytophan	0.25
L-Phenylalanine	0.10
L-Threonine	0.50
L-Valine	0.80
L-Methionine	1.10
L-Leucine	1.10
L-Isoleucine	0.70

In addition, arginine and histidine have been shown (Ministry of Agriculture, 1966) to be necessary for growing children.

Of these amino acids, L-lysine and L-threonine are absolutely essential, and the total requirement must be supplied by the diet. Some of the others can be synthesized in the body from other amino acids. Protein foods may therefore be graded according to the amounts of the essential amino acids they contain; this gives a measure of the biological value of the food. Animal proteins, with the exception of gelatin, contain all the essential amino acids, whereas vegetable proteins may lack one or more of them. Nevertheless it is important to realize that both animal and vetable proteins may be mixed in the diet.

Because protein cannot be stored in the body, is relatively poorly metabolized, and is required for the most effective gain in strength during training, drugs have been increasingly used to assist protein metabolism. Briefly, the hormone testosterone has two properties: first it is responsible for the normal development of the gonads and the secondary male sexual characteristics; second, it affects protein metabolism, allowing protein to be retained in the body, particularly in the muscles. This has led to the development of various agents in which the sexual aspect of the drug has been suppressed without lowering the anabolic properties.

These drugs, known collectively as anabolic steroids, have been used in clinical medicine for a long time. They have great value in convalescence after wasting illnesses. When used in the normal clinical dosage, they have very little effect on the reproductive organs or on secondary sexual characteristics of the patient while having a considerable effect on the recovery of weight and strength. However, this dosage has little effect on a normal individual as far as any increase in strength is concerned; therefore athletes using anabolic steroids during training have been tempted to increase the dosage very considerably. (The use of up to ten times the maximum clinical dosage has been reported.) When athletes have taken anabolic steroids together with a high protein diet, considerable increases in body weight have been found and the effects of a strength-training program have been dramatically increased. In one instance, an athlete increased his body weight by over 20 kg in 6 months, and his strength increased proportionately. An improvement like this is obviously of importance in any sport in which strength and body weight are important.

Although the sexual aspects of these drugs have been suppressed by the manufacturers and are of little significance when the drug is taken in a normal clinical dosage, these side effects are considerable when the drugs are taken in these vast doses. Thus, in men there are atrophy of the testes, an increase in the size of the breasts, deposition of fat in the female distribution, impotence, and sterility. In women, the reverse happens; there are enlargement of the clitoris, atrophy of the breasts, interference with the normal menstrual cycle, lowering of the voice, and development of body and facial hair. All these effects are reversible, and the individual slowly returns to normal after ceasing to take the drug. This, of course, includes a return to normal protein metabolism and, hence, to the former body size.

These drugs stop further growth if taken during the period of bone growth. There is also some evidence that they cause water retention and possibly permanent damage to the kidneys and liver. Despite these drawbacks there are those who will risk their health for the sake of a gold medal and will also risk disqualification from their sport, for all sporting bodies have now agreed to legislate against this use of drugs. Unfortunately, although it is possible to legislate against their use, it is virtually impossible to enforce the law because the drugs are taken during training, and at the time of competition it is impossible to detect with any certainty that they have been taken.

When considering the nutritional aspects of the development of strength and power, the caloric content of the diet is also important. The recommended (Ministry of Agriculture, 1966) daily intake for anyone in a sedentary occupation is 2500 cal, whereas anyone in a very active occupation will need

4250 cal/day. If the daily caloric intake is insufficient, there will be a loss of body weight and the individual's general health will suffer. Subjects working on a diet which provided only two thirds of their daily requirement showed listlessness, weakness, lack of ability to sustain work, and loss of sexual drive.

It has been said that strength can be increased by exercise. Whenever a muscle is subjected to progressive work which involves overload there will be an increase in strength, provided that the work stops short of the onset of local muscle fatigue. Various studies have been made into the relative merits of isometric, concentric isotonic, and eccentric isotonic exercises as far as strength gain is concerned. Berger (1962) showed that there was very little difference in the effects of isometric and isotonic exercises on the development of strength but that dynamic overload training is more effective than static training for improvement in the vertical jump. Chui (1964) investigated the effects of isometric and dynamic weight training upon speed of movement and found that there was no significant difference between the two. Hellebrandt and Houtz (1956) showed that strength gain depended upon the continual employment of overload and stressed the importance of the subject being motivated to that end.

In the field of corrective physical education the work of De Lorme and Watkins (1948) is important because they were the first to lay down the basic principles of progressive resistance training. MacQueen (1954) pointed out that different techniques could be used specifically for the development of muscle hypertrophy which differed from those used for the development of strength (a fact that has not been overlooked by body builders). Zinovieff (1951) reversed the progression used by De Lorme and Watkins by starting each session with the heaviest weight and then using progressively lighter weights. This technique became known as the Oxford techinque. McMorris and Elkins (1954) compared the Oxford and the original De Lorme techniques and came to the conclusion that the Oxford method produced a 5.5% greater increase in strength. Hettinger and Müller (1953) stated that strength could be increased by a daily sustained contraction of at least one third maximum for a minimum time of 6 sec. This work generated a new research interest in isometric training such as that of Morehouse (1967).

Recently, still another method of strength training has been introduced under the name of "isokinetics." In this technique a device is used that not only applies a resistive load to the muscle but can also be set so that the speed at which the movement is made is controlled. A number of papers have been published claiming excellent results from this method of training (Thistle et al., 1967; Dick, 1968; Perrine, 1968).

The fact that a muscle group can produce its greatest power when working against a load which lies between half and two-thirds of the maximum weight that can be moved has been used as a basis for power weight training at

Saint Luke's College, Exeter (Travers, 1969). In this technique the speed at which the exercise is carried out is recorded. Thus this technique approximates that of isokinetics but without the use of any apparatus other than conventional weights.

It is interesting to note that both isokinetics and power weight training involve the factor of speed and, hence, are more directed toward the development of power than raw strength. Since power is developed in the vertical jump, it is also important to note that Berger (1962) found that dynamic overload training was more effective than static training in improving the vertical jump. The relationship between strength and power is emphasized in research by Zorbas and Karpovich (1951), who showed that shoulder speed was increased in 300 weight lifters when compared with 300 nonlifters.

Modern technology has allowed more detailed measurements to be made of biophysiological parameters. Reference has already been made to the use of photoelectric timing devices for the measurement of limb speeds and to the use of devices for measuring the time of thrust. The most accurate measurements require even more sophisticated apparatus, such as the force platform. In its simplest form this consists of a baseboard fitted with strain gauges which will measure any thrust applied to the platform. The output of the strain gauges is fed to an amplifier and recording apparatus which is calibrated so that the thrust may be measured accurately. The apparatus is elaborate and costly and therefore is used only in laboratory experiments. In the field the measurement of strength and speed still relies on the use of dynamometers and stop watches.

REFERENCES

Asmussen, E.: Some physiological aspects of fitness for sport and work. *Proc. Roy. Soc. Med.*, **62**(11)Pt. 2:1160–1164 (Nov., 1969).

Bach, L. M. N.: Conversion of red muscle to pale muscle. *Proc. Soc. Exp. Biol. Med.*, **67**(3):268–269 (1948).

Berger, R. A.: Effects of dynamic and static training on vertical jumping ability. *Res. Quart.*, **34**(4):419–424 (1963).

Chui, E. F.: Effects of isometric and dynamic weight-training exercises upon strength and speed of movement. *Res. Quart.*, **35**(3):246–257 (1964).

Cooper, D. L.: Nutrition in athletes. From a paper delivered at the American Health Association Conference, Stillwater, Okla., 1958.

De Lorme, T. L., and A. L. Watkins: Techniques of progressive resistance exercise. *Arch. Phys. Med. Rehabil.*, **29**:263–273 (1948).

Dick, F. W.: Isokinetic exercise. *Brit. J. Sports Med.*, **4**(1):27–34 (1968).

Fick, R.: *Anat. und Mech. der Gelenke.* Teil 3, Allgemeine Gelenk und Muskel Mechanik, Fuscher, Jena, 1911.

Hellebrandt, F. A., and S. J. Houtz: Mechanisms of muscle training in man: experimental demonstration of the overload principle. *Phys. Ther. Rev.*, **36**(6):371–383 (1956).

Hettinger, T., and E. A. Müller: Muskelleistung und Muskeltraining. *Arbeitsphysiol.*, **15**:111–126 (1953).

Hill A. V.: The heat of shortening and the dynamic constants of muscle. *Proc. Roy. Soc. of London*, Series B, **126**:136–195 (1938).

Karpovich, P. V.: *Physiology of Muscular Activity*, 6th ed. W. B. Saunders, Philadelphia, 1965.

MacQueen, I. J.: Recent advances in the technique of progressive resistance exercise. *Brit. Med. J.*, **II**:1193–1198 (Nov. 20, 1954).

McMorris, R. O., and E. C. Elkins: A study of production and evaluation of muscular hypertrophy. *Arch. Phys. Med. Rehab.*, **35**:420–426 (1954).

Ministry of Agriculture, Fisheries, and Food: *Manual of Nutrition*. Her Majesty's Stationery Office Publication, 1966.

Morehouse, C. A.: Development and maintenance of isometric strength of subjects with diverse initial strengths. *Res. Quart.*, **38**(3):449–456 (1967).

Perrine, J. J.: Isokinetic exercise and the mechanical energy potentials of muscle. *J. Health Phys. Educ. Rec.*, **39**:40–44 (1968).

Ross, W. C., R. L. Wixon, H. B. Lockhart, and G. F. Lambert: The amino acid requirements of man. The valine requirement, summary and final observations. *J. Biol. Chem.* **217**:987–995 (1955).

Starling, E. H., and L. Evans: Davson and Eggleton (eds.) in *Principles of Human Physiology*, 14th ed. Lea and Febiger, Philadelphia, 1968.

Thistle, H. G., J. H. Hislop, M. Moffroid, and E. W. Lowman: Isokinetic contraction: a new concept of resistive exercise. *Arch. Phys. Med. Rehabil.*, **48**:279–282 (1967).

Travers, P. R.: *Fitness Training*, (In press, 1973).

Zinovieff, A. W.: Heavy-resistance exercises. The "Oxford technique." *Brit. J. Phys. Med.*, **14**(6):129–132 (1951).

Zorbas, W. S., and P. V. Karpovich: The effect of weight lifting upon the speed of muscular contractions. *Res. Quart.*, **22**(2):145–148 (1951).

Exercise and Endurance

6

P. CERRETELLI
University of Milan
Milan, Italy

Endure, as is well known, means "sustain without impairment or yielding." The aim of the present chapter is mainly to analyze the various mechanisms, both physiological and to a lesser extent psychological, that may limit the intensity and the duration of human endurance for muscular work. Because the factors limiting the ability to do work vary with the characteristics of both the individual and the exercise (aerobic versus anaerobic, isotonic versus isometric), it is useful for the present discussion to review:

1. The different types of muscular activity and their energy requirements, the various sources of energy available in the human body and their maximal amounts (maximal capacity) and rates of production (maximal power).
2. How the physiological characteristics of the subject (age, sex, training, working habits, ethnic peculiarities) may affect performance.

Energy Sources for Work

The energy sources for muscular work have been traditionally divided into *anaerobic* and *aerobic*. The primary process supplying the free energy necessary to do work has been identified as the splitting of the high energy phosphate bonds—adenosine triphosphate (ATP), adenosine diphosphate (ADP), phosphocreatine (PC), in general high energy phosphate ($\sim$P). These compounds are found in varying concentrations in all living cells and particularly in those, like muscle fibers, that are differentiated for contraction. They are the special form of chemical energy in which the energy set free by the oxidation of the substrate or by anaerobic glycolysis is stored so that it can be released to the tissues upon demand.

The amount of energy set free by the oxidation of 1 mole of glucose (starting from glycogen) is about 690 kcal; however, only 400 kcal/mole glucose is captured in the form of high energy phosphates and therefore available to perform work.

When oxidative resynthesis of the high energy phosphates is limited or blocked (such as in hypoxia or in anoxia), the energy necessary for the process may be derived from another energy yielding process, that is, anaerobic glycolysis. The production of free energy when 1 mole of glucose (starting from glycogen) is transformed into lactic acid (2 moles) is about 57 kcal; of these, 30 kcal may be utilized for the resynthesis of 3 moles of $\sim$P. Therefore only about 8%, $(57/690) \times 100$, of the energy that may be delivered by 1 mole of glucose when oxidized can be utilized through the anaerobic pathway.

When a series of nerve impulses reaches the muscle fiber, the splitting of ATP into ADP and inorganic phosphate (P_i) occurs together with a liberation of energy. Actin and myosin utilize the energy set free by the ATP splitting and combine into actomyosin, this process being the basis of muscle contraction.

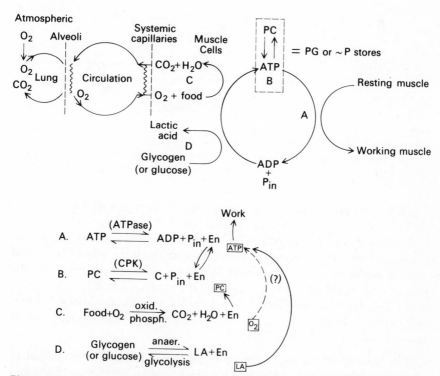

Figure 6-1. Schematic representation of the various energy sources for muscular work. A, B, C, and D correspond to the different reactions as indicated in the modified Lohmann scheme (see below).

Actomyosin, on the other hand, when activated with calcium ions (Ca), acquires an ATPase activity: a phosphate radical is split from ATP thereby releasing large quantities of energy, thus continuing the process. ADP is promptly reconverted into ATP by the simultaneous splitting of PC. The PC resynthesis follows with some delay. In aerobic conditions and at steady state, the effect of the outlined events (see the Lohmann scheme, Figure 6-1) is that the muscle ATP and ADP concentrations are constant while a decrease of the PC concentration occurs which is proportional to the oxygen uptake ($\dot{V}_{O_2}$) by the muscle (Figure 6-2).

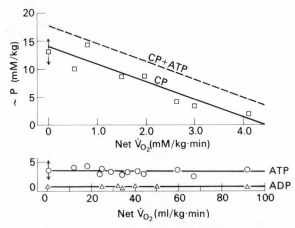

Figure 6-2. ATP, ADP, PC and total phosphagen (ATP + PC) (mMoles/kg) at steady state in the dog gastrocnemius as a function of the net O_2 uptake. [Modified from J. Piiper, P. E. di Prampero, and P. Cerretelli: Oxygen debt and high energy phosphates in gastrocnemius muscle of the dog. *Amer. J. Physiol.*, **215**:523–531 (1968).]

In the presence of oxygen the energy required for the resynthesis of PC is drawn from oxidative reactions without any lactic acid formation. In the presence of glucose but in the absence of oxygen, the PC and ATP resynthesis is obtained by way of anaerobic glycolysis with the formation of lactic acid and the production of energy (about 220 cal are delivered per gram of lactic acid produced) (Margaria et al., 1963c). Of the various reactions appearing in the Lohmann scheme (Figure 6-1), together with the qualitative features (for example, kinetics of the reactions), some quantitative aspects are of practical relevance. Among these are

1. The *capacity* of the single energetic mechanisms, that is, the amount of ATP and PC that may be split in the absence of an active resynthesis, and the maximal entity of the glycolytic process.
2. The *maximal rate* at which the different sources of energy may be made

available to the working muscles, that is, the maximal power that can be developed.

3. The *efficiency* of the transformation of one of the different sources of energy into the other, for example, from reaction B to A or from C to A of Figure 6-1.

Before describing the various features of the different reactions indicated in Figure 6-1, it may be useful to define the concept of oxygen debt.

The oxygen debt is the amount of oxygen taken up by the subject at the end of exercise in excess of the resting level. It obviously does not measure only the amount of energy (expressed as oxygen equivalent) made available to the subject by the body stores at the beginning of work (oxygen "deficit"), but also the amount of oxygen necessary for rebuilding the stores from which the energy was originally drawn, a process whose efficiency may be well below 100%. These energy sources may be "alactic" in origin (splitting of high energy phosphate bonds) and/or "lactacid." One may therefore speak of an alactic and of a lactacid oxygen debt.

The Alactic Mechanism

Reactions A and B of the Lohmann scheme may be considered jointly for practical purposes (since the efficiency of the ATP recharge by the PC splitting is about 100%) according to the following equation:

$$(\text{ATP} + \text{PC}) = \text{PG} \rightleftharpoons \text{G} + \text{P}_{\text{in}} + \text{Energy} \rightarrow \text{Work} \qquad (6.1)$$

where PG stands for phosphagen (Margaria, 1967), that is, the sum of the ATP and PC concentrations in muscle or total high energy phosphates, $\sim$P, and P_{in} is inorganic phosphate.

Since the amount of energy set free by the splitting of 1 mole of $\sim$P is about the same whether it is derived from ATP or PC, it is the amount of PG which should be known for the calculation of the so called "net" alactic oxygen debt built up by the muscles. The "net" fraction of the alactic debt corresponds to the amount of oxygen required to rebuild the PG stores depleted as a consequence of exercise and is proportional to the workload. Di Prampero et al. (1970b) have recently indicated that the "net" alactic oxygen debt ("net" $V_{O_2}^{\text{alact}}$) is a constant fraction of the oxygen uptake ($\dot{V}_{O_2}$) at steady state:

$$\text{"net" } V_{O_2}^{\text{alact}} = 0.4\, \dot{V}_{O_2}$$

The maximal capacity of reaction (6.1) in man may be evaluated once the PG muscle concentration at rest (25 mmoles/kg) is known on the basis of the following assumptions:

1. The total muscle mass of an average size man is 30 kg.
2. 80% of the resting muscle PG is split as a consequence of an exhaustive exercise.

From the above calculation the maximum "net" alactic oxygen debt turns out to be 2.24 liters of oxygen or 11.2 kcal. In fact, on the basis of a P/O ratio of 3, 18.7 kcal are required to rebuild 1 mole of ⃗P, whence 11.2 kcal are necessary to resynthesize the 600 mmoles (20 × 30) of ⃗P split.

The "actual" maximal energy output by the alactic mechanism varies with the type of exercise, as has recently been shown by di Prampero (1971). Very heavy exercise, exhaustive in 8 sec when started from rest, for instance, does not allow a depletion of more than 50% of the original PG stores. In order to produce an 80% depletion of the PG stores, the above indicated exercise must be performed starting from a steady exercise level requiring an oxygen uptake of about 60 ml/kg·min [Figure 6-3 (di Prampero, 1971)]. An alternate procedure for depleting the PG stores is that of reducing the workload, thus allowing a somewhat longer exhaustion time; an exercise exhaustive in 60–90 sec leads to an almost complete depletion of the alactic energy stores of the body.

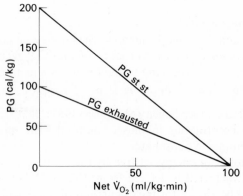

Figure 6-3. Phosphagen (PG) concentration in muscle in oxygen equivalent units (cal/kg) as a function of the oxygen consumption during steady state exercise (line "PG st st"). The line "PG exhausted" indicates the concentration of muscle PG at the end of an exhaustive burst of very heavy exercise of 8-sec duration, preceded by a steady exercise of the intensity indicated on the abscissa (schematic). Both PG and $\dot{V}_{O_2}$ are referred to 1 kg of body weight. [From P. E. di Prampero: The alactic oxygen debt: its power, capacity and efficiency. In B. Pernow and B. Saltin (eds.), *Muscle Metabolism During Exercise*. New York, Plenum Press, 1971.]

In practice, only the "gross" alactic oxygen debt is measured. The "net" value is obtained by introducing a correction of about 400 ml of oxygen, which must be subtracted from the overall "gross" value obtained, in order to make allowance for the contribution to the measured debt by the myglobin and hemoglobin oxygen stores of the muscles.

For the determination of the maximum "gross" oxygen alactic debt, a procedure has been suggested (Cerretelli et al., 1966) consisting of the following steps:

1. The subject performs an exhausting exercise of about 60–90 sec duration, the total energy requirement of which is known (En_{tot}).
2. The actual oxygen uptake during the exercise (En_{O_2}) is determined.
3. The amount of lactic acid produced (En_{LA}) is measured.

The term "gross" alactic oxygen debt may be obtained from the following equation:

$$\text{``gross''} \ V_{O_2}^{alact} = En_{tot} - (En_{O_2} + En_{LA})$$

The "net" oxygen alactic debt is obtained by subtracting about 400 ml of oxygen from the "gross" value. .

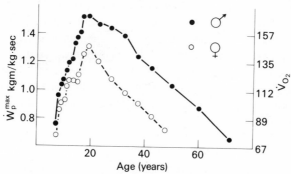

Figure 6-4. Maximum alactic anaerobic power ($\dot{W}_P^{max}$) expressed as mechanical power (kgm/kg·sec, left ordinate) and as oxygen consumption equivalent ($\dot{V}_{O_2}$, ml/kg·min, right ordinate) as a function of the age.

The maximal power that the subject can develop on the basis of splitting the PG has been shown to be the absolute maximal power that the body is able to develop. It is set by the kinetics of the PG splitting as indicated by di Prampero (1971). In the adult it amounts to about 50–60 kcal/min, corresponding to the power exerted by splitting 6 moles of PG per minute, or 200 mmoles/kg of muscle per minute (Figure 6-4). As the muscle PG stores that can be utilized for exhaustive work correspond to about 20 mmoles/kg, the muscle mass could theoretically exert its maximal power only over a period of about $\frac{1}{10}$ min or 6 sec. The maximal rate of PG splitting, together with the amount of PG in the body, set the maximal power and endurance for an anaerobic alactic exercise, such as sprint running, high or broad jumping, and so on.

The thermodynamic efficiency of the transformation of chemical energy (in the form of $\sim$P) into mechanical energy is of the order of 0.6 (Krebs and Kornberg, 1957).

The Aerobic Mechanism

Concerning reaction C of Figure 6-1, three specific aspects should be considered:

1. The kinetics of the readjustment of the oxygen uptake in the transition from a given metabolic level to a higher one.
2. The maximal level that can be attained by this process in the body at steady state and the efficiency of the oxidative process.
3. The properties and the availability of the substrate.

1. At the beginning of work, oxygen uptake undergoes an exponential increase characterized by a half time $(t\frac{1}{2})$ of about 30 sec as determined at the mouth of the subject by the "breath-by-breath" analysis (di Prampero et al., 1970b). The "true" kinetics of the process is faster $(t\frac{1}{2} = 17\text{--}20\text{ sec})$, however, when measured at the tissue level. This is shown, for example, by the experiments conducted on the isolated dog gastrocnemius muscle (Piiper et al., 1968) and by experiments based on the measurement of the transients of oxygen uptake when shifting from mild to heavier exercise (di Prampero et al., 1970b), a condition in which the oxygen uptake at the mouth reflects more closely the actual consumption occurring at the muscle level.

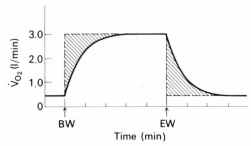

Figure 6-5. Oxygen uptake as a function of time at the onset of exercise (*BW*) and in the recovery phase (*EW*) (schematic).

In contrast to the oxidative processes, the mechanical power exerted by the muscles may attain a steady level in a very short time (1–2 sec) after the beginning of the exercise. Part of the energy necessary to carry out the work must be drawn, therefore, in the first 2–3 min of activity from tissue sources and, in aerobic conditions (that is to say, when the workload imposed on the muscles does not exceed that for which the maximal oxygen uptake is required), mainly from the PG stores. The body builds the so-called alactic oxygen debt, which has been defined in the previous section (Figure 6-5).

At steady state, the oxidative processes supply an adequate amount of energy for the activity of the muscles; the energy flux from reaction C to B and from B to A (Figure 6-1) is the same.

$$E\dot{n}_{O_2} = E\dot{n}_{P_C} = E\dot{n}_{ATP}$$

Under these conditions, that is, when the energy sources for the ATP re-synthesis are oxidative, the capacity of process C is practically indefinite.

2. The maximal power that can be exerted on the basis of reaction C corresponds to, and may therefore be measured from, the maximal oxygen uptake ($\dot{V}_{O_2}^{max}$) that the body is able to attain. In the adult untrained subject $\dot{V}_{O_2}$ corresponds, on the average, to about 40 ml of oxygen per kg of body weight per minute. However, this figure is subject to large variations in relation to several variables inherent both to the subject (age, sex, training, and so on) and to the environment (hypoxia, hyperoxia, heat, and so on).

The factors limiting the maximum oxygen availability and utilization at the muscle level are the following:

Lung factors
  1. Alveolar ventilation.
  2. Diffusion of the respiratory gases through the alveolocapillary membrane (transfer factor).
Blood factors
  3. Oxygen and carbon dioxide uptake by the blood.
Cardiocirculatory factors
  4. Thoracic circulation (cardiac output).
  5. Peripheral circulation.
Tissue factors
  6. Diffusion of oxygen from the capillaries to the cells.
  7. Oxygen utilization ability of the cell.

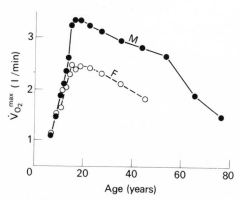

Figure 6-6. Maximal oxygen uptake (liter/min) as a function of age in untrained males and females. [From P. Cerretelli, P. Aghemo, and E. Rovelli: Aspetti fisiologici dell'-adolescente in relazione alla pratica dell'esercizio fisico. *Med. Sport,* **21**:400–406 (1968).]

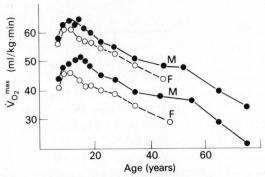

Figure 6-7. Maximal oxygen uptake as a function of age in ml/kg · min (lower curves) and in ml/kg of lean body weight per minute (upper curves) in untrained males and females. [From P. Cerretelli, P. Aghemo, and E. Rovelli: Aspetti fisiologici dell'adolescente in relazione alla pratica dell'esercizio fisico. *Med. Sport*, **21**:400–406 (1968).]

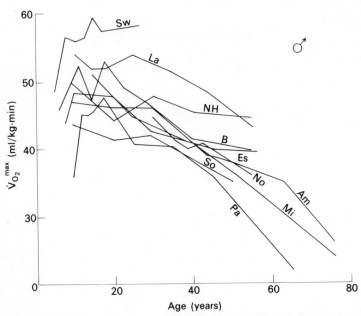

Figure 6-8. Average maximal oxygen uptake as a function of the age in males of different ethnic groups. *Sw*, Swedes; *La*, nomadic Lapps; *NH*, Nilo-Hamitics; *B*, Bantu; *No*, Norwegians; *Es*, Alaska Eskimos; *Am*, U.S. Americans; *Mi* and *So*, Italians; *Pa*, Pascuans. [From D. A. Steplock, A. Veicsteinas, and M. Mariani: Maximal aerobic and anaerobic power and stroke volume of the heart in a subalpine population. *Int. Z. agnew. Physiol.*, (1971).]

The pulmonary function does not appear to be the factor limiting the maximum aerobic performance in the healthy subject. This is clearly demonstrated by the constancy of the arterial pressures of carbon dioxide (P_{aCO_2}) and oxygen (P_{aO_2}) even during very heavy exercise. Should there be a limitation in the mechanics of breathing or in the transfer factor, an increase of P_{aCO_2} and a simultaneous drop of P_{aO_2} should occur, at least during heavy work. Cardiac output seems to be the primary limiting factor to the maximal oxygen uptake. However, within certain limits, the peripheral circulation and the tissue factors also may play some role in determining the ceiling for the oxygen uptake of the subject. Training, for instance, together with a higher maximal cardiac output induces a higher maximal arteriovenous oxygen difference, which may be related both to a better development of the capillary network of the muscle as well as to a higher concentration of mitochondria and respiratory enzymes in the muscle.

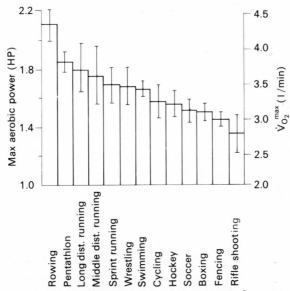

Figure 6-9. Maximal aerobic power (HP, left ordinate, and $\dot{V}_{O_2}$, liter/min, right ordinate) in different Olympic athletes. [From P. E. di Prampero, F. Piñera Limas, and G. Sassi: Maximal muscular power (aerobic and anaerobic) in 116 athletes performing at the XIX Olympic Games in Mexico. *Ergonomics*, **13**:665–674 (1970).]

The average maximum oxygen uptake in both absolute figures and per 1 kg of total and lean body weight is given in Figures 6-6, 6-7, and 6-8 as a function of the age for nonathletic subjects belonging to different ethnic groups (Cerretelli et al., 1968; Steplock et al., 1971) and in Figures 6-9 and 6-10 for a group of Olympic athletes (di Prampero et al., 1970c).

As to the efficiency of reaction C (Figure 6-1), it may be determined only when the P/O ratio (that is, the number of moles of $\sim$P resynthesized by $\frac{1}{2}$ mole of oxygen consumed) is known. This ratio, determined by muscle extracts as well as in isolated dog muscle, is about 3. A P/O ratio of 3 implies that the resynthesis of 3 moles of ATP requires the consumption of $\frac{1}{2}$ mole of oxygen (corresponding to 11.2 liters of oxygen, or 56 kcal).

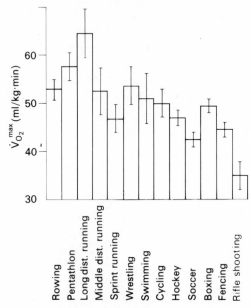

Figure 6-10. Maximal aerobic power (ml/kg·min) in different Olympic athletes. [From P. E. di Prampero, F. Piñera Limas, and G. Sassi: Maximal muscular power (aerobic and anaerobic) in 116 athletes performing at the XIX Olympic Games in Mexico. *Ergonomics*, **13**:665–674 (1970).]

Depending on the ΔG value of ATP, the efficiency of reaction C (Figure 6-1) may vary between $21/56 = 0.375$ and $30/56 = 0.535$. The total efficiency of processes A, B, and C (Figure 6-1) may then be calculated by multiplying 0.37 (or 0.56) by 0.6 (the efficiency of the transformation of chemical energy into mechanical energy), from which a maximum overall efficiency value ranging between 0.22 and 0.32 is obtained. This value compares rather well with the measured maximal efficiency value of an aerobic exercise, such as uphill walking, for which a value of 0.25 has been found (Margaria, 1938).

3. The possible fuel for muscular aerobic work is provided by carbohydrates, lipids, and proteins. Proteins contribute a very small fraction of the overall oxidative energy (about 3% of the resting metabolism, independent of workload) (Margaria and Foa', 1939).

Free fatty acids (FFA) are the major fuel in the postabsorptive human at rest, and during at least some forms of light work. This is shown by the low respiratory quotient values of the whole body and, more recently, by the relatively high conversion rate of ^{14}C-labeled tracers to carbon dioxide. More glycogen is used as the intensity of work increases; the respiratory quotient may approach values ranging from 0.9 to 0.95 under these conditions (when metabolism is 8–10 times higher than at rest). The contribution of glycogen seems to be proportionally less for a given workload in trained than in untrained subjects (Havel, 1971; Hermansen et al., 1967). When heavy exercise is prolonged for several hours, the glycogen stores (on the average 400 g in the young adult subject) may be completely depleted, and the contribution of the lipids to the overall energy requirement increases, as indicated by the drop of the respiratory quotient to values near 0.7–0.75 (Margaria, 1939). Endurance is limited, however, in the latter condition because carbohydrates are required in order to metabolize fatty acids in the Krebs cycle.

The Lactacid Mechanism

When muscles are stimulated to develop a power higher than that for which their maximal oxygen uptake is required, mechanism D outlined in the Lohmann scheme (Figure 6-1) comes into use. This reaction provides the aliquot of the energy necessary to keep the PG concentration constant at the level indicated by the upper line of Figure 6-3. (The abscissa of this graph should be slightly modified, as it should indicate the total energy requirement, that is, $\dot{V}_{O_2}$ + lactic acid production rate expressed as oxygen equivalent, rather than the $\dot{V}_{O_2}$ of the muscles).

The PG in such a case is resynthesized in part by reaction C (Figure 6-1), which provides the maximal possible flux of energy compatible with the physiological characteristics of the subject and the given set of environmental circumstances, and partially by process D, that is, by way of anaerobic glycolysis and the ensuing formation of lactic acid.

The occurrence of reaction D is clearly outlined by Figure 6-11 (Margaria et al., 1963c). The solid curve labeled $\dot{V}_{O_2}$ indicates the steady state oxygen uptake as a function of the workload in a subject running on a treadmill at different speeds and/or slopes, whereas line LA indicates the lactic acid production rate (not concentration) in grams per minute at each exercise level. It may be clearly seen that when $\dot{V}_{O_2}$ reaches the maximal value compatible with the cardiovascular characteristics of the subject, production of lactic acid in significant amounts begins. Below this level, LA production is negligible. This behavior is observed particularly when a large number of muscles or the whole body are involved in the exercise, for example, stepping up and down a bench (Shepard, 1968), cycling (Passmore and Durnin, 1955), and rowing (di Prampero et al., 1970a). It is obvious, however, that such a clear-cut onset of the anaerobic contribution to the overall metabolism of the working body cannot be found if only a limited group of muscles is at work. In the latter case, glycolysis would already be contributing a sizable amount of energy when the body as a whole had only attained a submaximal oxygen uptake level.

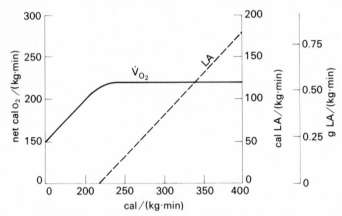

Figure 6-11. Steady state oxygen uptake (net = total − resting) and lactic acid production as a function of the work load (cal/kg·min). Whereas $\dot{V}_{O_2}$ is given in cal/kg·min, lactic acid production is given both in g/kg of body weight per minute and in its caloric equivalent on the basis of the ratio: 1 g LA ≃ 220 cal. Lactic acid production becomes significant only after $\dot{V}_{O_2}$ has reached its maximum level. [From R. Margaria, P. Cerretelli, P. E. di Prampero, C. Massari, and G. Torelli: Kinetics and mechanism of oxygen debt contraction in man. *J. Appl. Physiol.*, **18**:371–377 (1963).]

The incline of line LA of Figure 6-11 indicates the number of calories, computed as oxygen equivalent, that have been saved per unit of LA produced. In man, in physiological conditions, it has been calculated that 44 ml of oxygen (or 220 cal) are saved for every gram of LA produced. This constant was determined directly in man by Margaria and coworkers (1963c), and its value has been recently confirmed by experiments carried out on the isolated and perfused dog gastrocnemius (Cerretelli et al., 1969b).

A lactacid oxygen debt may be built also in the transition from rest to exercise when the oxidative reactions (C in Figure 6-1) lag behind the mechanical performance of the muscle. Under these conditions, such as in the 100-m dash, the subject may draw the energy for the exercise only from anaerobic reactions (A, B, and D) since, due to the delayed respiratory and circulatory readjustments, reaction C begins contributing oxidative energy only at the end of the performance.

The maximal capacity of the lactacid mechanism of the young adult (both male and female) appears to be 220–250 cal/kg of body weight. This value

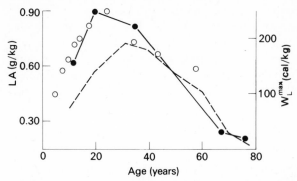

Figure 6-12. Maximum amount of lactic acid produced by the body (W_L^{max}) both in g/kg of body weight and in the corresponding caloric equivalent (ordinate at the right) as a function of the age in Italian males (●), Swedish females (○) and American males (---). [From P. Cerretelli, P. Aghemo, and E. Rovelli: Aspetti fisiologici dell'adolescente in relazione alla practica dell'esercizio fisico. *Med. Sport,* **21**:400–406 (1968).]

decreases significantly with aging [Figure 6-12 (Cerretelli et al., 1968)] and with changing environmental conditions, particularly in chronic hypoxia [Figure 6-13 (Cerretelli, 1967)].

The amount of the lactacid oxygen debt built by the subject as a consequence of a nonexhaustive anaerobic exercise can be calculated from the increment of LA concentration in blood. According to Margaria et al. (1971) an increase of 10 mg% in the blood LA concentration corresponds to building an oxygen debt (lactacid) of 3.5 ml/kg of body weight.

The maximal power that the human body may develop on the basis of the glycolytic mechanism has been determined by Margaria et al. (1964). It amounts to about 20–25 kcal/kg of body weight per hour, or to a $\dot{V}_{O_2}$ of

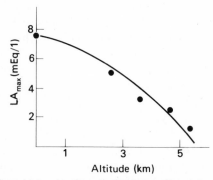

Figure 6-13. Lactic acid levels after maximum continuous performance at various altitudes. [Modified after H. T. Edwards: *Amer. J. Physiol.,* **116**:367 (1936).]

65–80 ml/kg·min, which is approximately 50–80% higher than the corresponding maximal aerobic power of the subject.

The efficiency of the resynthesis of PG by way of anaerobic glycolysis is not significantly different from that of the oxidative pathway. The efficiency of glycolysis as a whole for the general economy of the body is, however, very low; only about 8% of the potential energy of each mole of glucose can be utilized for rebuilding the primary source of energy for work.

Evaluation of the Most Common Physical Activities on an Energetic Basis

Once the energy giving processes available to the body for its working requirements are known in their qualitative as well as quantitative features, it is possible to analyze the various athletic performances and to attempt predictions about how the body is able to engage in them. All physical exercises may be grouped into categories for which similar energetic processes are required. It is useful therefore to classify into

1. First type: those exercises producing exhaustion of a group or all muscles in a very short time (from less than 1 sec up to about 20 sec).
2. Second type: those exercises bringing about exhaustion in a period ranging from about 1 to 10 min.
3. Third type: the exercises that can be prolonged from 10 to 15 min up to several hours.

Independent of the intensity of the exercise (power required) and of its duration, all exercises listed above may be classified as *uniform* or *intermittent*. Furthermore, each exercise is definitely characterized by a prevailing energy source, either anaerobic or aerobic.

For the exercises referred to as of the first type, a further distinction should be made between exercise involving a unique action (for example, high jump, pole vault, throwing) that may be sustained by one or more specialized muscle groups and exercises characterized by repeated identical actions involving all or most of the body musculature (for example, 100–200-m dashes, 110-m hurdles, track bicycling).

The unique or prevailing source of energy for exercises belonging to the first type is that defined as *anaerobic alactic*. It is, in fact, the splitting of high energy phosphates (PG) that permits the possibility of performing at very high power when the glycolytic and oxidative mechanisms are not available due to the delay with which they are activated. The best performers in these athletic specialties have a larger muscle mass, probably a significantly higher PG muscle concentration, and, consequently, a greater amount of PG in the body. These factors result in a higher maximal power and the possibility of enduring an "all out" exercise for a longer period of time at maximum power. These subjects need not necessarily have a high aerobic power. The most exhausting exercise that may be considered at the borderline between the first and second type is the 200-m dash, where, besides alactic sources, a sizable amount of glycolytic energy is required, as indicated by the relatively high amount of lactic acid produced (on the average 0.3 g/kg of body weight or 30% of the maximum lactacid capacity). In this exercise, as in all exercises of this type, the oxidative sources contribute only a minor fraction of the overall energy (in the case of the 200-m dash, less than 8%).

The Energy Cost of Sprint Running

Recently, on the basis of data dealing with maximal capacity of the anaerobic mechanism, an analysis has been made of the various contributions by the different energy giving mechanisms during very heavy exercises, those that lead to exhaustion in only a few seconds. The energy expenditure for an 80-m run performed in 10 sec by young trained nonathletic subjects was found to be 0.15 kcal/kg, that is, 1.88 kcal/kg·km (Margaria et al., 1963a). This value includes and averages three different energy components:

1. That required to sustain the acceleration at the start.
2. That required to overcome the air resistance.
3. That required to maintain the speed.

The first aliquot amounts to about 4 kgm/kg or 9.5 cal/kg when measured as mechanical work. If one assumes an efficiency of 0.25, the energy spent for the acceleration of the body may be calculated at about 0.038 kcal/kg of body weight. The air resistance (expressed as the energy requirement to overcome it) is about 0.3 cal/kg·m or 0.024 kcal/kg for the 80-m run. The energy consumption for the maintenance of the speed at steady state may then be calculated as

$$\frac{0.150 - 0.038 - 0.024}{0.080} = 1.08 \text{ kcal/kg·km}$$

a value of the same order of magnitude of those found at much lower speeds (8 km/hr).

Among exercises of the second type, the prolonged sprints are of particular interest (for example, 400-m run, 400-m hurdles, 100-m swim, 1000-m run, and bicycling). For such exercises the alactic anaerobic energy sources as well as the aerobic processes are evidently insufficient; the former due to their limited amount, the latter both for the delay with which they may become available to the body and for the limited power they provide. The most important role is played in this case by the anaerobic glycolysis. The subject at the end of the event (that is, at exhaustion) has completely exploited both his alactic and his glycolytic sources of energy, thus incurring his maximal alactic and lactacid oxygen debt.

The time course of his energy utilization is as follows: At the onset of work most of the contribution will be given by the alactic sources (Figure 6-14). Later, after a few seconds (2–10 sec, depending on the intensity of the exercise), most of the energy is supplied by the glycolysis, while a progressive increase of the energy output by oxidative mechanisms takes place. The level of performance will be the highest possible when the utilization of the anaerobic sources, particularly lactacid, is distributed uniformly throughout the exercise. In fact, once the maximal lactacid oxygen debt of the subject has been accumulated, the maximal power that the muscles will be able to develop drops to that allowed by the maximal oxygen uptake of the subject or, more precisely, somewhat below this level because an aliquot of the oxygen taken up by the body is utilized for the resynthesis of part of the lactic acid produced into glucose and glycogen.

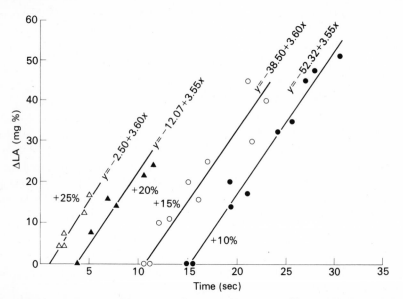

Figure 6-14. Increase of lactic acid (Δ LA) in blood in mg% as a function of the duration of the exercise in seconds. The four lines refer to four workloads and were obtained by changing the incline of the treadmill from 10 to 25%. In all experiments the speed was kept constant at 18 km/hr. [From R. Margaria, P. Cerretelli, and F. Mangili: Balance and kinetics of anaerobic energy release during strenuous exercise in man. *J. Appl. Physiol.*, **19**:623–628 (1964).]

It is thus important that the subject's phosphagen and glycogen stores be intact at the onset of the performance. This is very often neglected in practice, as is indicated by the unphysiological characteristics of the "warming up" procedures utilized by many athletes, which lead to considerable lactate production before the beginning of an event. The maximal endurance for exercises of this type will be achieved by athletes who, besides having a high maximal capacity in the anaerobic (alactic and lactacid) mechanisms, are characterized by a very high maximal aerobic power that will allow them to sustain a higher average power throughout the performance.

The energy source on which the body relies for performances of the third type (for example, marathon running, long distance running, skiing, cycling, swimming, skating) is the oxidative one. The higher the maximal aerobic power of the subject, the better his performance. In such cases the participation of the anaerobic energy sources, due to their limited capacity, may be considered almost negligible, except for the final sprint.

On the basis of data dealing with the energy cost of running obtained in the laboratory and by knowing the maximal oxygen uptake of the subject, it is possible to calculate the theoretical minimum time required for running a given distance. For example, assume the distance to be covered is 42 km (standard marathon run) and the net $\dot{V}_{O_2}^{max}$ of a subject is 80 ml per kg of body weight per minute, that is, 400 cal/kg·min. The energy requirement for running is known (Margaria et al., 1963b), amounting to 1 kcal (or 1000 cal) per kg of body weight per km, that is, 400 cal/kg per 400-m distance. The subject will therefore be able to cover, at most, 400 m̃/min on the basis of his aerobic mechanisms, and the shortest time required for the 42,000-m run will then be 42,000/400 = 105 min. Similarly, if instead of 80 ml/kg·min, the $\dot{V}_{O_2}^{max}$ of the subject were 60 ml/kg·min, the same distance would be covered in 140 min. The record* time for the marathon run is somewhat over 120 min, thus indicating an oxygen requirement of about 70 ml/kg·min, a very reasonable value for a well trained long distance runner (di Prampero et al., 1970c). It appears from these data that the subject is able to work at least 2 hr at, or near, his maximal oxygen uptake. The performance of the cardiovascular system, particularly that of the heart (cardiac output), must therefore be quite constant at its maximal level, irrespective of whether the heart rate increases considerably throughout the performance.

The Energy Cost of Walking, Running, Swimming, and Rowing

The energy cost of walking and running has been calculated both as a function of the speed and of the incline of the ground. Such values undergo only limited changes among subjects. This is due to the fact that such exercises are quite usual and therefore practically uninfluenced by style.

In Figure 6-15 the energy cost of walking is indicated as a function of the speed and of the incline. It appears that for every incline there is an optimal speed with a minimum energy requirement (Margaria, 1938). The energy cost of running has been calculated for both level and uphill running. It

---

* It would not be, strictly speaking, appropriate to set a record for the marathon run as the track is not standardized.

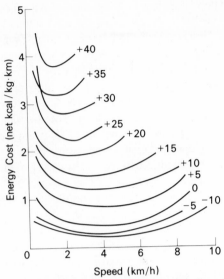

Figure 6-15. Net energy consumption in walking as a function of the speed and of the incline. [R. Margaria: Sulla fisiologia e specialmente sul consumo energetico della marcia e della corsa a varia velocita ed inclinazione del terrano. *Atti. Reale Acc. Naz. Lincei,* **7**:299–368 (1938).]

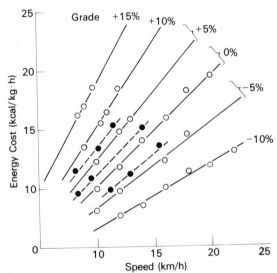

Figure 6-16. Energy cost of running on a treadmill as a function of speed and of slope; ○ athletes, ● sedentaries. [R. Margaria, P. Cerretelli, P. Aghemo, and G. Sassi: Energy cost of running. *J. Appl. Physiol.,* **18**:367–370 (1963).]

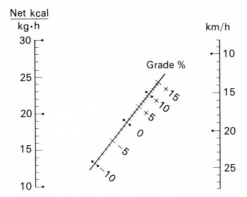

Figure 6-17. Nomogram for calculating the energy expenditure in running when speed and incline are given. [From R. Margaria, P. Cerretelli, P. Aghemo, and G. Sassi: Energy cost of running. *J. Appl. Physiol.*, **18**:367–370 (1963).]

appears that it is independent of the speed within a very wide range (Figure 6-16). Figure 6-17 (Margaria et al., 1963b) shows a nomogram from which the energy cost of running at different speeds and slopes of the ground may be calculated.

The mechanical efficiency of walking and running changes as a function of the incline of the ground, reaching a maximum value (about 25%) when the slope exceeds +20% [Figure 6-18 (Margaria et al., 1963b)]. Whereas in walking or running on the level or on a moderate slope most of the potential energy accumulated by the body at each step is immediately reconverted

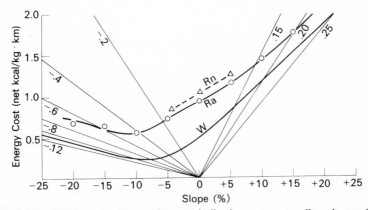

Figure 6-18. Net (corrected for resting metabolism) energy expenditure in running as a function of the incline of the ground in walking (*W*) and in running: athletes (*Ra*) and sedentaries (*Rn*). [From R. Margaria, P. Cerretelli, P. Aghemo, and G. Sassi: Energy cost of running. *J. Appl. Physiol.*, **18**:367–370 (1963).]

into kinetic energy and lost as heat, when the incline of the ground is high an increasing fraction of this energy is retained and utilized for lifting the body.

The energy cost of swimming at a given speed is very high as compared to that of walking. It does not seem to vary markedly as a function of the style, including underwater swimming. This is shown in Figure 6-19 where the energy cost of swimming is plotted as a function of speed and compared with that of other activities such as walking, running, bicycling and rowing (Cerretelli, in preparation).

Riding a bicycle at a given speed has an energy cost of less than 50% of running on a track. The reason for this "saving" of energy may be found in the fact that in cycling on a level plane, the subject does not work against gravity, and the energy is utilized only for overcoming the friction of the ground and the air resistance. This explains why cyclists can perform races of several hundred kilometers at 40 km/hr without intermission or may cover distances of 4000 km in 20 days or less without developing any significant symptom of fatigue.

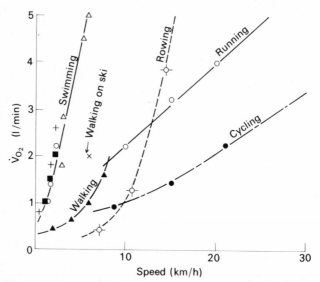

Figure 6-19. Oxygen uptake (liter/min) as a function of the speed (km/hr) for different exercises: +, underwater swimming; ○, back stroke; ■, breast stroke; △, crawl; -◇-, data refer to energy expenditure of a single rower in a "two with coxswain" shell. [From P. Cerretelli. Fisiologica del Lavoro e dello Sport. In preparation.]

Rowing involves the use of most body muscles (arms, legs, and back). It is therefore a very demanding exercise. Since the water resistance (R) opposing the shell displacement increases as an exponential function of the average speed (V_m), the energy output of the rower also must increase exponentially with increasing velocity (di Prampero et al., 1970a).

Intermittent Exercise

Several events, particularly team sports, require repeating a performance within a very short time or carrying out heavy activity with frequent intermissions. From the energetic point of view, such exercises require the participation of the various known energy sources to an extent which may vary considerably. There are situations in which the muscles are calling upon their alactic stores only. It is evident in such cases that the performance may be repeated several times without any significant deterioration, provided sufficient time (2–3 min) is allowed between two successive bursts of activity to pay the alactic oxygen debt. This is the case, for instance, for the throws and for the jumps.

Exercises which involve building a lactacid oxygen debt (for example, the 200- and 400-m dashes and several others included in the second type) cannot be repeated before the lactacid oxygen debt has been paid without incurring a severe decay in performance. The latter process, as was demonstrated long ago by Margaria et al. (1933), is rather slow ($t_{\frac{1}{2}} = 15$ min) and is generally not completed in less than 1 hr.

There are, moreover, sports that require alternating exercises of the third type with others of the first and second types. It is evident in this case that it would be more profitable for the subject in such situations to avoid building a lactacid oxygen debt. This could not be repaid in the short intervals allowed during the game, since it would require a considerable aliquot of energy that could otherwise be utilized for the performance. The subject should be taught to draw the energy for short bursts of activity, superimposed on a base of heavy aerobic work, only from alactic stores that can be quickly restored.

The Energy Cost of Isometric Exercise and its Limiting Factors

The oxygen supply to the muscles engaged in isometric contractions is considerably reduced, as is the blood flow, particularly when the tension exerted by the muscles exceeds 30% of their maximal potential tension. This critical tension level, however, seems to vary widely in different groups of muscles. Therefore, due to anaerobiosis, the determination of the oxygen uptake during a predominantly isometric exercise is not indicative of the total energy expenditure of the muscles. The energy balance during graded isometric contractions of the gastrocnemii in humans is indicated in Figure 6-20 (Cerretelli et al., 1970), where both oxygen uptake and LA production rates are given.

It appears that

1. The "net" total energy consumption for maintaining the muscle contraction increases linearly with the increase in tension (kg).

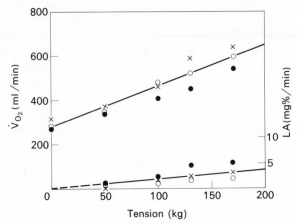

Figure 6-20. Oxygen uptake (total) and lactic acid production (LA) for maintaining different tensions by the two calves. [From P. Cerretelli, M. Fumagalli, and E. Camoni: Energetica della contrazione muscolare isometrica nell'uomo. *Arch. Fisiol.*, p. 51, XXII Congr. Ital. Physiol. Soc., Pavia, 1970.]

2. The anaerobic (lactacid) component accounts for about 25–30% of the total energy output for the muscle.
3. The energy cost for the onset of the contraction increases progressively with the development of increasing tension (Figure 6-21).

It is evident that endurance in isometric exercise is dramatically limited by the reduction of the local blood flow. Both heart rate (HR) and cardiac output ($\dot{Q}$) increase disproportionately to $\dot{V}_{O_2}$ (as compared to isotonic exercise) during steady isometric exercise [Figures 6-22 and 6-23 (Veicsteinas

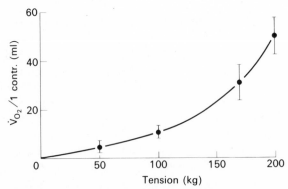

Figure 6-21. Oxygen consumption necessary for exerting a single contraction by the two calves at the tension indicated on the abscissa. [From P. Cerretelli, M. Fumagalli, and E. Camoni: Energetica della contrazione muscolare isometrica nell'uomo. *Arch. Fisiol.*, p. 51. XXII Congr. Ital. Physiol., Soc., Pavia, 1970.]

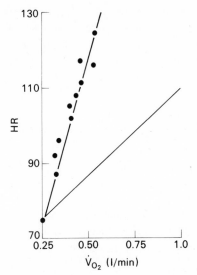

Figure 6-22. Heart rate versus oxygen uptake at steady state during isometric contractions of the calves. The thin line refers to walking. [From A. Veicsteinas, M. Fumagalli, E. Camoni, and P. Cerretelli: La gettata cardiaca nella contrazione muscolare isometrica nell'uomo. In preparation, 1971.]

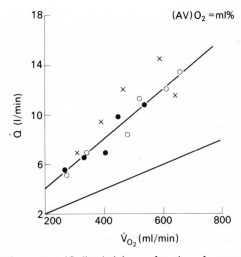

Figure 6-23. Cardiac output (Q, liter/min) as a function of oxygen uptake (ml/min) during steady isometric contractions of the two calves. Iso (AV) oxygen lines are also drawn. [From A. Veicsteinas, M. Fumagalli, E. Camoni, and P. Cerretelli: La gettata cardiaca nella contrazione muscolare isometrica nell'uomo. In preparation, 1971.]

et al., 1971)], while the arteriovenous oxygen difference seems to remain practically at the resting level. This enhanced heart activity has been attributed to a reflex action elicited by a sudden increase of the peripheral resistances brought about by the isometric contraction of a muscle area (Lind and McNicol, 1965). Arterial blood pressure also increases remarkably as a result of isometric exercises.

Some Considerations on the Factors Limiting Human Performance: Study of Records in Athletics

The world's records for running different horizontal distances provide some very interesting physiological data as was pointed out by Hill (1926) about 50 years ago.

A classical representation of some of these data is given by Lloyd (1966). He plotted the distances of various athletic running events as a function of the minimum time necessary to cover the various distances by the world record holder (Figure 6-24). A linear interpolation is then made through the points. Some of the points are located below the line, indicating relatively "low" performances which are likely to undergo an improvement in the near future. Lloyd also attributed a physiological significance to the parameters of the lines appearing in Figure 6-24 by relating, over different intervals, time of performance to distance covered in the range between 50 yards and 623 miles. The intercept on the ordinate of the lines would be indicative of the energy store of the tissues (oxygen debt), whereas the slope of the lines is the rate of the energy consumption and, for very long runs, practically the maximal aerobic power of the subject.

Another very useful representation is that in which running times or distances achieved in jumping or throwing events are plotted as a function of calendar time. From this graph it is possible to predict the future evolution of some of the records. In particular, the following deductions can be made (Cerretelli, in preparation):

1. The reduction of the performance times follows a simple exponential function.
2. The reduction of performance times is relatively more pronounced for the long lasting running events than for the sprints, indicating that the tissue energy sources on which the latter performances depend are much more constant among individuals than is the maximal aerobic power.
3. There are no signs that for most of the performances we are reaching an asymptote, that is, the theoretical limit.

According to Lloyd (1966) it is rather difficult to make predictions about the evolution of world records on physiological grounds. Basing the analysis on extrapolations, Lloyd predicts by the year 2000 an improvement of about .

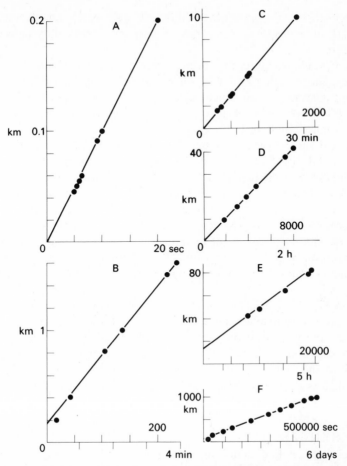

Figure 6-24. World records (1965) in running distances from 50 yards up to 623 miles. Distances in kilometers are plotted as a function of the record time required to cover them. The intercepts on the ordinates are in relation to the body energy stores, whereas the slopes are functions of the power developed by the subject. [From B. B. Lloyd: The energetics of running: an analysis of world records. *Adv. Sci.,* 515–530 (1966).]

5.5% in the sprints and of about 7.5% for the marathon run, which should be accomplished in about 2 hr.

Conclusions

As may be easily grasped from the previous description, exercise endurance depends on several predictable physiological factors, mostly in connection with the various mechanisms providing energy to the muscles. Among these factors, those that are built in the body, such as the phosphagen and glycogen stores, can contribute anaerobically only limited amounts of energy for work at a maximal rate, which is different in sedentary subjects and athletes.

As a peculiar feature, the sprinter athlete has a larger muscle mass and therefore more energy available, whence a higher maximal power. Also the different efficiencies with which various subjects transform chemical energy into useful work obviously affects the endurance for an all-out exercise.

Endurance for long lasting aerobic exercises is related not only to the maximal tissues oxygen availability (imposed individually by the maximal oxygen uptake of the body or by the blood flow to the muscles) but also to the availability of the fuel. A lack of glycogen in muscles limits performance because the lipids are, so to speak, a "dependent" fuel. Blood glucose contributes only a negligible amount of energy to the working muscles because it must be converted into glycogen before becoming available for metabolism; therefore, the most important endurance limiting factors are the glycogen concentration of the muscles before the beginning of the performance and the kinetics of glycogen synthesis during recovery by the known enzymatic reactions involved.

Besides physiological factors, other variables, particularly of psychological origin, are known to affect endurance for a given long lasting exercise. Among these are the morale of the athlete, his self-confidence with respect to the other competitors, a high level of achievement, a high personal motivation as well as the motivation deriving from belonging to a specific group. The latter factors obviously cannot increase the maximal power of the subject, but they can postpone the onset of the decay which is referred to as fatigue.

REFERENCES

Ambrosoli, G., P. E. di Prampero, and P. Cerretelli: L'influenza del contenuto in fosfageno (PC + ATP) sul rendimento meccanico del muscolo. *Boll. Soc. Ital. Biol. Sper.*, **45**:768–771 (1969).

Cerretelli, P.: Lactacid O_2 debt in acute and chronic hypoxia. In R. Margaria (ed.): *Exercise at Altitude*. Amsterdam, Excerpta Medica Foundation, pp. 58–64, 1967.

Cerretelli, P.: Fisiologia del Lavoro e dello Sport (in preparation).

Cerretelli, P., F. Cuttica, and B. Caru': Aerobic and anaerobic energy capacity and power in the aged. *Proc. 7th Int. Cong. Gerontol.*, pp. 529–532, 1966.

Cerretelli, P., P. Aghemo, and E. Rovelli: Aspetti fisiologici del'adolescente in relazione alla practica dell'esercizio fisico. *Med. Sport*, **21**:400–406 (1968).

Cerretelli, P., and P. E. di Prampero: High energy phosphate resynthesis from anaerobic glycolysis in muscle. *J. Physiol.*, **204**:115–116 (1969a).

Cerretelli, P., P. E. di Prampero, and J. Piiper: Energy balance of anaerobic work in the dog gastrocnemius muscle. *Amer. J. Physiol.*, **217**:581–585 (1969b).

Cerretelli, P., M. Fumagalli, and E. Camoni: Energetica della contrazione muscolare isometrica nell'uomo. *Arch. Fisiol.*, XXII Congr, Italian Physiol. Soc., p. 51, Pavia, 1970.

Craig, A. B.: Limitations of human organism. *J. Amer. Med. Assoc.*, **205**:734–740 (1968).

di Prampero, P. E.: The alactic oxygen debt: its power, capacity and efficiency. In B. Pernow and B. Saltin (eds.): *Muscle Metabolism during Exercise*, New York, Plenum Press, pp. 371–382, 1971.

di Prampero, P. E., F. Celentano, G. Cortili, and P. Cerretelli: A biomechanical analysis of rowing. *Proc. Reg. Congr. I.U.P.S.*, No. 123, Brasov, 1970a.

di Prampero, P. E., C. T. M. Davies, P. Cerretelli, and R. Margaria: An analysis of O_2 debt contracted in submaximal exercises. *J. Appl. Physiol.*, **29**:547–551 (1970b).

di Prampero, P. E., F. Piñera Limas, and G. Sassi: Maximal muscular power (aerobic and anaerobic) in 116 athletes performing at the XIX Olympic Games in Mexico. *Ergonomics*, **13**:665–674 (1970c).

Edwards, H. T.: Lactic acid in rest and work at high altitude. *Amer. J. Physiol.*, **116**: 367 (1936).

Havel, R. J.: Influence of intensity and duration of exercise on supply and use of fuels. B. Pernow and B. Saltin (eds.) In *Muscle Metabolism During Exercise*, New York, Plenum Press, pp. 315–325, 1971.

Hermansen, L., E. Hultman, and B. Saltin: Muscle glycogen during prolonged severe exercise. *Acta Physiol. Scand.*, **71**:129–139 (1967).

Hill, A. V. Muscular Activity. Herter Lectures, 1924. Baltimore, Williams and Wilkins, 1926.

Krebs, H. A. and H. L. Kornberg: *Energy Transformations in Living Matter*. Berlin, Springer Verlag, 1957.

Lind, A. R. and G. W. McNicol: Cardiovascular responses to static and dynamic exercise. *Ergonomics*, **8**:379 (1965).

Lloyd, B. B.: The energetics of running: An analysis of world records. *Adv. Sci.*, 515–530 (1966).

Margaria, R.: Sulla fisiologia a specialmente sul consumo energetico della marcia e della corsa a varia velocità ad inclinazione del terreno. *Atti Reale Acc. Naz. Lincei*, **7**:299–368 (1938).

Margaria, R., Die Verwertung von Kohlenhydraten und ihre Unentbehrlich— keit bei Muskelarbeit. *Arbeitsphysiol.*, **10**:539–552 (1939).

Margaria, R. Energy sources for aerobic and anaerobic work. In R. Margaria (ed.): *Exercise at Altitude*, Amsterdam, Excerpta Medica Foundation, pp. 15–32, 1967.

Margaria, R., H. T. Edwards, and D. B. Dill: The possible mechanisms of contracting and paying the oxygen debt and the role of lactic acid in muscular contraction. *Amer. J. Physiol.*, **106**:689–715 (1933).

Margaria, R., and P. Foa': Der Einfluss von Muskelarbeit auf den Stickstoffwechsel, die Kreatin und Säureausscheidung. *Arbeitsphysiol.*, **10**:553–560 (1939).

Margaria, R., P. Cerretelli, F. Mangili, and P. E. di Prampero: Le coût énergétique durant la course. *Proc. 1st Eur. Congr. Sport Med.*, Prague, pp. 497–499, 1963a.

Margaria, R., P. Cerretelli, P. Aghemo, and G. Sassi: Energy cost of running. *J. Appl. Physiol.*, **18**:367–370 (1963b).

Margaria, R., P. Cerretelli, P. E. di Prampero, C. Massari, and G. Torelli: Kinetics and mechanism of oxygen debt contraction in man. *J. Appl. Physiol.*, **18**:371–377 (1963c).

Margaria, R., P. Cerretelli, and F. Mangili: Balance and kinetics of anaerobic energy release during strenuous exercise in man. *J. Appl. Physiol.*, **19**:623–628 (1964).

Margaria, R., P. Aghemo, and G. Sassi: Lactic acid production in supramaximal exercise. *Pflügers Arch.*, **326**:152–161 (1971).

Passmore, R., and J. V. G. A. Durnin: Human energy expenditure. *Physiol. Rev.*, **35**:801–840 (1955).

Piiper, J., P. E. di Prampero, and P. Cerretelli: Oxygen debt and high energy phosphates in gastrocnemius muscle of the dog. *Amer. J. Physiol.*, **215**:523–531 (1968).

Shepard, R. J., S. M. Benade, C. T. M. Davies, P. E. di Prampero, R. Hedman, J. E. Merriman, K. Myhre, and R. Simmons: *Bull. World Health. Org.*, **38**:757–764 (1968).

Steplock, D. A., A. Veicsteinas, and M. Mariani: Maximal aerobic and anaerobic power and stroke volume of the heart in a subalpine population. *Int. Z. angew. Physiol.* (1971).

Veicsteinas, A., M. Fumagalli, E. Camoni, and P. Cerretelli: La gettata cardiaca nella contrazione muscolare isometrica nell'uomo (in preparation) 1971.

Psychological Aspects of Physical Activities

7

Gunnar Borg
University of Stockholm
Stockholm, Sweden

Research in physical activity includes many psychological problems that are of interest to the fields of sport and physical education, ergonomics and human factors engineering, and medicine and rehabilitation. There are many reasons why the psychological aspects of various physical activities should be studied. One theoretical reason is that, according to general scientific classifications, performance problems in physical activity belong to the same "descriptive level" and "explanatory level," in a macro-micro-continuum from sociology to biophysics, as do most other psychological problems. Since psychology is a behavioral science and deals with studies of human performance, there will be an overlap with work physiology. The psychology of physical activities is then one branch within the broad field concerning the scientific study of human physical activities, a scientific field for which I have tentatively proposed the name "ergology."

Another reason that psychological problems are of interest in this field is that physical activities may be looked upon as configurations or "gestalts" depending on a complex interaction of many factors. Not only physiological, morphological, and biochemical factors are involved but also psychological ones such as perceptual and information processes, decision making, memory storage and other cognitive factors, psychomotor coordination, learned movement patterns and technique, various motivational factors to participate and perform, emotional factors, and personality traits. Some of the important aspects are the relationships between physical stress and physiological and mental functions, the variations in psychological performances with physical arousal and fatigue, and the importance of physical fitness for a healthy life.

A physically stressing situation to which a subject tries to adapt himself may be studied with regard to perceptual, performance, and physiological responses. These three different kinds of stress indicators, or effort continua,

141

complement one another. When studying sport achievements or performances in daily work (for example, after improvements made in industrial work tasks according to human factors criteria), it is important to know the "costs" at which the individual is working. Besides a study of the technical aspects and the physiological responses of the man at work, the psychological "costs" in the form of perceived exertion, subjective stress, and fatigue should be studied to enable us to understand the individual better.

We should try to identify different intensity levels in a perceptual continuum and see how they are related to one another and to the corresponding levels in the performance and physiological continua. In psychophysical studies most interest has been focused on minimum and maximal thresholds, on differential thresholds, and on the type of functions describing the variation between these limits. However, in everyday life there are other intensity levels of interest, such as various adaptation levels, preference levels, forced adaptation levels, and stress zones. When we try to adapt ourselves to a work situation, the load must not be so high that we come too near the stress zone in relation to our present maximal working capacity. To identify which industrial task is too strenuous for the individual, the perceived "difficulty" of the work can be obtained and used as a stress indicator. Measurements of apparent force and perceived difficulty can also be used for a quantitative evaluation of the degree of physical stress and can thus complement the physiological measures.

General Studies of Subjective Force and Perceived Exertion

Toward the close of the 1950s in Umeå, Sweden, we started to study subjective force and perceived exertion during physical work by means of modern psychophysical methods. One factor that led us to start this empirical research was a clinical observation that the decrease in physical working capacity experienced by an individual did not seem to correspond to the decrease determined by physical work tests. When a lumber worker came to the hospital complaining that his working capacity had gone down at least 50%, the laboratory tests revealed a decrease of only 20 or 30%. This discrepancy could not be interpreted as simulation, but seemed to be a general perceptive problem connected to a nonlinear relationship between perceived exertion and physical performance. Since a decrease of physical working capacity as perceived by the subject is one of the most important reasons to see a doctor, we wanted to study this problem further.

Psychophysical methods have been developed, especially by S. S. Stevens (1957, 1966), for a quantitative evaluation of the intensities of perceptions. These methods allow for determinations on a "ratio level," that is, the scales may roughly be considered as equidistant scales with a zero point; this permits descriptions of the relation between subjective and objective intensities in terms of mathematical functions. Many sense modalities have been studied, and a power function seems to be the most general expression for describing how subjective intensity varies with physical stimulus intensity.

Experiments have been performed to study how subjective force during short-time work (less than one minute) on a bicycle ergometer varies with the pedal resistance. In several experiments that used ratio production methods such as halving and doubling, where the subject had to set a variable intensity so it was perceived to be half as intense or twice as intense as a certain standard stimulus, power functions with an exponent of about 1.6 seemed to give good descriptions of the variation of subjective force with physical workload. The same results have been obtained with estimation methods where randomly presented workloads had to be judged by the subjects in terms of percentage of a certain standard workload or in relation to their notion of a maximal load (Borg and Dahlström, 1959, 1960; Borg, 1962, 1972).

In studies of subjective handgrip force, positively accelerated functions with an exponent of about 1.7 have been found (Stevens and Mach, 1959). An exponent of 1.6 also was found for apparent foot pressure in a study by Eisler (1962). A new type of method was applied in a study by Borg, Edström, and Marklund (1970) where the stimulus intensity was varied as a function of time, and the subject's task was to report how he perceived the variation. When the workload on the bicycle ergometer was changed as the 0.5 power of time, the variation was judged to be about linear. The exponent of the corresponding psychophysical function is 2.0. For hard work of longer duration (more than 1 min), the stress on the circulatory and respiratory systems is an important factor determining perceived exertion. The expression of the psychophysical functions might therefore be somewhat different for work of longer duration than for work of short duration. However, in several studies Borg (1962) found positively accelerated functions with an exponent around 1.6 for the increase of perceived exertion with workload in an ordinary test of physical working capacity, where the workload is increased in a stepwise fashion, as in the tests utilized by Sjöstrand (1947) and Wahlund (1948). Hueting and Sarphati (1966) also obtained positively accelerating functions in their studies of "fatigue" (in this case "fatigue" has about the same connotation as "exertion") during an ordinary work test. For practical purposes, however, they applied linear regression curves to their data.

The nonlinearity between subjective and objective intensities should be kept in mind. If we want to adapt work intensity to a subject and avoid this acceleration so that we can obtain subjectively equal increases of load, the objective work intensity ought to increase by smaller and smaller steps. The results are also of interest when considering how man experiences changes in his physical working capacity. Because of the shape of the psychophysical function, a decrease in an individual's objective maximal working capacity by a certain percentage causes a greater perceived decrease than that decrease perceived when exertion has involved a certain submaximal workload.

Borg and Edgren (1972) studied the subjective adaptation to heavy physical work on a bicycle ergometer in two groups of subjects, one male group ($n = 7$) and one female group ($n = 7$). In the beginning each subject had to set the workload corresponding to his perception of half (50%) of his maximal exertion. Then, during the first 15 sec of the trial, the subject adjusted the workload so that it corresponded to his perception of half his maximal exertion, as it was perceived at the outset. Once each minute the subject adjusted the workload to the same subjective intensity. The idea was that the subject should produce a workload of just the right intensity to keep the perceived intensity the same throughout the time period. In Figure 7-1 the results are shown for both the male and the female groups. There was some uncertainty in the starting data so that, because the number of subjects is fairly small, the results have to be interpreted with caution. However, it is quite obvious that the subjective adaptation gives rise to the strongest change right at the beginning of the work and that the best function for describing the workload change over time, keeping the subjective intensity constant, is an exponential function.

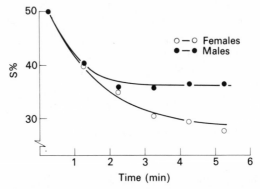

Figure 7-1. Adaptation curves for one group of males ($n = 7$) and one group of females ($n = 7$). S is the produced physical intensity corresponding to an equal subjective intensity. The figure shows relative values in percentage of a maximal value (see text) with the curves anchored at the first trial.

In another series of experiments the subjects had to estimate the change in the subjective intensity over time when the workload was kept constant. The adaptation curves obtained in this manner closely resembled those from the production experiments; they increased according to positively accelerated functions but were the inverse of the curves shown in Figure 7-1 (Borg and Edgren, 1972).

Differential Studies of Perceived Exertion

For practical and differential purposes, the "ratio-scaling methods" described above are not very applicable. Simple rating methods of a category type have therefore been developed to obtain values of perceived exertion. The first scale that was widely used consisted of 21 points, where the *odd values* were anchored with verbal expressions such as "very light" and "rather laborious" (Borg, 1962). This scale has been used to study perceived exertion during an ordinary work test with a stepwise increase in the workload involving various groups of normal people and patients. A very high correlation, $r = 0.85$, was found between ratings on this scale and heart rates (Borg, 1962).

The scale that has been most frequently used during recent years is the Ratings of Perceived Exertion (RPE) scale which works in the same manner as the 21-point scale. The RPE scale consists of 15 grades from 6 to 20 and is constructed to obtain a very close correlation with heart rate. For healthy middle-aged men the heart rate at moderate to high intensities may be roughly predicted from the RPE values simply by multiplying by 10. Before a subject is tested, he is given simple instructions to rate the degree of exertion as accurately as possible according to the scale, which is presented to him in a quarto format. The subject answers by saying a number and by pointing with his finger at the perceived scale value.

The ratings of perceived exertion increase in a fairly linear manner with the workload and, thus, also with the heart rate. High correlations are always found in normal groups of subjects, when "normal" variation of physical stress is used from light to hard work. Most of the correlations are between 0.80 and 0.90 (Borg et al., 1968; Skinner et al., 1969; and Borg, 1971b). In groups of patients the correlation goes down and varies from 0.50 to 0.70, depending on the heterogeneity of the group with respect to the various factors affecting the degree of exertion.

There are marked differences in physical working capacity among people of different ages, body composition, and so on. For various kinds of sub-maximal work similar differences are found in physiological responses to physical stress, so that young and fit people react with less physical stress than old and less fit people. The same result is also obtained in psychological responses, such as perceived exertion. Thus, women react with a stronger response of perceived exertion than men for the same physical work. However, when relative values are used, so that the intensity of the response is set in relation to the capacity of the individual, no sex differences are found.

In a study by Borg and Linderholm (1967), both male and female subjects of various ages had to go through a physical work test with a stepwise increase in the workload each 6 min according to methods used by Sjöstrand (1947) and Wahlund (1948). Ratings of perceived exertion according to the

21-point scale were obtained at the same time as heart rates. The female groups rated the exertion to be higher in relation to workload than did the male groups, but there were no significant differences between the sexes.

In the same study Borg and Linderholm (1967) found fairly great differences between age groups with respect to the relation between perceived exertion and heart rate. For workloads of different intensities the heart rate did not change with age. The ratings of perceived exertion, however, increased for the same workloads fairly linearly with age. Since we know that physical working capacity decreases with age, the ratings give a better and more direct indication of the "real" change in physical stress with age than do heart rates. The maximal heart rate decreases with age in a fairly linear fashion (Robinson, 1938; I. Astrand, 1960; Strandell, 1964; and Borg and Linderholm, 1967). For subjective work intensities, according to the ratings, the heart rate decreases with age as the maximal heart rate decreases. This result validates the use of ratings and the use of relative heart rates. As indicators of physical stress, the ratings do not have to be corrected for age, but the heart rates do. The "same" degree of stress is thus indicated by the same rating value; however, by decreasing heart rates with age according to special equations for the various relative intensities (for example, for 66% of the range above the resting value), the age-independent interindividual reference level in heart rate, that is, the relative heart rate (RHR) can be obtained.

$$RHR_{0.66} = 150 - 0.5(A - 20)$$

where 150 for the 20 year olds is set as a reference level and A is the age in years (Borg and Linderholm, 1967; Borg, 1970b).

As we have seen, a difference exists between various age groups in the relationship between heart rate and perceived exertion. There also exists a difference due to body composition and activity level. In a study of work on a bicycle ergometer Skinner et al. (1969) showed that, at the same submaximal workloads, active subjects had lower heart rates and lower ratings than did sedentary subjects. In addition, heavier subjects had a lower heart rate than lean subjects, but there was no difference in ratings. When work was compared on an absolute basis, there were differences which seem to be related to the level of fitness and body composition. When related to working capacity, however, these factors were not of measurable importance.

The effect of training on perceived exertion in physical work has been studied using a group of Swedish soldiers (Linderholm, 1967). After a period of conditioning, the subjects' ratings of exertion for a given workload were lower than before the conditioning program. The same result was found in studies by Docktor and Sharkey (1971), Ekblom and Goldbarg (1971), and Borg et al. (to be published). Data from Borg et al. are shown in Figure 7-2. Under the same workloads both heart rates and ratings go down in about the same manner so that the relation between heart rates and ratings is unaffected. In the study by Ekblom and Goldbarg (1971), the ratings were lower after training for a given level of oxygen uptake but were the same when related to the "relative" (per cent of maximum) oxygen uptake.

In a bicycle ergometer study involving a representative sample of men born in 1913 in Göteborg, Sweden (Grimby et al., 1972), perceived exertion was measured using the method proposed by Borg (1970b) together with several physiological variables. The authors found that the ratings of physical stress gave some additional information and that the error of measurement was comparatively small, or, as they state: "It is worth noticing that the standard deviations for perceived exertion are of similar magnitude as those for the heart rates."

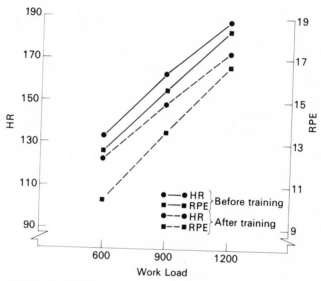

Figure 7-2. Heart rates (HR) and ratings of perceived exertion (RPE) at three different workloads before and after a period of physical training.

A few studies have also been performed investigating different types of work. Experiments by Noble and Borg (reported by Borg, 1970b, and Noble et al., to be published) have shown that jogging is perceived to be easier than walking at the same moderate-to-high speed and that heart rate is higher for jogging than for walking at the same subjective intensities (ratings). Ekblom and Goldbarg (1971) found that the ratings of perceived exertion for given levels of oxygen uptake were higher during arm work than during leg work, as well as during cycling when compared with running or swimming. In a study they did on autonomic nervous system blocking agents, the positive correlation between heart rate and ratings was altered.

Some Clinical Studies

In some Swedish hospitals the discussed method of obtaining category ratings of perceived exertion during a work test (see pages 145–147) is now used routinely. Results from thousands of patients have been obtained and analyzed with regard to the medical syndromes in question. Three main groups of patients have hitherto been analyzed (Borg and Linderholm, 1970): patients with coronary heart disease, patients with arterial hypertension, and patients with the vasoregulatory asthenia syndrome. In comparison with a healthy control group of the same age, the group with vasoregulatory asthenia had a higher heart rate (HR) at particular rating values (R) (that is, they rated the exertion to be less in relation to the heart rate), especially at low intensity levels. This result is shown by the two upper lines in Figure 7-3. Results of a similar nature were also found in the group with arterial hypertension. However, the patients with coronary heart disease rated the exertion to be higher in relation to heart rate, especially at high intensity levels, than a healthy control group of the same age. (See the two lower lines in Figure 7-3.) For all the patient groups studied there was a smaller increase in heart rate in relation to a given increase in the rating of perceived exertion. The differences found between the groups of patients and the control groups are of differential diagnostic interest.

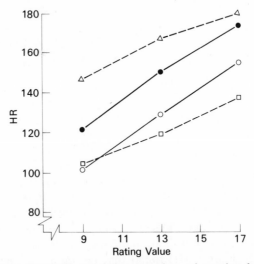

Figure 7-3. Heart rates (HR) in relation to ratings of exertion for two groups of patients and two healthy control groups of the same age as the patients. *Upper dashed line:* patients with the vasoregulatory asthenia syndrome; *upper full line:* the corresponding control group (age about 30 years). *Lower dashed line:* patients with coronary insufficiency; *lower full line:* the corresponding control group (age about 60 years).

In a study of physical working capacity and of the relation between heart rate and perceived exertion (Borg et al., 1969), clients at a rehabilitation center in the United States went through a test on a bicycle ergometer involving a stepwise increase in the workload. The group had about 40% lower physical working capacity, according to the workload at a pulse rate of 150 beats/min, than did two different groups of students used as reference groups. The clients also rated the exertion to be higher for the same workloads than the normal reference groups. It seems probable that the main reason for the result is the effect of institutionalization and bad conditioning programs.

The influence of hypnotic suggestions on perceptual and physiological responses to a bicycle ergometer task was studied by Morgan et al. (1971). In this study the subjects had to work under a certain constant workload and were told that they were going to exercise under light, moderate, and heavy workloads. The results of the study showed that hypnotic suggestion evoked perceptual and physiological changes that led the authors to conclude that "complex somatopsychic phenomena govern perceptual and physiological responsivity to muscular exertion."

A Bicycle Ergometer for Physiological and Psychological Studies

None of the existing bicycle ergometers satisfies all the demands of general usefulness required in physiological and psychological studies. It is, for example, very difficult now to determine muscular strength for short-time work, to perform intermittent work with short pauses and fast changes of the stimulus conditions, or to work steadily while continuously varying the load. When we want to determine terminal thresholds for dynamic muscular strength, the power variation should be large enough to avoid ceiling effects. It should also be possible to increase the workload linearly—or according to some other suitable function—with the pedalling time and to regulate it by means of a reliable automatic device.

The ergometer should also be very flexible in the variation of required power increase or decrease per unit of time in order to make it possible to adapt the experimental conditions to the great differences that exist among individuals with respect to muscular strength, endurance capacity, perceived exertion, and work motivation. This flexibility of the ergometer is especially desirable if the working conditions are to be manipulated during the experiment so as to bring about subjective conformity in the working conditions. It is also important that these requirements be met in psychophysical experiments, where changes of subjective force and perceived exertion are studied with ratio-scaling methods.

The new bicycle ergometer (Borg, Edström and Marklund (1971)), which is a modification of the one designed by Holmgren and Mattsson (1954), fulfills the above mentioned requirements. Of the ergometer's two main components, the pedalling unit is identical with the latest version described by Holmgren and Mattsson, except for the flywheel, which has a rotating mass of 40 kg × m² by means of which "dead phases" during pedalling are eliminated. The regulator unit is constructed to regulate the generator load up to 7000 kilopound meters per minute (kpm/min) (about 1.150 watt) with transistors as the basic components of the unit. The potentiometer, which controls the power level, is constructed to give a continual change of power with the pedalling time, either linearly or according to a power function with one of the following exponents: 0.40, 0.50, 0.66. The speed of the precision motor, attached to the axle of the potentiometer, is adjustable permitting different rates of power increase (or decrease) from 0 to 500 kpm/min per sec. The regulator unit also consists of a potentiometer, which controls a mechanism for fast resetting of the power level, and automatic starting and cut-out devices.

This ergometer is particularly useful for performance tests of physical working capacity, for example, the cycling strength test (CST) (Borg, 1962) and the cycling strength and endurance test (CSET) (Borg, 1968), and also for psychophysical determinations of subjective force and perceived exertion (Borg, Edström and Marklund, 1970).

Two Individually Adapted Performance Tests

Some of the commonly used work tests on the bicycle ergometer in Sweden are those designed by P.-O. Astrand (1952), I. Astrand (1960), and Astrand and Ryhming (1954), by Sjöstrand (1947) and Wahlund (1948), and by Tornvall (1963). The first two tests utilize heart rate during submaximal work as a direct indicator of physical stress and as an indirect estimate of working capacity. The third type of test is of maximal character and gives information about performance capacity.

The CSET (Borg, 1962; 1968) is a pure performance test and takes into consideration the advantage of an interindividually constant testing time. The test consists of a series of intermittently determined thresholds, usually 10, with one determination per minute. At each determination the workload is continuously increased from an initially rather low level to a level where the individual is unable to pedal any further. The initial level of a forthcoming determination is directed by the final level of the preceding one, thus a feedback system is built into the test to keep the testing time fairly constant for each individual. The strength thresholds form a work curve which is analyzed with respect to level, regression, and residual variation, the curve gives information about the individual's dynamic muscular strength, endurance capacity, and motivation for physical work.

The reliability and validity of the CSET are high. In several studies significant correlations have been obtained with various field criteria, such as wages in lumber work ($r = 0.62$), ratings of military fitness of infantry men ($r = 0.55$), and results from athletic competitions (Borg 1962; Borg and Stockfelt, 1966). In Figure 7-4 two CSET curves are shown for a group of male soldiers, one before a conditioning program and one after about 1 month of training.

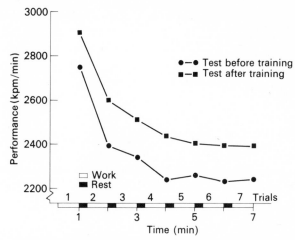

Figure 7-4. Two CSET curves (see text) consisting of thresholds for maximal performances on bicycle ergometer, one curve before training and one curve after training.

The principles for a test, called the individually adapted work test (IAT), which utilizes stepwise-increased workload changes in accordance with the subject's heart rate as well as his ratings of perceived exertion, have recently been developed by Borg (1966) and Borg, Edgren, and Marklund (1970a). The test gives a behavioral measurement of physical working capacity in the form of the highest workload under which a subject is able to work for 4 min. The subjects have to work for the same duration on a series of subjectively equal workloads instead of on physically equal loads.

To be able to keep the testing time fairly short (about 10 min), the test is divided into two main parts. The first part consists of a work period of 6 min and is subdivided into three phases of 2 min each. Heart rate and ratings of perceived exertion are registered at the end of each phase and are used to determine the workload for the next phase. The workload is successively increased from phase to phase so that, after the first 6 min, the subject should have reached the highest workload at which he is able to continue for another 4 min. The magnitude of the workload adjustment at the end of each steering phase depends on how near the individual's heart rate and rating of perceived exertion are to the expected values for the actual sample of subjects. The initial level is determined by anamnestical, morphological, and other available laboratory data. Preliminary studies have produced good results with respect to the relation between the observed time and the expected testing time of 10 min, and high correlations have been found with other work tests of maximal character as well as with external criteria of physical performance capacity.

A Study of the Transition from Short-Time Work to Prolonged Work

To study the transition from short-time (mainly anaerobic) to prolonged (mainly aerobic) work, determinations of terminal thresholds were made using the bicycle ergometer (Borg et al., 1972). Thirty male students took part in the experiment, which was arranged so that the subjects had to work as long as they could during short work periods. The workload was increased continuously until they could not pedal any more. The rate of the workload increase was varied from 10 to 100 kpm/min per sec. The results, presented in Figure 7-5, show how the strength thresholds vary with the time used per trial (for each rate of workload increase). The dashed line is based on a rough correction of the thresholds due to the slight additive influence of the fly-wheel (40.1 kg × m²).

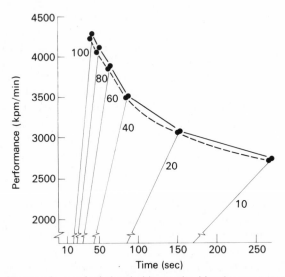

Figure 7-5. Changes in terminal thresholds on the bicycle ergometer showing the transition from short-time work (mainly anaerobic) to prolonged work (mainly aerobic). The rate of the workload increase was varied from 10 to 100 kpm/min · sec.

As can be seen from Figure 7-5, the curve falls linearly with time in the beginning; however, it changes direction after 1 min and levels off more and more, indicating a physiological transition from anaerobic to aerobic work. This result was also supported by changes in the correlations between the thresholds and external measurements of endurance capacity (such as results from a skiing competition and a cross-country race) and muscular strength (such as force of handgrip and shoulder thrust). The bicycle ergometer has now been improved to permit studies of threshold changes in a range from 1 to 500 kpm/min per sec. One tenable hypothesis is that an S shaped function will be found in which the inflection point may be connected to the transition from anaerobic to aerobic work.

Work Motivation

An important concept in the field of motivation is the concept of "drive," which is included in many theoretical systems (for example, Woodworth, 1918; Hull, 1943, 1951; Miller and Dollard, 1941; and Brown, 1961). Closely connected to the concept of drive is that of "arousal." The activation theorists, such as Duffy (1934, 1962), stress that behavioral arousal can be observed by means of a variety of measurements and that arousal varies in a continuum from sleep to a very excited state. Another theoretical proposition concerning arousal states that performance increases from a low point, when arousal is low, to a high point, at an intermediate level of arousal, and then declines as arousal increases still further, that is, in accordance with an inverted U-shaped relation where the optimum is dependent upon the complexity of the task (Yerkes and Dodson, 1908).

The theory of achievement motivation developed by Atkinson and Feather (1966) asserts that the strength of motivation to achieve, as expressed in performance level, is a multiplicative function of the motive strength, the subjective probability of goal attainment (expectancy), and the incentive value of success. The incentive is assumed to be an inverse linear function of expectancy. The relationship between "motivation" and "expectancy" follows an inverted U-shaped curve with an optimum level of motivation occurring when expectancy = 0.50 (Atkinson, 1958). The assumed positive relationship between the motive to achieve and the level of performance is shown to be reduced when another motive (for example, monetary need) is involved. When motivation to achieve and to avoid failure are simultaneously aroused, their algebraic sum constitutes the resultant motivation.

A model for the quantitative analysis of work motivation was suggested by Borg (1962, 1964a), and by Borg, Edström, and Marklund (1967a). In this model, "work motivation" is a construct indicating the extent to which the individual utilizes his endowments (for example, motor and circulatory organs) for maximum performance.

A physical performance is expected to depend on work motivation, technique, and physical endowments, which can be estimated from morphological and physiological measurements (Borg, Edström, and Marklund, 1967a). For simple physical performance (for example, work on a bicycle ergometer), the difference between an observed performance and a performance predicted on the basis of physical endowments constitutes a residual which makes estimation of work motivation possible, since the technique used can be assumed to influence only a small portion of the total performance variance. In Figure 7-6 the principles for calculating work motivation are shown. A and B are two individuals, one with a high and the other with a low work motivation.

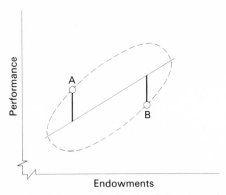

Figure 7-6. The figure shows how motivation-loaded performances may be predicted from nonmotivation-loaded endowments. According to this model of work motivation, quantitative measurements of motivation are obtained; for example, *A* represents a subject with a high work motivation and *B* a subject with a low motivation.

Some investigations have been performed on work motivation using three different kinds of motivation indicators: (1) perceptive, such as perceived exertion, (2) performance, such as motivation-loaded maximal performances, and (3) physiological, such as heart rate and lactate acid concentration. In experiments by Borg and Edström (1964, 1967) CSET performances were studied in connection with "high" and "low" motivation induced through instructions. During low motivation the subjects were instructed to work about half their maximal capacity. Significant differences in performance during "high" and "low" motivation were obtained in level, slope, and residual deviation of the CSET curve. A tendency toward a larger relative deviation and a smaller total slope was found during "low" motivation than during "high." A positive correlation ($r = 0.57$) was found between the motivation-loaded personality trait validity (implying good energy resources) according to the Marke-Nyman Temperament scale (Nyman and Marke, 1962) and the slope of the CSET.

Different types of actual physical performances (for example, maximal work during a specified time and CSET measurements) were subtracted from those predicted on the basis of different indicators of physical endowments (for example, workload at a heart rate of 170 and morphological measurements indicating muscularity). The differences were used as quantitative measurements of motivation for physical performance in a study by Borg, Edström, and Marklund (1967a). The obtained motivation measurements showed high correlations with one another although they were derived by quite different methods. Two sets of measurements of motivation with high intercorrelations were discerned: one set included relations between measurements concerning anaerobic work and another concerning aerobic work.

In experiments on monetary reward (Borg et al., 1971) the results showed that motivation-loaded maximal performances, derived using the CSET method, increased with increased reward and that this effect was positively related to monetary need, as measured with a behavioral indicator. The change of performance with changes in the amount of monetary reward followed a negatively accelerating course. The same course was obtained for changes in performance with the same number of trials when a constant reward was given.

Some Particular Aspects with Regard to Training

In exercise prescriptions it is sometimes hard to determine the intensity of the exercise that is most suitable for a certain individual. One good indicator of the intensity of the exercise is, of course, the heart rate. However, some people have difficulty in counting the heart rate or, if they can, soon become "pulse-counters" who cannot do anything without counting pulse rates. Thus they focus their interest too much on this activity and become somewhat too preoccupied with it. A complement of pulse counting is the subjective feeling of exertion. We should not underestimate people's ability to regulate work intensity in relation to the effort they feel they are making. Normally we do this when exercising. When exercise is felt to be too demanding, a person slows down until he has recovered enough to increase the intensity again.

If we want to supplement exercise prescriptions in the form of statements concerning physical conditions (such as distance, time, speed, and so on) and physiological responses (for example, pulse rates) with subjective estimates of the perceived exertion, we should train patients to rely on the perception of the exertion that is just right for them. In this connection it is important to know that different kinds of physical activities might cause different degrees of subjective exertion in relation to heart frequency. If it is important to avoid high heart frequencies, lack of knowledge concerning these things might be somewhat dangerous. In a training period after an illness it is important to check the effect of the training. This, however, often cannot be done in a laboratory, so there is need for a very simple test that anyone can use. From the point of view of motivation it is also important to be able to check one's working capacity fairly often and follow the change due to training.

A simple fitness test can then be associated with an ordinary day-to-day activity such as walking, in which the technique required to execute the movements is habitual. The difficulty in controlling the speed at which one moves is especially great in maximum exertion. For this reason maximum exertion is avoided so that the circulatory organs are not burdened "unnecessarily." The individual is, instead, allowed to walk at a moderate pace or jog slowly for a certain distance, for example, 1 km (kilometer). The course should be relatively flat and suitable for a normal stroll. It is important here that subjects walk at a constant speed. This is not likely to be a problem as long as they keep to a normal "walking distance" and do not have to stress themselves too much. The time required to cover the distance together with the pulse rate is taken immediately after completing the course. After a short rest period, the performance is repeated, this time with slightly greater effort, though not as much as maximum effort. In this manner, two (or more) time and pulse recordings are obtained that differ somewhat from one another. In the calculation of fitness using this method, a measurement is thus obtained from the pulse-speed diagram in the form of the speed for a certain reference level of pulse rate. This value can be compared with previous or subsequent values or with the values of other individuals.

In this test the dependent-independent variable system is changed in an unusual way compared with ordinary tests. Speed is not used as an independent variable but is, instead, permitted to vary from subject to subject, depending upon the subjective speed determined by the instruction and the experience of the individual.

Studies are now under way utilizing this test. Preliminary results show that the test is useful and that the possibility of maintaining a constant speed is good. Figure 7-7 shows the small speed fluctuations in a group of male subjects ($n = 11$) who walked 1000 m at two different speeds according to the instructions (1) to walk at a normal and just right speed and (2) to walk as fast as possible, but at a constant speed. Since the validity is to some degree self-evident, we would suggest the use of the test as a simple "home test" which would allow for a constant check of endurance fitness and thus may also motivate persons to engage in further training.

To evaluate the effect of physical training on certain psychological functions, such as perceived exertion, we need a model like the one presented in Figure 7-8. In the figure S stands for physical intensities with measurements of physical performances being expressed in S units. Response values are plotted along the vertical axis. In psychophysical experiments we cannot make any direct comparisons of the raw values, but have to use some kind of relative response values. To make this possible the maximal or terminal (t) values are anchored at the corresponding stimulus intensities. Two curves are

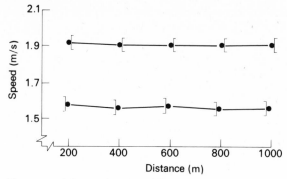

Figure 7-7. Mean speed fluctuation (including the standard error at each checking point—after 2000 m) for a group of male subjects ($n = 11$) walking 1000 m at two self-determined speeds according to two different instructions.

presented in the figure: curve 1 shows the *R-S* relation before training and curve 2 shows the *R-S* relation after training. According to the model the maximal physical intensities are set to be subjectively equal, and the range from zero (or a very low value related to the absolute threshold) to the terminal is used as a frame of reference. The intensity of a response (for example, subjective force) depends upon its position within the subjective range, which in turn depends upon the stimulus range in question and the type of *R-S* function.

If a man, for example, has trained his muscular strength so that the heaviest weight he can lift has increased from S_{t1} to S_{t2}, the subjective feeling of how heavy a submaximal weight S_x is should diminish according to Figure 7-8.

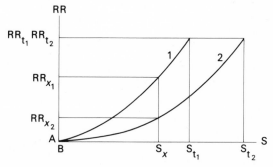

Figure 7-8. The figure shows a model for interprocess comparisons including evaluations of the effects of training. Relative response values (*RR*) are plotted against stimulus intensities (*S*). S_{t1} is the terminal threshold (for example, the heaviest weight a person can lift) and S_{t2} the same kind of threshold but after a period of training. In the figure *A* and *B* show the starting point of the curves. Sx is a submaximal intensity level that gives rise to the subjective response RR_{x1} before training, and RR_{x2} after training.

Mathematically the model may be described in the following way. In the general stimulus response function $R = a + k(S - b)^n$, where R is the intensity of the response, a and b are basic intensity levels showing the starting point of the function, S is the stimulus intensity, k is a constant, and n is the exponent. The constant k is derived from (Borg, 1961, 1970a):

$$k = \frac{R_t - a}{(S_i - b)^n}$$

Two individual curves may then be drawn in the same diagram showing the differences between two occasions, or two subjects, on a series of submaximal intensity levels. Relative response values may then be calculated in the following manner:

$$R_x = \left(\frac{S_x - b}{S_t - b}\right)^n$$

This method of calculating relative response values may also be of value in other kinds of interprocess comparisons, for example, when physiological raw values might be misleading as indicators of the intensity of physical stress or disease.

Self-Appraisal and Physical Fitness

The way an individual perceives himself is an important personality characteristic. Many psychologists have worked with "self-concepts" and "self-theories," for example, Mead (1934), Horney (1950), Rogers (1951, 1959), and Stephenson (1953). In the self-theories, personality disturbances are set in relation to the difference between the "self" as an individual sees it and his "ideal" self. Another important comparison is the difference between the "self" as perceived by the subject and his characteristics as described by ordinary test methods. Such a comparison provides a basis for analyzing the difference between the "self" evaluated by the individual (subjectively) and the corresponding attributes as they "really are" (objectively). The concept of "reality conception" is now introduced in this connection and is generally defined as the difference between subjective and objective measurements.

An accurate self-appraisal is of great importance for good adaptation to modern society. This is true of physical as well as mental attributes and capabilities. A person taking part in a training program after a severe infarct or a minor sickness may underestimate his actual capacity, and thus avoid all kinds of strenuous activities. By doing this he becomes more and more unfit and unable to manage an occupation or take part in leisure time activities. Or, he may overestimate his capacity and stress himself too much.

The way a subject appraises his own muscular strength and endurance capacity in relation to his measured capacity has been studied in a group of 70 middle-aged men who took part in a study of some physical characteristics, conditioning, and coronary risk factors (Bar-Or et al., to be published). A simple rating method was developed to get measurements of self-appraisal. The method functioned well, and positive correlations were found between self-appraisals and ergometer measurements of working capacity, with most correlations being between 0.30 and 0.40. The correlations were low but significant and may be used in some predictive studies. Obviously there is, however, much room for many individuals to get to know their own capacity better. This is important with respect to exercise prescriptions, so that the right meaning of the prescription is given and comprehended by the individual.

The Relation Between Physical Activation, Exertion, Working Capacity and Some Psychological Functions

Since the time of the Greek philosophers there has been an interest in the relation between Psyche and Soma. According to modern philosophy man cannot be divided into two separate parts, mental and physical; the psychological and the physiological functions are, on the contrary, integrated into a complex configuration. In modern medicine the existence of psychosomatic diseases shows very clearly the interdependence of these two "entities"; somatic disturbances have psychological effects and vice versa. The Greek expression "Mens sana in corpore sano" seems more valid today than ever.

According to anecdotal sports information and the general experiences of many people, a positive correlation exists between physical fitness and mental capacity. Curiously enough, very few studies of an empirical nature have attempted to substantiate this claim. However, a few studies have been carried out concerning the relation between physical activation, exertion, and certain psychological functions. In some of these studies physical work has been used to manipulate the degree of "arousal" and its effect on psychological functions. In accordance with the activation theories of an inverted U relationship between arousal and performance, the best performance occurred during a moderate degree of arousal. Elliott (1964) found that auditory time was shortest under a moderate degree of arousal. Sjöberg (1969) also found evidence to support the inverted U relationship in a reaction time experiment where activation was manipulated by work on a bicycle ergometer. In the studies by Borg, Edström, and Linderholm (1966) and Borg (1969), certain small changes were found in psychomotor and memory functions after moderate to hard physical work. The function most sensitive to physical stress was hand-arm steadiness, which began to deteriorate shortly after the onset of light physical stress and deteriorated further and further according to a somewhat positively accelerating function (Borg, to be published).

On the basis of findings from a few experimental studies and some field experiments there seems to be a small but positive correlation between physical fitness and mental functions such that people who are more physically fit are also more stable with respect to many psychological characteristics. Most people also agree that good physical fitness has a positive, therapeutic effect and gives a feeling of well-being, which might be one of the most important effects of physical exercise.

REFERENCES

Astrand, I.: Aerobic capacity in men and women with special reference to age. *Acta Physiol. Scand.* **169**:1–92 (1960).

Astrand, P.-O.: *Experimental Studies of Physical Working Capacity in Relation to Sex and Age.* Copenhagen, Munksgaard, 1952.

Astrand, P.-O. and I. Ryhming: A nomogram for calculation of aerobic capacity (physical fitness) from pulse rate during submaximal work. *J. Appl. Physiol.* **7**:218 (1954).

Atkinson, J. W.: Towards experimental analysis of human motivation in terms of motives, expectancies, and incentives. In J. W. Atkinson, (ed.), *Motives in Fantasy, Action, and Society.* Princeton, N.J., Van Nostrand, pp. 288–305, 1958.

Atkinson, J. W. and N. T. Feather (eds.): *A Theory of Achievement Motivation.* New York, Wiley, 1966.

Bar-Or, O., J. S. Skinner, E. R. Buskirk, and G. Borg: Physiological and perceptual indicators of physical stress in 41 to 60-year-old men who vary in conditioning level and in body fatness. To be published.

Borg, G.: Interindividual scaling and perception of muscular force. *Kungl. Fys. Sällsk. Förh.*, **12**:117–125 (1961).

Borg, G.: *Physical Performance and Perceived Exertion.* Lund, Gleerup, 1962.

Borg, G.: Bestämning av motivationens inverkan på fysisk prestation. *Nord. Psykiat. Tidskr.*, **18**(6):591–596 (1964a).

Borg, G.: A note on some psychophysical problems. *Educ. Psychol. Res. Bull. Umeå Univ.*, No. 4, 1964b.

Borg, G.: Om bestämning av fysiska "maximalarbeten" och möjligheten att predicera dessa utifrån subjektiv ansträngning. *Rapp. Pedagog. Psykol. Inst., Umeå Univ.*, No. 6 1966.

Borg, G.: Ett flexibelt arbetsprov med styrning av arbetsbetingelserna. *Psykol. Unders., Klin.-psykol. Lab., Umeå Univer.*, No. 5, 1967.

Borg, G.: The three-effort continua in physical work. *Proc. XVIth Int. Congr. Appl. Psychol.*, Amsterdam, pp. 394–397, 1968.

Borg, G.: Den fysiska ansträngningens inverkan på reaktionstid, flickerfusion och handstadighet. *Report from the PA-Council*, Stockholm, pp. 0023, 1969.

Borg, G.: Relative response and stimulus scales. *Rep. Inst. Appl. Psych., Univ. Stockholm*, No. 1, 1970a.

Borg, G.: Perceived exertion as an indicator of somatic stress. *Scand. J. Rehabil. Med.*, **2**–**3**:92–98 (1970b).

Borg, G.: The perception of physical performance. In R. J. Shephard (ed.), *Frontiers of Fitness*, Springfield, Ill., Charles C Thomas, pp. 280–294, 1971a.

Borg, G.: Psychological and physiological studies of physical work. In W. T. Singleton and D. Whitfield (eds.), *Measurement of Man at Work*, London, Taylor and Francis, pp. 121–128, 1971b.

Borg, G.: A ratio scaling method for interindividual comparisons. *Rep. Inst. Appl. Psychol.*, *Univ. Stockholm*, No. 27, 1972.

Borg, G., N. Cavallin, C.-G. Edström, and G. Marklund: Motivation and physical performance. *Rep. Inst. Appl. Psychol.*, *Univ. Stockholm*, No. 19, 1971.

Borg, G., and H. Dahlström: Psykofysisk undersökning av arbete på cykelergometer. *Nord. Med.*, **62**:1383–1386 (1959).

Borg, G., and H. Dahlström: The perception of muscular work. *Umeå Vetensk. Bibl. Skr.*, **5**:1–26 (1960).

Borg, G., and B. Edgren: A study on adaptation to short-time work on bicycle ergometer with some implications for the validation of ratio estimations, 1972. To be published.

Borg, G., B. Edgren, and G. Marklund: A flexible work test with a feedback system guiding the test course. *Rep. Inst. Appl. Psychol.*, *Univ. Stockholm*, No. 8, 1970a.

Borg, G., B. Edgren, and G. Marklund: A simple walk test of physical fitness. *Rep. Inst. Appl. Psychol.*, *Univ. Stockholm*, No. 18, 1970b.

Borg, G., B. Edgren, and G. Marklund: The effect of training on heart rate and perceived exertion in physical work. To be published.

Borg, G., and C.-G. Edström: Motivation och fysisk prestation. *Rapp. Pedagog.-Psykol. Inst.*, *Umeå Univ.*, No. 1, 1964.

Borg, G., and C.-G. Edström: Om några motivationsindikatorer vid fysiskt arbete. *Psykol. Unders.*, *Klin.-Psykol. Lab.*, *Umeå Univ.*, No. 1, 1967.

Borg, G., C.-G. Edström, and G. Marklund: Arbetsmotivation. Differensen mellan observerade och förväntade fysiska prestationer. *Psyk. Unders. Klin.-Psykol. Lab.*, *Umeå Univ.*, No. 6, 1967a.

Borg, G., C.-G. Edström, and G. Marklund: En cykelergometer för fysiologiska och beteendemätningar. *Psykol. Under.*, *Klin.-Psykol. Lab.*, *Umeå Univ.*, No. 10, 1967b.

Borg, G., C.-G. Edström, and G. Marklund: A new method to determine the exponent for perceived force in physical work. *Rep. Inst. Appl. Psychol.*, *Univ. Stockholm*, No. 4, 1970.

Borg, G., C.-G. Edström, and G. Marklund: A bicycle ergometer for physiological and psychological studies. *Rep. Inst. Appl. Psychol.*, *Univ. Stockholm*, No. 24, 1971.

Borg, G., C.-G. Edström, and G. Marklund: Effects of the rate of the work load increase on terminal thresholds for physical work. *Rep. Inst. Appl. Psychol.*, *Univ. Stockholm*, No. 25, 1972.

Borg, G., K. Egerman, E. Freeman, and T. Gust: A study of physical and perceived exertion. *Rep. Pennsylvania Rehabil. Center*, Nos. 4 and 6, 1969.

Borg, G., and H. Linderholm: Perceived exertion and pulse rate during graded exercise in various age groups. *Acta Med. Scand.*, Suppl. 472:194–206 (1967).

Borg, G., and H. Linderholm: Exercise performance and perceived exertion in patients with coronary insufficiency, arterial hypertension and vaso-regulatory asthenia. *Acta Med. Scand.*, **187**:17–26 (1970).

Borg, G., B. J. Noble, and M. A. Sherman: A perceptual indicator of physical stress. Paper presented at Annual Convention of the American College of Sports Medicine, Pennsylvania State University, May 2, 1968.

Borg, G., and T. Stockfelt: The cycling strength test (CST) som prediktionsinstrument vid prövning av skyttsoldater. *MPI Rapport 1966*, p. 46.

Brown, J. S.: *The Motivation of Behaviour*. New York, McGraw-Hill, 1961.

Docktor, R., and B. J. Sharkey: Note on some physiological and subjective reactions to exercise and training. *Percept. Mot. Skills*, **32**:233–234 (1971).

Duffy, E.: Emotion: An example of the need for reorientation in psychology. *Psychol. Rev.*, **41**:184–198 (1934).

Duffy, E.: *Activation and Behaviour*. New York, Wiley, 1962.

Eisler, H.: Subjective scale of force for a large muscle group. *J. Exp. Psychol.*, **64**:253–257 (1962).

Ekblom, B., and A. N. Goldbarg: The influence of physical training and other factors on the subjective rating of perceived exertion. *Acta Physiol. Scand.*, **83**:399–406 (1971).

Elliott, R.: Physiological activity and performance. *Psychol. Monogr.*, **78**:587 (1964).

Grimby, G., M. Aurell, J. Bjure, B. Ekström-Jodal, G. Tibblin, and L. Wilhelmsen: Work capacity and physiological responses to work. The Men Born in 1913 Study. Department of Clinical Physiology I, and Unit of Preventive Cardiology, Medical Clinic I, University of Göteborg, Sweden. To be published.

Holmgren, A., and K. H. Mattsson: A new ergometer with constant work load at varying pedalling rate. *Scand. J. Clin. Lab. Invest.*, **6**:137 (1954).

Horney, K.: *Neurosis and Human Growth*. New York, Norton, 1950.

Hueting, J. E., and H. R. Sarphati: Measuring fatigue. *J. Appl. Psychol.* **50**(6): 535–538 (1966).

Hull C. L.: *Principles of Behaviour*. New York, Appleton-Century-Crofts, 1943.

Hull, C. L.: *Essentials of Behaviour*. New Haven, Yale University Press, 1951.

Linderholm, H.: Experience from training of conscripts. *Försvarsmedicin*, **3**:188–201 (1967).

Mead, G. H.: *Mind, Self and Society*. Chicago, University of Chicago Press, 1934.

Miller, N. E., and J. Dollard: *Social Learning and Imitation*. New Haven, Yale University Press, 1941.

Morgan, W. P., B. L. Drinkwater, S. M. Horvath, and P. B. Raven: Perceptual and metabolic responsivity to standard bicycle ergometry following various hypnotic suggestions. Paper presented before the Canadian Association of Sports Sciences and the American College of Sports Medicine, Toronto, Ontario, Canada, 1971.

Noble, B., G. Borg, and M. A. Sherman: A perceptual indicator of physical stress and the reliability and validity of various measurements of physical working capacity. To be published.

Nyman, G. E., and S. Marke: *Sjöbrings Differentiella Psykologi: Analys och skalkonstruktion.* Lund, Gleerup, 1962.

Robinson, S.: Experimental studies of physical fitness in relation to age. *Arbeitsphysiologie,* **10**:251 (1938).

Rogers, C. R.: *Client-Centered Therapy.* New York, Houghton Mifflin, 1951.

Rogers, C. R.: A theory of therapy, personality and interpersonal relationships as developed in the client-centered framework. In S. Koch (ed.), *Psychology: A Study on Science, III,* New York, McGraw-Hill, pp. 184–256, 1959.

Sjöberg, H.: Psykisk prestationsförmåga och fysiologisk aktivering. Unpublished thesis, Psychological Institution, University of Stockholm, 1969.

Sjöstrand, T.: Changes in the respiratory organs of workmen at an ore smelting works. *Acta Med. Scand.,* **196**:687–699 (1947).

Skinner, J. S., G. Borg, and E. R. Buskirk: Physiological and perceptual characteristics of young men differing in activity and body composition. In B. Don Franke (ed.), *Exercise and Fitness—1969,* Proceedings of a symposium presented in Champaign-Urbana Campus, April 25–26, 1969.

Stephenson, W.: *The Study of Behaviour.* Chicago, University of Chicago Press, 1953.

Stevens, J. C. and J. D. Mach: Scales of apparent force. *J. Exp. Psychol.,* **58**:405–413 (1959).

Stevens, S. S.: On the psychophysical law. *Psychol. Rev.,* **64**:153–181 (1957).

Stevens, S. S.: Matching functions between loudness and ten other continua. *Percept. Psychophys.,* **1**:5–8 (1966).

Strandell, T.: Heart rate, arterial lactate concentration and oxygen uptake during exercise in old men compared with young men. *Acta Physiol. Scand.,* **60**:197 (1964).

Tornvall, G.: Assessment of physical capabilities. *Acta Physiol. Scand.,* **58**:201 (1963).

Wahlund, H.: Determination of the physical working capacity. *Acta Med. Scand.,* **132**, suppl.:215 (1948).

Woodworth, R. S.: *Dynamics of Behaviour.* New York, Columbia University Press, 1918.

Yerkes, R. M., and J. D. Dodson: The relation of strength of stimulus to rapidity of habit-formation. *J. Comp. Neurol. Psychol.,* **18**:459–482 (1908).

The Medical Examination

Part II

SECTION EDITOR:
J. KRÁL
Charles University

The Organs, Systems, and Functions

8

J. Král
Charles University
Prague, Czechoslovakia

A medical examination is essential for a subject prior to his participation in a performance test using submaximal or maximal loads. Its aim is (1) to determine whether the subject is healthy and (2) to evaluate the subject's aptitude for taking part in physiological and performance tests. If we are examining a *sample population*, those persons who are not healthy or have some congenital abnormality should be excluded. If we are studying some group of not completely healthy persons in order to determine the advisability of their participation in physical activities, a preliminary medical examination is naturally indispensable. In youth, we are interested in determining not only the state of health but also the biological age, that is, whether body development and maturity correspond to chronological age. In older age groups, generally in persons over 40 years of age, we must be concerned about the cardiovascular system, which may be overloaded by a submaximal or maximal test. Therefore, a very careful observation of the ECG during the whole test is essential.

The medical examination before a subject takes part in performance tests should be concluded by a statement from the physician that the examined person is able to undergo possibly exhausting functional testing.

Justification

The state of the individual's health must be determined very carefully with respect to the probable load to be imposed by the impending exercise, since stationary states of illnesses may be activated by exercise. These findings, though not important in the daily life of the subject, must be reexamined, and a precise diagnosis made. At older ages special attention must be given to the cardiovascular system of the subjects. An insufficiency in the system may appear only after exercise has begun. Therefore, a special medical examination which includes a work test should be given before beginning exercises involving greater workloads.

The medical examination presupposes that every person involved has previously been subjected to x-ray screening of the chest. This screening procedure guarantees that no person with pulmonary tuberculosis or bronchial carcinoma will be subjected to a performance test. If this screening has not been done, an x-ray of the chest becomes an obligatory part of the medical examination.

Medical History (Form A)*

.When taking a medical history, it is necessary to be aware of any deception on the part of those who would like to participate in exercise but who should not tolerate illness or discomfort during physical effort. On the other hand, others may engage in deception because they are compulsorily obliged to participate in exercise and do not wish to do so. Such knowledge is especially valuable when asking the question "Do you feel healthy?" (6.0).

If this question is answered negatively, it is necessary to determine why the subject does not feel healthy. If the negative statement is true, the performance test will probably not be carried out and thus all the following examination becomes unnecessary, except when the medical examination is being done before a functional test of an ill person.

The Amount and Kind of Sleep (7.0). For adults, 7–8 hr of sleep daily are necessary. If this is not possible, longer sleep on Saturday and Sunday can provide some compensation. Not only are the number of hours of sleep per week of importance but also the kind of sleep; agitated sleep, with dreams, sweating in the night, and so on may evoke a suspicion of some illness.

Smoking Habits (8.0). It is important when evaluating the influence of smoking to know how long the habit has lasted and in what form and amounts nicotine has influenced the organism.

Alcohol (9.0). It is also necessary to determine the amount and kind of alcohol intake if one is to interpret certain findings accurately.

Coffee (9.4). To estimate the influence of coffee on certain circulatory findings it is necessary to determine the individual's daily intake.

Medicine or Drugs (10.0). Regular intake of various medicines or drugs could influence different functions of the organism. To evaluate findings correctly, it is therefore necessary to know what kinds of medicines the examined person is taking regularly.

Different Complaints (11.0). Pain in the locomotor system (joints, muscles, and tendons) may be of different origins and may make it impossible for an individual to perform certain kinds of functional tests. Frequent headaches

* The numerals in parentheses throughout the chapter refer to certain sections of the medical examination found in Part VII, Section 2, pages 458–68.

could diminish the level of performance, as well as could the regular ingestion of medicine.

Abdominal pains may be caused by certain illnesses (for example, appendicitis, gastric or duodenal ulcer, colitis, hernia, and so on). They also may be induced by running (so called "stitch in the side").

Difficulties in the heart region may be of a different kind. Pain in young people is not ordinarily produced by diseases associated with the heart. Rather, it may emanate to the cardiac region from the abdomen or may be of nervous origin. Pain near the heart in older persons is primarily caused by coronary insufficiency. Irregularities in the contractions of the heart may be experienced as a transitory arrest of the heart, palpitations, or as an irregular pulse.

Difficulties of breathing which appear during muscular activity could be of circulatory or of pulmonary origin. Chronic or acute bronchitis, asthma, and, on rare occasions, other illnesses are usually responsible for these difficulties.

Eyesight (12.0). Knowledge concerning a participant's nearsightedness or farsightedness and color blindness or night blindness is an important prerequisite in determining his ability to participate in sport, especially games. Participants, however, very frequently deny having these deficiencies. At times, frequent blinking will indicate that a person is nearsighted, even though he denies having to wear glasses.

Hearing (13.0). Hearing is not so important for participation in sport activity, with the exception of high degrees of, or complete, deafness.

Handedness (14.0). Handedness is very important for players of different games. For our purposes it is not important if the lefthandedness is inborn or acquired.

Past and Present Diseases (15.0). Past diseases may have some consequences for present performance. Present diseases may reveal that the examined person cannot be placed in the category of healthy subjects. In this case any recommendation concerning participation in a performance test must be carefully considered.

Major Surgery (16.0). Major surgery refers to abdominal, thoracic, cerebral, and other similar operations.

Major Injuries (17.0). Major injuries are denoted by fractures, large wounds, and so on.

Unconsciousness (18.0). A loss of consciousness may be caused by a trauma (for example, a blow to the head) or by noninjury-related occurrences such as vasomotor collapse.

Questions for Women. Menstruation (20.0), pregnancies (21.0), deliveries (21.1), and miscarriages (21.2) are to be recorded, because they may have an influence on physical performance. A present or past gynecological disease (22.0) can especially influence results on a performance test.

Family History

All hereditary states and diseases of parents must be delineated. Other diseases in the family also ought to be mentioned. The physician can then more easily detect the first signs of some hereditary disease.

Physical Examination

Use the system of coding of age in decimals (see Appendix A, page 537). To measure *height* (23.0) the subject stands on a horizontal platform barefooted, with the heels together, stretching upwards to his fullest extent. The lower border of the right orbit and the upper margin of the external auditory meatus ought to lie on the same horizontal line. The shoulders should be relaxed and the arms and hands stretched straight downward. Care must be taken to ensure that the angle of the anthropometer does not deviate from the perpendicular line and that its arm is horizontal.

The *weight* (24.0) of the subjects in the group to be tested should be taken approximately at the same hour of the day, after emptying the urinary bladder, but not after a heavy meal.

Body Development in Youth

The degree of development can be estimated through a comparison of an individual's height and weight with the average attained at a particular age in a given country or ethnic group (see later) and from the development of the genitals and pubic hair in boys and in girls from breast and pubic hair development.*

All ratings are on a scale from 1 to 5, and thus the standards for pubic hair can be made the same in both sexes. If a composite sex-character development rating is required, pubic hair ratings can be averaged with the genital ratings for boys, and with the breast ratings for girls. Naturally, the ratings can be assigned with more accuracy if a longitudinal study of a child is available, since they are really based on the occurrence of change from a previous state. However, fair accuracy is attainable even when the child is seen only once. Pubic hair ratings are perhaps easier to give than genital and breast development ratings under these circumstances.

The appearance of the breast bud is as a rule the first sign of puberty in the female, though the appearance of pubic hair may sometimes precede it. Stage 4 development of the areolar mound does not occur in all girls; in probably about a quarter it is absent and in a further quarter relatively slight. Furthermore, the areolar mound, when it does occur, often persists well into adulthood; it seems to be at least as much a matter of adult physique as a passing stage of adolescent development.

* For a description of the stages in the development of the genitals, pubic hair, and axillary hair, see Part VII, Section 4C, pages 516–18.

Areolar diameter enlargement continues from stage 2 to stage 5 but proceeds faster in the early stages. Accurate breast development ratings on a cross-sectional basis may be very difficult, but in longitudinal work the general increase in breast size enables stages 3, 4, and 5 to be assigned fairly confidently.

Abnormalities

Eyes (26.0). Abnormalities may be strabismus, conjunctivitis, or other conditions that require wearing spectacles or contact lenses. With respect to vision, one may be nearsighted or farsighted. Nearsightedness between 6–10 diopters may be dangerous in the case of weight lifting or other exercises which result in an increased intrathoracic pressure, because of the possibility of retinal detachment.

Ears (27.0). Abnormalities may be deafness, "cauliflower ear" in wrestlers, exostoses in swimmers, and so on.

Nose (28.0). Deformity of nasal bones of the septum may exist, mostly in boxers and rugby players.

Skin (29.0). Abnormalities may be warts, hemangioma, eczemas, and so on.

Mouth and Throat

Tonsils (30.1). These are ordinarily examined only through direct inspection. Hypertrophy, caused mainly by chronic tonsillitis, is the most common finding. If a tonsilectomy has been performed, scars are seen. Acute tonsillitis (angina) is a contraindication for any participation in sport or performance testing.

Teeth (30.2). The most common problems are decay or prosthesis in older persons. The mucous membrane of the *tongue* or *gum* may be pale, red, or covered with apthae, and so on.

Neck

Lymphadenopathy (31.1). This condition may be detected by inspection or palpation, mostly in the cervical chain, axilla, inguinal region, and so on. If it is found, further examinations must be carried out to determine its significance.

Thyroid Gland (31.2). The thyroid gland is usually normal or may exhibit a slight diffuse enlargement. This enlargement may be irregular, and due to solitary nodules. The gland, however, may be small and unusually hard. If there are signs of thyropathy (trembling of the fingers, staring and protruding eyes, tachycardia, and so on) a further examination must be made. An increased metabolism may completely change the result of a functional test.

Thoracic Region

Chest (32.0). The configuration of the chest is mostly normal, vaulted, or flat. The most common deformities are funnel chest and pigeon breast.

Lungs (33.0). By percussion and auscultation, pleuritis sicca or exsudativa, bronchitis, tuberculosis, and so on may be detected. Screening x-ray examination is compulsory.

Cardiovascular System (34.0)

Heart. By palpation (34.1), the impulse of the apex may not be detected, may be normal, or may be forceful. The latter is mostly of emotional origin, especially in young people, but may in some cases signify a hypertrophy of the heart. In this case, the localization of the impulse is outside the midclavicular line.

By palpation, thrills (34.2) may also be detected. They are mostly localized in the apex area, but may also be on the whole surface of the heart area. Their localization may be in presystole or diastole.

In *auscultation* (34.3), heart sound abnormality refers to (1) first or second sounds that are too loud or too soft, (2) murmurs, and (3) additional sounds. A list of the most frequent changes in auscultation is given in Appendix D, pages 540–41.

Pulse Rate (34.5). Pulse rate at rest is calculated after 5 min in a supine position by auscultation in the heart area or by palpation of the radial artery. Normal values differ with age. The values obtained by Montoye et al. are shown in Table 8-1.

Table 8-1 Pulse Rate

	Age in Years							
	10	15	20	25	35	45	55	65
Males	83.5	80.6	73.9	76.0	75.0	76.0	76.0	72.9
Females	89.0	82.5	80.7	78.0	79.0	79.0	78.2	75.9

The rhythm may be regular or irregular with respiration. There may be extrasystoles (premature beats), bigeminy, complete arrhythmia (atrial fibrillation), and so on.

Blood Pressure (34.6). A mercurial manometer should be used to measure systolic and diastolic blood pressure.* A cuff 14 cm in width should be applied evenly and firmly to either arm after removing impeding clothing. The lower edge of the cuff should be about 2 cm above the antecubital space with the rubber bag centered over the brachial artery. When inflated the cuff should not compress the underlying tissue. It should be rapidly inflated to a point 20–30 mm Hg (millimeters of mercury) above the pressure at which the radial pulse is obliterated. The stethoscope should be applied immediately below the edge of the cuff over the area where the brachial artery pulse is palpable. Cuff pressure should then be permitted to fall at a rate of not more than

* See *WHO Tech. Rep. Ser.* No. 231, 1962, pp. 4 and 5.

2–3 mm Hg per pulse beat. The first appearance of an audible pulse beat is recorded as the *systolic pressure*. As the cuff pressure falls further, the sounds will suddenly become muffled and eventually disappear. Until it becomes clear which phase (that is, muffled sounds or disappearance of sounds) more correctly represents the diastolic value, both pressures should be recorded as *diastolic pressure*.

Blood pressure (systolic and diastolic) increases with age. Normal upper limits in adults are considered to be 140/90 mm Hg.

Abdomen (35.0)

If no dullness is found by percussion and no resistance or pain by palpation, the subject may be considered to be normal. Possible abnormalities are hepatomegaly, splenomegaly, enlargement of the gallbladder, and hernia (36.0). The presence of hemorrhoids (37.0) should also be recorded if a rectal examination is done.

The Shape of the Spine (38.0)

In the anteroposterior (sagittal) plane, the spine may have a normal curvature, may be more rounded in its thoracic part (often found in cyclists), or may have a greater lordosis in the lumbar region (often seen in figure skaters). Changes in the vertebrae and in the intervertebral discs may cause a straight back.

Deviations in the frontal plane (scoliosis) may be found in the thoracic or in the lumbar segments of the spine. With higher degrees of round back, lumbar lordosis, or scoliosis, an x-ray examination of the spine is indispensable. Other abnormalities may be scapulae alatae, block of some vertebrae, and so on.

Extremities (39.0)

Upper Extremity (39.0). Abnormalities may be either congenital or acquired after injury. Chronic lesions (for example, tennis elbow) ought to be recorded.

Lower Extremity (40.0). In older persons the patency of arteries can be detected by palpation of the posterior tibial artery and the dorsalis pedis artery. Varicose veins may be a great handicap and even dangerous for some sportsmen (for example, cyclists). The degree of dilation of the veins and the absence of phlebitis must be recorded.

Interdigital epidermophytosis, if neglected, may impair a person's ability to participate in sport, not only because of its specific effects but also because of its systemic influence.

Nervous System (41.0)

Possible abnormalities are paresis or paralysis of some muscle groups, neuritis, and so on.

Mental State (42.0)

While taking the medical history and during the examination, abnormal answers or behavior may reveal an abnormal mental state.

Reproductive System (43.0)

The testicles of the boys have already been examined during the procedure for determining the degree of maturity. During this examination an incomplete descent of one of the testicles may have been found. If this is the case, a surgical intervention may be necessary depending upon age. The examination of genitals may also reveal hermaphroditism, which naturally must be examined by specialists.

Laboratory Data

The findings obtained by inspection, palpation, percussion, and auscultation must be supplemented by laboratory findings.

Urinalysis (44.0)

The presence of *protein* is an indication for further examination. Different methods may be used. Because a positive finding may be pathological, it is necessary to perform a microscopic examination. Red cells or casts (hyalin or granular) may signify a lesion of the kidneys or the urinary tract but may also be found in apparently healthy persons after strenuous exercise.

Sugar level in the urine may be determined by reduction in a test tube or by using the paper method. Finding sugar in the urine of young people is rare, although it may often be present in elderly persons. A finding of sugar in the urine does not necessarily preclude participation in a performance test, but further examination is definitely required, including a glucose tolerance test.

Vital Capacity (45.0)

Apparatus. Hutchinson's spirometer, gasometer, or spirograph.

Test Description. The examined person is tested while standing. After a maximal inspiration he expires air from his lungs into the apparatus until the point of complete expiration has been reached. This expiration should be repeated three times at about 15-sec intervals. The maximal value from these three expirations is recorded.

Evaluation of Results. The value of vital capacity (VC) depends on several factors, namely, height, weight, age, and sex. In order to determine whether the measured value is higher or lower than the so called "ideal vital capacity," which corresponds to the height, weight, age, and sex of the examined person, the "index of vital capacity" is calculated. The measured value is adjusted for body temperature and pressure saturated with water vapor, BTPS (special tables are commonly used).

$$\text{Index of VC } \% = \frac{\text{Measured VC} \times 100}{\text{Theoretical VC}}$$

The theoretical value of vital capacity can be calculated by different formulas. The most commonly used is Anthony's formula; the value of the theoretical basal metabolism found in Harris-Benedict's tables is multiplied by 2.3 for men and 2.1 for women.

Forced Expiratory Volume (FEV) (46.0)*

Conditions. Subjects may be seated or standing, coats and ties or any other restrictive clothing are removed, and smoking is prohibited for at least half an hour before the test.

Instruments. A number of instruments providing accurate quantitative records with ordinary air-flow rate (under 400 liters/min) are available. Calibration of the spirometers and flow meters is necessary, a description of the method being provided by the supplier. Repeated evacuations of the spirometer bell or bellows into a large Tissot gasometer usually provide a very accurate check on the volume delivered. Drum speed can be checked by a stop watch.

Procedure. The recording technique depends somewhat on the instrument employed, but the considerations mentioned below should be kept in mind. As previously noted, the subject may be seated or standing. The procedural routine should be standard, including the verbal instructions and practical demonstrations to the subject. The following is an example of a routine commonly used when performing FEV with spirometric recording.

1. The spirometer is set and the mouthpiece attached while the subject is seated and told: "This is a test of your lung capacity which you will perform in several trials."
2. The mouthpiece is inserted while the subject is told: "This is a clean mouthpiece, which is held between the teeth and lips. Hold it firmly but please don't bite it."
3. The technician then says: "In a moment I'll ask you to take as deep a breath as you possibly can. When I say 'blow,' you will breathe out all the air in your chest as rapidly and completely as possible. You have to do it as rapidly as possible, all at once."
4. The technician demonstrates a full inspiration and expiration. When ready, the technician starts the kymograph and instructs the subject, "Take a deep breath, ready, blow!"
5. The technician should watch for nose and mouth air leaks and for pinching

* Rose, G. A., and H. Blackburn: *Cardiovascular Survey Methods.* Geneva, WHO, 1968.

of the mouthpiece or tubing and continue to encourage a complete expiration by admonishing the subject to "keep blowing, keep blowing."

6. Two curves of good quality are required, without cough or artifact, similar in contour and agreeing within 5% in total capacity (FEV). Without curves for inspection, the standard routine consists of one practice procedure followed by two recorded tests.

The test often precipitates coughing and sputum raising or, in some subjects, air trapping. At least half a minute should elapse between tests. In rare cases the subject will not be capable of understanding instructions; if so, the technician should demonstrate the complete test with mouthpiece in place. Technician training must take place in "real life" situations and should be carried out under the supervision of an experienced person. When possible, one technician should specialize in the procedure for the field study. The production of clean (smooth) repeatable curves is adequate evidence of good technique.

Measurement of Expiratory Curves

A wisely used method of measuring spirometry curves is that of the combined United States Army and Veterans Administration Study (Kory et al., 1961). Figure 8-1 illustrates the measurement of the total vital capacity, forced expiratory volumes at 0.75 and 1.00 sec ($FEV_{0.75}$, $FEV_{1.00}$). Average values of the two "technically best" curves, as described, are tabulated. Plastic rules or protractors may be devised to facilitate and improve reliability of measurement (Rosner et al., 1967).

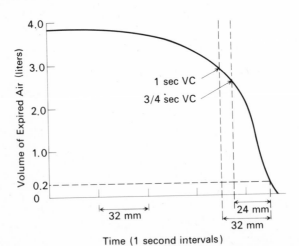

Figure 8-1. Forced expiratory volumes, forced vital capacity, and 3/4-sec and 1-sec timed capacities. Drum velocity, 32 mm/sec. [Reproduced, with permission, from Kory et al. (1961).]

Blood (47.0)

Hemoglobin (47.1), cholesterol in the blood (47.2) and the sedimentation rate (47.3) may be determined by several methods. Because there may be small differences when using different methods, the name of the method must be indicated.

Electrocardiogram (ECG) (48.0)

The subject should be in a supine position on a comfortable couch wide enough to support the upper limbs without any tendency to slip over the edge. The room should be warm and the subject should be at ease. It may be necessary to inquire whether he wishes to empty his bladder. Electrode jelly should be rubbed well into the skin at contact areas and muscular tremor and AC interference must be avoided. (Be sure to attach original ECG.)

After 5 min rest, take the standard leads, V_1–V_6 chest leads, and unipolar limb leads. Repeat the tracing if possible during work on a bicycle ergometer. If this is not possible repeat it after the subject's performance of 30 knee bends in 30 sec. Record the time elapsed between the end of exercise and taking the ECG. (Be sure to attach original ECG.)

Heart Volume Determination

Apparatus. Radiographic apparatus and ancillary equipment.

Description. Three variables are necessary for the calculation of cardiac volume. They are obtained by teleroentgenography in the frontal and sagittal planes with the patient lying down (see Figures 8-2, 8-3, and 8-4). For the film in the frontal plane, the cassette is placed close to the heart in front of the sternum; for the sagittal film it is placed directly against the left side of the thorax. The films are exposed in rapid succession, independently of the cardiac cycle, but in the same respiratory phase (that is, during shallow inspiration). To preclude a Valsalva effect, the subject's mouth remains open. No significant variations in volume occur between the prone and the supine position. In the prone position the frontal area is larger, whereas the antero-posterior diameter is smaller than in the supine position. In the prone position the heart is in broader contact with the anterior chest wall. Its volume, how-

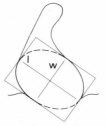

Figure 8-2.   Vertical and horizontal diameter of the heart.

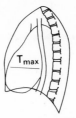

Figure 8-3. The longest anteroposterior diameter (T_{max}).

ever; is not greater than in the supine position, as might be wrongly assumed from the frontal view alone. Therefore, the two required film exposures can be made either in the prone or in the supine position. Before the picture is taken the person will swallow a spoonful of barium to show the posterior outline of the heart exactly.

Calculations. The formula for determining heart volume is based on the assumption that the volume of a body of any shape is equal to the sum of the surface area of a parallel projection of the body and its mean linear expansion in the direction of the projection. The surface area is obtained from the ortho-diagram. The mean expansion (depth) in the direction of the projection can only be measured indirectly, as it depends upon the shape of the body. The mass of the heart is most closely represented by a spheroid body (sphere ellipsoid) and a constant (K), which is characteristic for the shape of the heart. Thus the Rohrer-Kahlstorf formula is

$$\text{Volume} = K \cdot Fa \cdot T_{\text{max}}$$

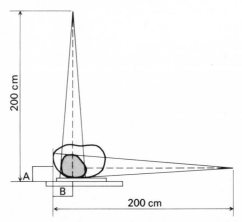

Figure 8-4. Technique for radiographic examination of the heart in frontal and sagittal planes in prone position to get the pictures shown in Figures 8-2 and 8-3. In adults (*A*) frontal plane, 10 cm ; (*B*) sagittal plane, 20 cm.

where K equals 0.63, Fa is the frontal (anteroposterior) orthodiagram, and T_{max} is the greatest depth of the lateral (sagittal) orthodiagram.

Heart area can be determined either by planimetry or according to the formula of the area of an ellipse.

$$Fa = \frac{\pi}{4} \cdot l \cdot w$$

where l = the length and w = the width of the area (Figure 8-2). The difference between the calculated and the planimetrically measured area is less than 3%. On substituting teleroentgenography for the orthodiagraphic method, the projectional error must be corrected. Assuming a focus-to-film distance of 2 m in the frontal and lateral pictures, with a uniform heart-film distance of 10 cm for the frontal and 20 cm for the lateral picture, the following formula applies.

$$Vol = 0.63 \cdot \frac{\pi}{4} \cdot \frac{200 - 10}{200} \cdot l \cdot w \cdot \frac{200 - 20}{200} T_{max} = 0.40 \cdot l \cdot w \cdot T_{max}$$

where l is the length and w is the width of the Moritz' cardiac quadrangle, and T_{max} is the largest horizontal (depth) diameter of the heart. In children the distance between film and heart is smaller and therefore the error of the projection is larger. The constant (K), for instance, in children 10 years old is 0.42 and in children 6 years old, 0.44.

The relative heart volume is expressed as the product of heart volume and body weight: HV/kp. A sample calculation follows for a subject with body weight $(kp) = 74$, $w = 11.0$, $l = 13.0$ cm, and $T_{max} = 14.0$. Thus

$$HV = 0.40 \cdot 11.0 \cdot 13.0 \cdot 14.0 = 801.80 \text{ ml}$$

which means that

$$HV/kp = 800/74 = 10.8$$

General Guide and Comments

The heart volume measurement allows estimations to be made of the influence of training on the work and load carrying capacity of men generally and of athletes in particular. The accuracy of the method has been reexamined several times. Its error in comparative studies is between 3 and 5% in the model, in living subjects, and in cadavers.

The blood group of the individual is obtained in specialized laboratories. Often this examination has already been completed and is recorded on the subject's identity card.

In Youth. Chronological age often does not correspond with biological age. Therefore, in youth a more precise determination of age is necessary. For this purpose the following determinations are carried out:

1. The determination of biological age from height and weight (Wetzel, Kapalín, Tanner, Hebbelinck and Borms, and so on).
2. The determination of skeletal age from the x-ray of the wrist (see pages 516–18)
3. The determination of the degree of maturity (see pages 518–24).

The Measurement of Functions

9

ALLAN J. RYAN
The University of Wisconsin
Madison, Wisconsin

It must be acknowledged immediately that information obtained by presenting a subject with a questionnaire will probably be less extensive and reliable than that which could be collected from the same subject by a trained interviewer. Questions that require some evaluation by the subject are often answered less reliably than when asked directly by someone who can rephrase them or ask supplementary questions to clarify the answers. Interpretation of the questionnaire responses by the reviewer must, therefore, be undertaken with considerable caution. If the opportunity is afforded, it would be highly advisable for the examining physician to review the answers given to see whether the questions were answered fully and with adequate understanding of their meaning.

Personal Data and Athletic History

Personal Data (1.0–3.4) *

The guide to the classification of work included in Part VII, Section 1, the Physical Fitness Measurement standards, should be most helpful to the subject and physician in classifying the subject's occupation correctly. Since many possible types of work are not included among the examples, additional interpretation by both the subject and physician may be required. Evaluation of the subject's response to the question relating to responsibilities at work will be difficult, at best, since many persons who actually have little responsibility either see themselves as having a great deal or would like to indicate that this is the case. The reverse is less likely to be true.

Athletic History (4.0–5.7)

The question as to whether a subject is a "competitive" sportsman or not is one that could yield several interpretations. In one sense this question could

---

* The numerals in parentheses throughout the chapter refer to the item numbers of Sections 1 and 2, Part VII.

be taken to refer to his attitude when engaging in sports; in another, it could be taken to mean that he engages in sports where one or more persons compete with one or more others; or finally, it might be assumed that it referred to participation in regularly organized competitions on either an individual or team basis.

The differentiation between amateur and professional in sports varies from country to country and even from sport to sport within the same country. Criteria which may be used in arriving at a classification include accepting prizes of substantial monetary value, receiving expenses, accepting subsidies, dividing profits from gate and other receipts, and receiving a salary for participation. Persons receiving any or all of the above, except for the last, have at one time or another or in one or another place been considered amateurs. In some sports, persons who are declared professionals in one sport may be considered amateurs in another. Professionals have also been reinstated as amateurs in some sports on presenting evidence that they are not and do not intend to receive remuneration of any kind for their participation.

The Medical Examination

The Medical History (6.0–22.0)

Some subjects may experience difficulty in understanding the terminology and relating the questions in the history of diseases (15.0) to personal experience. The examiner should take time to make a review of the answers to be sure that the subject understood the questions. The word "anginas," for example, might be related to heart disease by the subject even though the word "tonsillitis" is placed next to it in parentheses.

There would probably be some difficulty on the part of the layman in deciding what constitutes "major" surgery (16.0) and "major" injury (17.0) since physicians themselves are not always in agreement on these points.

In evaluating the menstrual history (20.0) there are many possibilities for variance depending on how women understand the questions and their own feelings about their personal situation. The duration is taken by some to mean only the number of days on which there is moderate to heavy flow. Regularity is a rather vague concept to many women who do not keep track of the number of days elapsing between the onset of each period.

The Physical Examination (23.0–43.3)

The examiner is asked to record the time of day at which the examination is performed. Body functions, such as respiration, circulation, digestion, and so on, are subject to rhythmical variations that follow an approximately 24-hr cycle (Dubois, 1959). Pulse, blood pressure, respirations, and core temperature may vary considerably during one cycle. In comparing one individual or group with another, some allowances might have to be made if the mean differences of local times of the day at which they were examined varied significantly.

Height (23.0). Evaluation of height depends on knowing whether standard procedures were employed for measuring persons who are unable to stand erect as well as those who are. For persons who are confined to a wheelchair or who have lost both lower extremities, sitting height is a significant measure.

Weight (24.0). Evaluation of recorded weights is dependent on knowing the type of instrument used for weighing. Since other anthropometric measurements are not being recorded, gross weight would be of much less significance than fat-free weight. A good approximation of this can be obtained by using a Lange calipers to measure anywhere from one to six skinfold thicknesses (Engle and Shelesnyak, 1934). The recording of both the gross and fat-free weights would offer significant information relating to an individual's general physical fitness.

Genital Development. Description of the stages of genital development in boys and men and of breast development in girls and women is given in Section 4C of Part VII. Recording these different stages of development of the secondary sex characteristics provides a better index of maturity than chronological age. This becomes important in comparing elementary school age children with regard to such performance characteristics as strength, endurance, coordination, and so on. Although there is relatively little information available from mass studies of different populations in many countries about the typical ages at which boys and girls undergo these changes, considerably more is known about the ages of onset of menses in girls. These data indicate that not only are there significant differences among the various areas of the world but even among countries in the same area; moreover, within these regions, significant changes have taken place within recent years, apparently as the result of changing environmental conditions (Engle and Shelesnyak, 1934; Burch et al., 1967).

Spine (38.0). Assessment of the results of the external examination of the spine, which in this profile appears to be limited to inspection, will be extraordinarily difficult if x-ray films and other data derived from a functional examination are not available. Any judgment based on an incomplete examination of the spine may be very misleading. The "normal" appearance is perhaps envisioned as an ideal carriage based on the observation of western European white man. In some populations, such as the pygmies of central Africa, this type of carriage might not be seen in anyone of the entire group surveyed. However, any deviation of the formation or positioning of the spine from what appears to be typical for the group under surveillance should call for the addition of such supplementary information as can be obtained to clarify its significance. In "round back," for example, it should be specified whether a pure kyphosis or a kyphoscoliosis is present. The former would suggest certain forms of arthritis, emphysema, Scheuermann's disease, and perhaps other conditions. The latter suggests the presence of so-called "idiopathic kyphoscoliosis," which affects young persons, or a disease such as tuberculosis of the spine.

Exaggerated lumbar lordosis may be indicative of anthropologic variations as in the steatopygous pygmies, a poor posture, an abnormality of development such as spondylolisthesis, a previous spinal injury, or some disease of the spine. A straight back would be a characteristic finding with Still's disease but might also be indicative of a recent injury or some other disease of the spine. Scoliosis may be the result of a short lower extremity, an old injury, a vertebral anomaly, or disease of the spine, in addition to the causes already mentioned for kyphoscoliosis.

Abnormalities of the Eyes, Ears, Nose, and Skin (26.0–29.0). Depending on the method used to ascertain visual acuity, information may be obtained as to vision of a close or distant object, depth perception, or distortion of the visual image by astigmatism. By linking the visual acuity with a diagnosis of some abnormality in the eye, some indication of the individual's overall state of health may be obtained, as in the case of a person with vision impaired for both near and far objects who has diabetic retinopathy. If glasses or contact lenses are worn and the corrected vision is recorded as well, some indication may be given of the severity of the visual defect.

Hearing acuity is not an item which is specifically requested in the Standards. If a diagnosis of deafness is recorded, some indication should be given as to whether nerve or conductive deafness is present and of the degree of hearing loss. A person deaf from birth may lack the ability to speak intelligibly. It would be appropriate to make a note of this as well.

Abnormalities of the nose may be significant for functional purposes, as in the case of obstruction of breathing, and for psychological reasons, where all or part of a nose is missing. It must be assumed that with diagnoses that imply obstruction, such as deviation of the septum, nasal polyps, and so on, some difficulty in respiration must result, even though this may be compensated for to some extent by mouth breathing.

Abnormalities of the skin will not, for the most part, indicate whether there might be impairment of physical fitness. Severe disorders, such as pemphigus, are associated, however, with profound systemic effects and may result in death. Another condition that may affect functional capacity substantially under conditions of high temperature and humidity is ichthyosis. System disorders such as dermatomyositis, scleroderma, and lupus erythematosus may manifest skin changes which are striking and may be associated with substantial reductions in functional capacity.

Mouth and Throat (30.0). Except in the case of acute throat infections, conditions found in the mouth and throat will rarely affect the overall state of physical fitness. Chronic tonsillitis may exert an unfavorable systemic effect, if such a condition can be imagined as the result of repeated acute infections rather than a steady state. There is no pathologic significance to tonsillar hypertrophy unless it is accompanied by other evidences of lymphoid hyperplasia throughout the body, in which case a generalized infectious state or malignant disease involving the lymphatic system might be suspected. In either case, profound temporary or permanent alterations of the level of fitness might be expected.

The presence of decaying teeth may have significance for the state of the subject's nutrition as well as for the general state of oral hygiene. A diet high in carbohydrates might be suspected. Malnutrition, due to pain on mastication of solid food is a possibility. Abscessed teeth may cause serious systemic effects, but the presence of a chronic, nonspecific "toxic" state leading to arthritis and other systemic manifestations has been generally rejected at the present time (the theory of a so-called "focus of infection"). A person who is edentulous and lacks a prosthesis may suffer from chronic malnutrition, although this depends on the type of diet available.

The Neck (31.0). The presence of lymphadenopathy may signify local infection as in a dental abscess, systemic infection as in mononucleosis, a malignant disease primarily in the lymphatic system as in Hodgkin's disease, or metastatic disorders as in lung cancer. The significance of such enlargement, therefore, depends on an exact diagnosis, and this should be provided if available. Calcification may be present in nodes where caseation has occurred, as in tuberculosis. The presence of a generalized lymphadenopathy in the body should probably be noted in this place because no other provision is made to record it on the form.

Diffuse enlargement of the thyroid gland may be associated with simple goiter, which occurs especially in parts of the world where the water supply is deficient in iodine. It may, however, especially in older persons, be associated with struma lymphomatosa (Hashimoto's disease), a late stage in some individuals of diffuse toxic goiter. Toxic goiter may be characterized by a diffuse enlargement of the thyroid, generally not as great as in simple goiter or struma, or by a nodular enlargement. Since it is almost invariably accompanied by characteristic eye changes and other signs and symptoms, its differentiation from the two former conditions and from nontoxic nodular goiter is not difficult.

Nontoxic nodular goiter may present a single nodule of variable size, ordinarily an adenoma of the thyroid, or multiple nodules made up of many adenomata. Symptoms associated with overproduction of thyroxine may be present even though a truly toxic state is not reached. A single nodule may be of malignant character, and clinical differentiation from a benign one may be impossible. Ordinarily the irregular enlargement of the malignant thyroid gland presents a type of hardness and/or fixation to surrounding structures which aids in the diagnosis.

Conditions of the thyroid more rarely encountered are thyroglossal cyst, where the ectopic thyroid can be formed at or above the level of the hyoid bone, other ectopic growths in the neck, or the small very hard struma of Riedel. Depending on the amount of functioning thyroid tissue present, these conditions may have significance for fitness, as demonstrated by changes in the metabolic rate of the body.

Rarely, a parathyroid enlargement may be palpated close to the thyroid gland. Bronchial cleft cysts and nerve sheath tumors are infrequently found but must be considered in a differential diagnosis of an unusual mass in the neck.

The Chest (32.0). Deformities of the chest may be due to congenital defect or malformation, injury, surgery, or disease. The extent of functional deficit depends on the interference with respiration and cardiac function. Some abnormalities are apparent by inspection, but others reveal themselves only by the symptoms they produce or by an x-ray examination. Absence or fusion of ribs is usually not of functional significance itself but may represent one part of a syndrome, such as Turner's, that produces other changes in the body of great importance. Ribs removed surgically will regenerate if the periosteum is left intact. Ribs may be removed with the periosteum to produce a collapse of the rib cage for therapeutic purposes, as in thoracoplasty for pulmonary tuberculosis and other lung diseases.

The deformity of funnel chest, which is due to a retraction of the sternum beginning early in life, may produce significant functional disorders if uncorrected because of the interference with the cardiovascular circuit and the reduction of lung volume. Pigeon breast, on the other hand, is infrequently the cause of functional deficits. The deformity due to kyphoscoliosis from various causes and the "barrel chest" of the emphysematous individual have already been mentioned.

Retraction of the ribs and restriction of movement on one side of the chest may result from adhesive and constructive pleuritis following emphysema or hemothorax. The reduction of pulmonary capacity is usually substantial and may not be completely corrected by decorticating the lung. Restriction of movement on one side without rib retraction may be caused by pneumonia, emphysema, hydrothorax, hemothorax, or paralysis of the phrenic nerve. In each case, additional diagnostic measures are necessary to clarify the responsible cause.

Respiratory System (33.0). Examination of the lungs by percussion and auscultation may lead to the suspicion of certain disease states but will seldom indicate reliably the exact diagnosis. In the absence of other supporting information, the assessment of possible impairment of functional capacity must remain temporarily obscure. One might expect to be able to detect complete absence of breath sounds over one lung, due either to its having been removed or to its being blocked or covered by some substance which has also collapsed it. A lung blocked by a bronchial obstruction will return a high-pitched percussion note, whereas one which is collapsed will return a dull or flat one.

The presence of fluid over a lung produces a flat note; air over fluid gives a hollow note above a flat note, depending on the respective levels of each component. Air over fluid may also produce a succussion "splash" when the chest is moved sharply from side to side. A pneumothorax will return a high-pitched note. Tactile and vocal fremitus will vary with the degree of inflation of the lung and with the presence or absence of a fluid or other tissue barrier to the direct transmission of the sound.

The presence of rales on auscultation may be indicative of the presence of fluid in the alveoli with or without collapse of some of these elements. Accurate diagnosis based on discrimination of particular types of rales is probably impossible, but fortunate guesses occur. Intermittent regular impairment of breath sounds in the course of the respiratory cycle, as in "cogwheel breathing" may be indicative of a partial functional or organic bronchial obstruction.

Cardiovascular System (34.0). Palpation of the anterior chest wall to ascertain the heart size may give significant information. The location of the apical impulse, if it can be felt, may give some indication of heart size; however, it must be emphasized that, as an otherwise unsupported piece of information, this may be very misleading. Failure to feel the apical impulse may be due to the presence of a small heart, low blood pressure, or a pericardial effusion. The presence of an unusually forceful impulse is not necessarily an indication of heart disease or even of high blood pressure. Failure to outline the borders of the heart by percussion may be due to a small heart size or to emphysema.

The presence of a "thrill" on placing the flat of the hand across the precordium is usually evidence of the presence of organic heart disease. It is invariably accompanied by a murmur of some sort which may help to clarify the cause of the disorder. The most common causes of such a "thrill" (vibration of the chest wall) are congenital and rheumatic heart diseases.

Heart Murmurs (34.4). The classification of heart murmurs is elaborated in Part VII of the Standards. A disquisition on the significance of the quality of heart sound and murmurs would require almost a textbook on cardiology and will not be attempted here. Suffice it to say that heart sounds of poor quality (that is, weak intensity) ordinarily indicate the presence of heart disease and that murmurs due to organic disease are intensified by exercise whereas functional murmurs tend to disappear.

The rhythm as well as the rate of the apical heart beat and pulse are significant. Where the rhythm is irregular a pulse deficit (difference between apical and pulse rates) may be suspected. Both rates should be checked simultaneously in such a case. A low resting pulse rate in the absence of other evidence of heart disease indicates ordinarily that the subject is a well-conditioned athlete. A rapid resting pulse, in the absence of any evidence of systemic or cardiac disease, indicates a deconditioned state of the subject. For the interpretation of the significance of different cardiac rhythms the reader is again referred to textbooks on cardiology.

So-called "low blood pressure" has no significance unless it accompanies an acute or chronic disease state, such as adrenal insufficiency. Systolic pressures as low as 80 mm of mercury may be normal for subjects of very small stature who exhibit poor general development. Systolic blood pressures may be lowered in acute or chronic fatigue states, but this is only temporary.

Elevation of the systolic blood pressure may occur as the result of acute emotional stress. This may be accompanied by some elevation of the diastolic pressure as well, but usually not to the same degree. Persistent elevation of the systolic and diastolic pressures, especially the latter, is indicative of chronic cardiovascular disease. The differentiation of the cause may be significant from the standpoint of progress and is important for treatment, but the deleterious effects on structure and function resulting from prolonged hypertension are common to each cause. Elevation of blood pressure in the upper extremities while pressure is low in the lower extremities is indicative of either coarctation of the aorta or an aneurysm of the aorta below the level of the subclavian artery. In the case of coarctation, a delay in the appearance of the femoral pulse compared to the radial is characteristic.

The pulse pressure ordinarily widens with exercise. It decreases with cardiac disease or in states of shock. The presence of a low pressure indicates a general functional deficit in the subject with few exceptions.

Abdomen (35.0). It may be assumed that in the examination of the abdomen inspection, auscultation, and palpation will be employed in that order. Inspection should focus at first on the shape of the abdomen. A scaphoid abdomen may indicate malnutrition (excluding severe deficiency states such as kwashiorkor, which causes enlargement of the liver and ascites) but may also be normal in small, poorly developed subjects. A distended abdomen may indicate the presence of fluid, a cyst or tumor, enlargement of an organ such as the liver, intestinal obstruction, or merely constipation or a distended urinary bladder. The interpretation of isolated masses in the abdomen becomes a matter of evaluating consistency, mobility, local tenderness, and other factors in relationship to the anatomic location of the mass in question. In this respect, auscultation may be very helpful. The presence or absence of bowel sounds, continuous murmurs or souffles, or a fetal heart beat may be helpful in establishing a diagnosis.

Scars found on the abdomen do not necessarily indicate particular surgical procedures or whether or not organs may be missing in whole or in part. Incisions are made for exploratory purposes sometimes and may be closed without any definitive procedure being undertaken. Within such limits, certain surmises may be reasonably accurate, even lacking other information.

A transverse scar with absence of the umbilicus usually means a hernia of that part has been repaired, although this may be only incidental to some other procedure. A right McBurney scar may indicate some procedure involving the appendix, removal or drainage. An incision paralleling the inguinal ligament and slightly above it usually means that an inguinal hernia has been repaired.

The presence of a fistula or an opening connected with a hollow viscus, such as a colostomy, is indicative of some recent or past disease state that may be active or inactive. The fistula may have occurred spontaneously or have been created by surgical artifice. Functional deficits cannot be assured unless one knows the general condition of the individual.

Hemorrhoids (37.0). The determination of the presence or absence of hemorrhoids is properly a part of a rectal examination. Since a complete rectal examination is not included in the Standards, it must be assumed that only an external inspection will be made. This can be deceptive because large hemorrhoids may be present but not seen unless they are proctoscoped. A single thrombosed external hemorrhoid may be seen easily and may indicate the presence of an internal component, a fissure, or both. The presence of hemorrhoids may be an isolated phenomena, but it may also be connected with increased intraabdominal pressure due to constipation, obstructing tumors of the bowel, cirrhosis, pregnancy, and other conditions.

Hernia (36.0). Congenital hernias (indirect inguinal, umbilical, epigastric) and acquired ones (direct inguinal, femoral, incisional) may be observed by inspection or detected only on palpation. A hernia that is not reducible may be incarcerated or strangulated. If the latter, other signs of a crisis will not be lacking. An incarcerated hernia may be asymptomatic and not produce any disorder, but it may convert spontaneously to a strangulated hernia at any time. Very large abdominal hernias (usually incisional) may contain most of the abdominal contents, which sometimes cannot be returned to the abdominal cavity proper because its size has diminished.

The Extremities (39.0 and 40.0). In order to determine the presence or absence of functional deficits, the chief considerations are the absence of any part, loss of a normal range of motion, evidence of incoordination, preservation of adequate circulation, muscle tone (including any evidence of spasticity), relative strength, preservation of deep tendon reflexes, and any disturbance of normal sensation. Any or all of these factors may be affected by virtue of a congenital defect, a disease, or an injury. Some defects may produce little or no loss of function for the part as a whole, whereas others may be responsible for a complete deficit.

Assessment of the functional state of the extremities usually depends on the analysis of the relationship of one or more abnormalities to a local condition producing a deficit, a systemic condition causing a local or more generalized deficit, or both. For example, loss of range of motion in a joint may be due to a local injury, to a generalized arthritis, or to a systemic disease such as scleroderma. Paralysis may be the result of loss of central or peripheral innervation of the involved muscles or even of a spastic condition where innervation is not properly balanced. Diagnostic measures other than inspection, palpation, and range of motion tests may be necessary. The reader is referred to texts dealing with orthopedics, kinesiology, and neurology.

The significance of failure to detect the posterior tibial and dorsalis pedis pulses on the foot has to be interpreted in terms of skin color and temperature of the involved extremity. A functional deficit with exercise should be expected. Arterial circulation may be functioning at a critical level, short of complete failure.

The presence of varicose veins does not necessarily mean that disability is present. Pain and swelling of the lower extremities may occur on long standing or on effort. The presence of dark pigmentation of the skin with atrophy and/or ulceration indicates an advanced state of decompensation of the venous circulation in the extremity. Chronic swelling, aggravated by walking with external bandaging, is indicative of chronic insufficiency of the deep veins.

The presence of interdigital fungus or secondary infection may be an indication of an abnormal amount of perspiration from the feet. The various fungi that may cause such a condition are ubiquitous, and their invasion of the skin is a reflection not of contagion but of temporarily lowered skin resistance, due primarily to excess moisture, warmth, and minor traumata.

The Nervous System (41.0). Abnormalities may result from congenital defects, damage due to metabolic disorders such as phenylketonuria and kernicterus, late effects of infectious disease such as poliomyelitis, trauma, surgical procedures, or to as yet unknown causes manifested by such syndromes as idiopathic epilepsy. Some of these conditions are incompatible with a state of good physical fitness, but others may not be, depending on the extent and localization of the involvement. The parapalegic who has lost normal function in the lower part of his body due to a meningomyelocele may be a skilled athlete, performing in wheelchair sports.

Assessing the significance of any neurologic disorder depends, therefore, not on making a diagnosis but in an exact as possible description of the functional limitation imposed by that disorder on the subject. The deficit may be physical, psychological, or both. Although mental testing is not included as part of this examination, the ability of the subject to respond directly and clearly to the history portion (assuming that no language problem is involved) may be taken as one piece of evidence of his mental capacity and orientation. Disorders of personality are much more difficult to identify and evaluate. They may easily be missed on a single examination by an examiner who has received no history of such a disorder and who has never had any contact with the subject previously.

The Reproductive System (43.0). Examination of the external genitalia may give some information of value regarding testicular function in the male subject. The presence of two testicles of good size and consistency in the scrotum offers a reasonable assurance of the "maleness" of the subject in question. In some cases, however, infertility may be present. The absence of one or both testicles from the scrotum is not, however, evidence of a lack of "maleness," because one or both may be found in the inguinal canal or even inside the abdomen. If they remain very long beyond the age of puberty in this position, they become nonfunctional. The loss of both testes as the result of trauma or surgical removal, if it occurs after full growth has been achieved, does not create a state of "femaleness" but rather the special condition of the castrated male, who manifests a generally male habitus but exhibits certain female traits.

External examination of the female genitalia offers little assurance of the "femaleness" of the subject, unless it is supplemented by other information indicating ovarian function. In determining the "femaleness" of any subject, the phenotype, genotype, and mental orientation must be considered in addition to the presence or absence of female sex organs (Editorial, 1967).

The evaluation of subjects demonstrating true or pseudohermaphroditic states is an extremely complex matter. In classification, it is better that such subjects should not be forced into either male or female categories but should be considered in a separate category of intersexual individuals. The implications of such conditions for physical fitness depend on the nature of the genetic disorder because certain disorders, such as Turner's syndrome, are associated with physical defects or characteristics which would produce impairments to overall fitness.

Laboratory Data (44.0–52.0)

A variety of methods are available for the performance of the procedures which are recommended in Part VII of the Standards. Variations in mean and range values occur among different procedures. For this reason, the method used should be stated where possible next to the value recorded. Some procedures are more sensitive than others. Time and expense may be critical factors in the selection of certain procedures. No one procedure is therefore recommended above others.

Urinalysis (44.0). The evaluation of proteinuria depends on the amount of protein in the specimen, the character of the protein, and the circumstances under which the specimen was obtained. The presence of a small amount of protein in the urine, up to 30 milligram percent (mg%), may have no significance or may be a sign of beginning or moderate kidney damage. Clarification of the significance of proteinuria depends on its presence in repeated specimens, tests of kidney function, and perhaps direct examination of the kidneys by cystoscopy, pyelography, or biopsy. The consistent presence of moderate to large amounts of protein in the urine (100–300 mg%) ordinarily indicates severe kidney damage. The nature and severity of the damage depend on supplementary examinations. One procedure that is suggested on the examination form, Section 2C of Part VII, is microscopic examination of the urine. The presence of red blood cells, casts, and especially casts containing red blood cells in the centrifuged specimen is strongly suggestive of kidney damage.

The protein ordinarily found in the urine is albumin. A protein precipitate following the addition of sulfosalicylic acid, which then disappears on heating but coagulates on boiling, is of low molecular weight (about 40,000) and is known as Bence-Jones protein. It may be indicative of certain systemic disorders such as multiple myeloma.

Protein may appear in the urine of some individuals who have a low threshold for its excretion on prolonged standing or walking. This condition is known as orthostatic albuminuria; it does not have any functional significance ordinarily. The appearance of albumin, casts, and red cells in the urine has been noted following vigorous activity, especially competition, in athletes (Alyea and Parish, 1958). The significance for the particular subject depends on additional studies to clarify the anatomical status and function of the genitourinary tract. A significantly high occurrence of abnormalities has been found in boxers who manifested postbout hematuria (Kleiman, 1960). Mental stress without physical exertion is apparently also capable of producing temporary albuminuria in some individuals who have apparently normal kidneys. Both myoglobin and hemoglobin may be found in the urine following very severe physical stress (Howenstine, 1968).

The appearance of small quantities of reducing substances in the urine in a casual specimen may be of no significance at all. Clarification of the meaning depends on obtaining repeated specimens, both fasting and postprandial, and determining blood sugar levels under both conditions. A glucose tolerance test may then be indicated. Although glucose is the substance most commonly found, fructose, and galactose may be responsible for producing a positive reaction of a reducing substance in the urine. Differentiation depends on specific tests to identify these other sugars. The presence of galactose indicates a genetic metabolic disorder.

Vital Capacity and Forced Expiratory Volume (45.0 and 46.0). Although a person who has a small vital capacity may be significantly lacking in physical fitness, it is not necessary to have a much larger than average capacity to demonstrate very good levels of physical fitness. A reduced forced expiratory volume is almost invariably associated with significant bronchopulmonary disorders, such as chronic bronchitis and emphysema. This would almost certainly signify a reduction in the level of physical fitness of the subject below his expected norm. Cigarette smokers will have a reduced respiratory flow rate, the degree of reduction depending on the amount smoked and the time they have been smokers.

Blood Values (47.0). The normal range of hemoglobin as determined by the modern electric colorimeter is 12.0–17.0 g for males and 11.0–15.0 g for females. By the Sahli method, values are somewhat less, and the percent of possible error is greater. Increases in the amount of hemoglobin may result from acclimation to decreased barometric pressure, as in persons living or competing at moderate to high altitudes (Buskirk et al., 1967), or as the result of diseases such as polycythemia and Ayerza's disease. In the case of the former, physical fitness and performance are affected only to the extent that athletes will not reach sea-level efforts in endurance events. In the latter, serious functional deficits result from the other pathologic changes characteristic of these two disease states.

Decrease in hemoglobin values may result from genetic defects (hereditary spherocytosis), blood loss (hemorrhage, menorrhagia), nutritional deficiency states (iron, protein), infectious disease (streptococcus infections), liver and splenic disease (Banti's syndrome), and toxic reactions (lead poisoning). Generally speaking, anemia is associated with reduced functional capacity, with the amounts of decrease depending on severity. Other factors associated with the specific condition responsible for the anemia may decrease this capacity even further. To predict the extent to which functional capacity may be reduced, identification of the disorder and estimation of its severity is necessary.

A false impression of the total amount of hemoglobin available in the blood may be obtained from the analysis of a single blood sample if the subject is dehydrated. Assessment of the hematocrit (normal 40–54% in males and 37–40% in females), blood volume, and color index may be necessary to complete the evaluation. Sickling of the red cells is characteristic of a variable percentage of persons of African Negro descent. Of those with this trait, a certain number will undergo periodic crises during which large numbers of their red cells are lysed, bringing about a temporary but often chronic lowering of blood hemoglobin.

The significance of slight to moderate elevations of total serum cholesterol is debatable (Wright and Frederickson, 1970), as far as the effects on accelerating the production of atherosclerosis in humans is concerned or as evidence of the status or progress of arteriosclerosis in any one individual. The ranges

Table 9-1 Ranges of Serum Cholesterol

Age, years	Mean, mg%	90% Range, mg%
1–30	180	110–250
30–39	200	150–280
40–49	245	160–325
50–59	250	140–340

shown in Table 9-1 may be accepted as normal for the age groups indicated. Total plasma lipids of all ages fall in the range of 400–1000 mg% (Frankel et al., 1970). Marked fluctuations in these levels may occur from day-to-day and even during the same day in individual subjects, depending on diet and physical activity. A condition of familial hypercholesterolemia is recognized and is usually associated with deposits of cholesterol aggregates in the skin.

Normal values for the erythrocyte sedimentation rate depend on the method used. The values in Table 9-2 may be considered normal for the two methods most commonly employed (Frankel et al., 1970). The presence of anemia causes an acceleration of the rate when the Wintrobe method is employed but not with the Westergren technique.

Table 9-2 Erythrocyte Sedimentation Rates

Method	Mean, mm/hr	Range, mm/hr
WINTROBE		
Male adults	4	0–7
Female adults	10	0–15
Children	5–10	1–15
WESTERGREN		
Male adults		3–5
Female adults		4–7

A tendency to sickling in the blood will decrease the rate of erythrocyte sedimentation as will also polycythemia. More rapid than normal rates are nonspecific indicators of the presence of infectious disease. Very rapid rates do not necessarily indicate a more severe disorder than when the rate is moderately increased. The change of the rate under observation and treatment is used in conditions such as rheumatic fever to chart the progress of the disease.

Of the many possible other determinations which might be carried out on blood samples, perhaps the most useful would be those for glucose (in subjects showing repeated presence of reducing substances in the urine) and for urea nitrogen (in subjects demonstrating persistent proteinuria in significant amounts). Levels of serum calcium, phosphorus, and alkaline phosphatase might be expected to show significant changes in subjects with certain skeletal disorders and malfunctions of the parathyroid gland.

The Electrocardiogram (48.0). The significance of changes from normal patterns for rest and exercise in the electrocardiogram is a complex matter, requiring not only knowledge of the variable conductance of electrical impulses across the myocardium but also considerable experience and exercise of sound judgment in interpretation. The reader is referred to works dealing with cardiology and electrocardiography for advice in these matters. The method by which the tracing is made should be known to assist in interpretation.

Optional Skeletal Age. The assessment of measurements of skeletal age is dealt with extensively in Part VII, Section 4C, Article 83. The significance of these assessments is that in young persons, when taken in conjunction with observation of the development of the secondary sex characteristics, a more accurate picture of their stages of development can often be obtained than from the chronological age.

Heart Volume. This determination is dealt with in detail in Part VII. Increases in heart size occur as the result of regular vigorous exercise or of heart or circulatory disease. The determination of the responsible causes depends on the interpretation of other data such as the electrocardiogram and the evaluation of the clinical status of the subject. Increase in heart size associated with physical activity is due to an increase in the thickness of the heart muscle and dilatation of the heart chambers. Although the volume of the heart decreases when regular exercise stops, it does not return to the baseline because that portion of the enlargement due to the increase in myocardial thickness tends to persist for some time.

Blood Groups. The distribution of subjects among the standard blood groups or according to other classifications such as the presence or absence of the Rh factor has no known significance at the present time in relationship to physical fitness. Some attempts have been made to relate blood groups to the occurrence of certain disease states, but the existence of such associations appear only from a statistical standpoint at the present and may prove illusory.

Conclusion

When the examining physician makes the decision at the conclusion of the examination of the subject whether he may or may not participate in stress testing and to what degree, he must take into account the personal and activity history as well as the physical examination and the laboratory tests. Drugs such as reserpine, propanolol, guanethidine, quinidine, nitroglycerine and other vasodilators, procaine amide, digitalis, catecholamines, ganglionic blocking agents, insulin and psychotropic drugs are in current use. Because of the possible unfavorable effects that may be induced by exercise when they are present, especially on the cardiovascular system, and because the specific conditions for which they are being taken must be considered, careful judgment must be made and specific precautions taken if subjects using them are to be tested.

Further and more extensive evaluation than that provided for in the sections on physical and laboratory examinations in Part VII of the Standards may be indicated in subjects who appear to be suffering from any of the following conditions:

1. Any acute or chronic infectious disease or a recent generalized infection.
2. Diabetes which is not well controlled.
3. Marked obesity.
4. Severe neurosis or psychosis.
5. Central nervous system disease.
6. Musculoskeletal disease involving the spine and the lower extremities.
7. Active liver disease.
8. Renal disease with nitrogen retention.
9. Severe anemia.
10. Significant hypertension.
11. Signs and symptoms of coronary artery insufficiency.
12. Significant cardiomegaly.
13. Arrhythmias of the three following types: second-degree atrioventricular blocks, ventricular tachycardia, and atrial fibrillation.
14. Significant disease of the heart valves.
15. Congenital heart disease without cyanosis.
16. Thrombophlebitis.
17. A strongly apprehensive or extremely negative view regarding exercise and its possible detrimental effects.

Extreme caution should be employed in testing subjects who manifest any of the following conditions:

1. Active or recent myocarditis.
2. Recent pulmonary embolism.
3. Congestive heart failure.
4. Third-degree atrioventricular block.
5. Presence of fixed-rate pacemaker.
6. Aortic aneurysm.
7. Ventricular aneurysm.
8. Liver decompensation.
9. Congenital heart disease with cyanosis.

It is inadvisable that such persons be subjected to stress testing at all except for reasons directly connected with their treatment, including rehabilitation.

All previously sedentary individuals should be started very slowly and progressed very gradually until their clinical response to testing can be evaluated. In the case of doubt regarding the ability of a subject to continue the test, it should be stopped immediately and restorative procedures instituted.

BIBLIOGRAPHY

Alyea, E. P., and H. H. Parish, Jr.: Renal response to exercise—primary findings. *J. Amer. Med. Assoc.*, **167**:807–813 (June 4, 1958).

Burch, T. K., J. J. Macisco, Jr., and M. P. Parker: Some methodological problems in the analysis of human menstrual data. *Int. J. Fertil.*, **12**:67–76, (Jan.–March, Pt. 2, 1967).

Buskirk, E. R., J. Kollias, E. Picon-Reatigue, R. Akers, E. Prokop, and P. Baker: Physiology and performance of track athletes at various altitudes in the United States and Peru. The International Symposium on the Effects of Altitude on Physical Performance. Chicago, The Athletic Institute, pp. 65–71, 1967.

Dubois, F. S.: Rhythms, cycles and periods in health and disease. *Amer. J. Psychiat.*, **116**:114 (Aug., 1959).

Editorial: Sex of athletes. *Brit. Med. J.*, **1**:5532, 185–186 (Jan. 28, 1967).

Engle, E. T., and M. C. Shelesnyak: First menstruation and subsequent menstrual cycles of pubertal girls. *Hum. Biol.*, **6**:431–453 (Sept., 1934).

Frankel, S., S. Reitman, and A. C. Sonnenwirth (eds.): *Gradwohl's Clinical Laboratory Methods and Diagnosis*, 7th ed. St. Louis, C. V. Mosby, 1970.

Howenstine, J. A.: Exertion-induced myoglobinuria and hemoglobinuria. *J. Amer. Med. Assoc.*, **173**:443–499 (June 4, 1960).

Kleiman, A. H.: Athlete's kidney, *J. Urol.*, **83**:321–329 (Apr., 1960).

Wright, I. S., and D. T. Frederickson (eds.): Primary prevention of the atherosclerotic diseases. Report of the Inter-Society Commission for Heart Disease Resources, *Circulation*, **42**:55–95 (Dec., 1970).

GENERAL REFERENCES

Physical Diagnosis

Adams, F. D.: *Physical Diagnosis*, 14th ed. Baltimore, The Williams & Wilkins Co., 1958.

Leopold, S. S.: *The Principles and Methods of Physical Diagnosis*, 2nd ed. Philadelphia, W. B. Saunders, 1957.

Major, R. H., and H. H. Delp: *Physical Diagnosis*, 6th ed. Philadelphia, W. B. Saunders, 1962.

Zatuchni, J.: *Notes on Physical Diagnosis*. Philadelphia, F. A. Davis Co., 1964.

Cardiology and Electrocardiography

Friedberg, C. K.: *Diseases of the Heart*, 2nd ed. Philadelphia, W. B. Saunders Co., 1956.

Hurst, J. W., and R. B. Logues: *The Heart, Arteries and Veins*. New York, McGraw-Hill Book Co., Blakiston Division, 1966.

Lamb, L. E.: *Electrocardiography and Vectorcardiography*. Philadelphia, W. B. Saunders Co., 1965.

Luisada, A. A. (ed.): *Examination of the Cardiac Patient*. New York, McGraw-Hill Book Co., Blakiston Division, 1965.

Laboratory Methods and Findings

Bauer, J. B., P. G. Ackerman, and G. Toro (eds.): *Bray's Clinical Laboratory Methods*, 7th ed. St. Louis, C. V. Mosby Co., 1968.

Frankel, S., S. Reitman, and A. C. Sonnenwirth (eds.): *Gradwohl's Clinical Laboratory Methods and Diagnosis*, 7th ed. St. Louis, C. V. Mosby Co., 1970.

Lynch, M. J., S. S. Raphael, L. D. Menor, P. D. Spone, and M. J. H. Inwood: *Medical Laboratory Technology and Clinical Pathology*. 2nd ed. Philadelphia, W. B. Saunders Co., 1969.

Ravel, R., *Clinical Laboratory Medicine*. Chicago, Year Book Medicine Publishing Inc., 1969.

The Validity of Stressful Activities

10

OUAY KETUSINH
Sports Science Center
Bangkok, Thailand

As a preliminary to any test for physical fitness involving vigorous exertion, a comprehensive program of medical examination is not only advisable but often indispensable. This is especially true for persons in middle age and older groups, that is, those over 40 years old, in whom some latent, symptomless defect may exist that would preclude severe exertion. A sudden physical load might precipitate a failure of the diseased tissue or organ, which could lead to debility, illness, or even death. Younger individuals are not exempt from such dangers either. Children especially must be treated with caution. For one reason, their organism is still immature and may be unable to cope with the extra load imposed by the tests; for another reason, they may be harboring some disease which has not yet been uncovered.

The following are examples of pathological conditions and diseases that may contraindicate tests involving stressful physical activities: in an elderly person, hypertension (high blood pressure), arteriosclerosis (hardening of arterial walls), degenerative heart disease, and emphysema; in a younger individual, congenital heart disease, rheumatic heart disease, nephritis (inflammation of the kidney), and hepatitis (inflammation of the liver). Discovery of these affections in time will avoid damage to the health of the subjects and avert serious or even fatal accidents.

In other cases, revelations made by the medical examination may not be sufficiently serious to contraindicate physical tests, but they may serve to call for caution in the testing and in some cases to explain why the results obtained from some procedures are substandard.

The Medical History

Before starting the actual examination the physician usually takes down the medical history of the testee. It is imperative that questions should be answered seriously and truthfully. A false statement may not only puzzle the examiner but may actually lead to wrong interpretations and dangerous misjudgment. Some information may serve to warn of possible dangers ahead or may point to the origin of certain defects that will be uncovered in the later phases.

Some habitual indulgences are of special interest to the physician. For example, a prolonged history of heavy smoking (more than 10 cigarettes a day) or drinking (more than 4 oz. of whisky, liquor, or gin daily) will indicate the need for a special search for vascular disorders (affections of the blood vessels), particularly in the limbs and the heart. The toxic substances associated with drinking and smoking tend to cause the walls of the blood vessels to degenerate and ultimately lead to blocking of the blood flow. One not uncommon result is seen as "intermittent claudication," in which the patient develops severe pain in the legs on walking even for a short distance; the pain disappears after rest but reappears on resumption of walking. When blood vessels of the heart (the coronary blood vessels) are affected, the incapacitation is severe and may be fatal.

Even the consumption of coffee and tea, harmless in moderation, may be significant when excessive. Caffeine, the primary active ingredient of coffee and tea, is a fairly potent alkaloid and strongly affects the central nervous system. Results of excessive use are usually seen as sleeplessness, nervousness, and temperamental instability. In some sensitive individuals an irritable, "nervous heart" may manifest itself as palpitation (consciousness of the heart's pumping) and a sense of fatigue even on slight exertion. All these symptoms may adversely affect the outcome of any test of physical ability. Another effect of the two beverages, particularly frequent in the case of sensitive persons, is constipation. This may affect the tests indirectly by causing gas in the abdomen and general debility accompanied by vague aches and pains in the joints and muscles.

Past illnesses may be of importance because some of them may render the individual prone to the development of specific diseases later. Thus, an attack of pleuritis (inflammation of the covering membrane of the lungs) may be followed by tuberculosis, and tonsillitis (inflammation of the tonsils) by rheumatic valvulitis (inflammation of the heart valves) or rheumatic arthritis (inflammation of the joints). A person who has suffered severe hepatitis (inflammation of the liver) is likely to develop portal cirrhosis (hardening of the liver) sooner or later, and one who has had a head injury at birth may develop epileptic seizures in later life.

Other illnesses may result in irreversible injury to the tissues or organs concerned. Thus, chronic bronchial asthma often leads to emphysema (dilation of the wind pipes), resulting in impaired oxygenation of the blood and poor physical capacity for the patient; cardiac failure may be the ultimate result, due to an impediment of the blood flow through the lungs. Some forms of arthritis cause injury to the tissues of the joint so as to limit its movement or even cause fixation, so that movement is no longer possible.

Certain diseases demand a marked limitation or even postponement of physical exercise to facilitate the proper recovery of the patient's health or even his survival. These include most forms of heart disease in the so-called acute (severe and dangerous) stages in which exertion may bring about a serious aggravation of the disease or even sudden death. Acute affections of the liver and the kidney also demand particular caution in connection with physical exercise because an overload may easily lead to failure of the organs.

Some chronic diseases may not contraindicate a fitness test but nonetheless demand caution in its use. Diabetes mellitus is a common example. Actually physical exercise is widely recommended as an important element in the therapeutic treatment of diabetes, helping the body to burn up excess sugar. But the exercise must be carefully controlled so that it does not endanger the delicate balance of sugar metabolism. A specialist should decide upon any exercise program. The same is true for a person suffering from chronic nephritis. Although exercise may be of help by accelerating blood circulation and stimulating perspiration, an excess may further injure the impaired kidney and hasten renal failure.

Diseases affecting the formation of blood or the digestion and absorption of food may result in a prolonged state of debility which will affect the scores on the physical activity tests. Malaria, helminthic infection (intestinal worms), and chronic gastroenteritis (inflammation of the stomach and intestine) are problems often encountered in many parts of the world. Major surgical operations such as gastrectomy (excision of the stomach), pulmonectomy (excision of the lung), and nephrectomy (excision of the kidney) may also cause prolonged debility. The loss of important organs or parts of organs also demands caution in subjecting a person to the physical activity tests even if he or she does appear healthy. Certain injuries, such as those due to accidents, may leave scars or deformities that hinder mobility and thereby impede the execution of certain aspects of some of the tests.

In the case of a female the menstrual history is particularly important. It informs the physician of the onset of the menstruation, its regularity or irregularity, and other features; on the basis of this information, the condition of general as well as sexual health may be inferred. Thus, the unusually large amount of blood lost in a case of hypermenorrhea may result in secondary anemia, which will cause poor performance on the tests, whereas dysmenorrhea may lower a woman's vitality through recurrent bouts of pain and nervous tension. A woman in menopause is apt to suffer from psychic as well as physical strains due to the changes in the hormonal system, and repeated pregnancies and deliveries may cause a laxity of the muscular walls in such a way as to preclude severe strains and set definite limits to exertion. All these conditions may not only affect test scores adversely but may also render conducting the tests in some way or other undesirable or impracticable.

The family history is always interesting and important in the eyes of the physician. Many diseases are hereditary and in younger persons may still exist in a stage that is undetectable by routine examination. A "positive" family history may occasion and direct a more thorough search and lead to discovery of the ailment in time to arrest or cure it. Of special importance are some hereditary heart defects and blood diseases. A history of cardiovascular accidents in the family should arouse wariness in the tester; although these afflictions are not hereditary in the strict sense of the word, the tendency appears to be prevalent among members of the same family.

Physical Examination

Height and weight should always be taken as a routine. Together these two serve as the simplest index of fitness, of nutritional status, and of general health. The overweight person is more often unfit than fit. The substatured and underweight are obviously malnourished now or have been at some previous stage. A change in body weight toward the "normal" or "standard" is an improvement, whereas a change in the opposite direction is a deterioration. This is particularly true in the case of children and youths.

The so-called secondary sex characteristics, such as the development of the breasts and the external genitalia and the distribution of hair and of subcutaneous fat, serve as prime indicators of the functional condition of the endocrine system concerned with sexual functions, for example, the sex glands, the pituitary body, and the adrenal glands. Over- or underactivity of these glands will cause abnormalities that will enable the physician to recognize the underlying trouble. The physical ability of the individual may be profoundly affected, positively or negatively, according to which gland is affected.

Skeletal defects, such as scoliosis (forward curvature of the spine) and lordosis (lateral curvature of the spine) are common in children. They are usually due either to faulty postural habits or—now less frequently—to rickets, both of which are amenable to treatment if instituted in time. In adults, especially in the aged, recent changes in skeletal form may be indicative of some serious bone disease. In any case, the efficiency of the person is likely to be more or less affected.

The eyes and ears need to be attended to, as they play specific roles in motion and locomotion. Defective eyesight or the loss of an eye lowers visual acuity or narrows the visual field, respectively, whereas an inflammation of the middle ear may affect the sense of direction and of equilibrium. In either case, the agility of the person may be markedly lowered. The hygienic condition of the mouth cavity is very revealing. It not only gives an idea about the health habits of the individual but also has some remote significance. For example, a "furred tongue" often points to poor digestion, and stomatitis (inflammation of the oral mucous membrane) is one common result of constipation. Decayed teeth and inflamed gums not only indicate improper care but also indicate the possibility of valvular heart disease so common in children and young adults. A similar ominous warning is given by an inflamed tonsil, especially when the inflammation is of the chronic purulent type with repeated exacerbations. In such a case of chronic tonsillitis, the lymph nodes (lymph glands) on the corresponding side of the neck or angle of the jaw may be enlarged and palpable. Such glandular enlargement in any part of the body is a sign of chronic infection in the vicinity or may be a danger signal for some sort of malignancy. To be absolutely sure, a biopsy must be taken.

The thyroid, the gland in the front part of the neck on both sides of the larynx (voice box), is often visibly enlarged. A slight enlargement, especially in teenage individuals and when free of accompanying symptoms, may be of little or no significance, belonging to the class of "adolescent goiter" which usually recedes by itself. On the other hand an enlargement, even though slight, that is accompanied by symptoms such as nervous irritability, wasting, or exophthalmos (protuberance of the eyeballs) may indicate the presence of hyperthyroidism (excessive activity of the thyroid) or toxic goiter; these conditions need active treatment and severe physical strain is contraindicated. The diametrically opposite condition is hypothyroidism (deficient activity of the thyroid) in which the person may present a picture of inactivity or inertia with little inclination to participate in any kind of physical activity. In this instance, testing is not contraindicated, but poor results are to be expected. In either case, a thorough laboratory examination will be needed to substantiate the diagnosis.

The general form of the chest is very instructive. The normal is that of an ovoid, flattened on the front and the back. In a "flat chest," the flattening is exaggerated. From the front the thorax looks unusually broad, but from the sides it appears thin and compressed. A "barrel chest" is almost round and is common in cases of chronic asthma. A "keeled chest" appears very much like that of a chicken or a dove, where the sternum (breast bone) protrudes markedly. A "funnel chest" presents the opposite picture, with the sternum sunken below the level of the ribs. These common abnormalities may be combined with deformities of the spine or may simply be due to some bad postural habits; some forms, however, may result from respiratory diseases in childhood. If the abnormality is severe, it may adversely affect test performance.

Inspection of the chest by percussion (tapping with the fingers), sometimes in combination with palpation, may permit the detection of deep-seated abnormalities inside. Thus, a dull note may indicate a consolidation resulting from tuberculous infection or a lung tumor. A hollow note may denote cavity formation or a pneumothorax (leakage of air into the thoracic cavity), whereas a flat note usually points to pleural effusion (fluid collection inside the chest).

A more delicate method of examination is auscultation, that is, listening with the stethoscope. It is especially useful in the case of the lungs and the heart. Some diseases produce definite changes in, or "additions" to, the normal sounds. For example, over the lungs may be heard the "friction rub" which is caused by pleuritis or fibrosis of the lungs. "Ronchi" are heard in asthma, "crepitation" in inflammation or edema of the lungs, and "tubular breathing" in a case of consolidation.

The heart, the most important organ concerned with exercise, needs a thorough examination, not only by auscultation but also by other methods. Thus, inspection may detect a displacement of the apex beat (tip of the heart) or an abnormal heaving of the chest wall, both of which may be the result of an enlargement of the heart. Thrills, a sense of vibration conveyed to a palpating hand, may indicate a flabby, dilated heart and may be sufficient ground for postponing testing. Auscultation may detect earlier and finer abnormalities, such as minor diseases of the heart valves and even congenital defects which may be symptomless. These are recognized by the presence of murmurs and other changes in the heart sounds. Considerable experience is required to form a correct diagnosis because some changes may be just functional, that is, caused by some temporary alteration in the working of the organ, such as accentuation in a case of mental excitement, whereas the same feature may also be encountered in a case of illness such as hyperthyroidism or some other toxicity.

The pulse is the most useful indicator of the heart's condition and level of function. It is easily studied, for example, by "feeling," and yet with practice will yield very useful information. Every worker in the field of exercise and sports should learn to feel the pulse properly. The recommended technique is to place the first three fingers of the palpating hand on the radial artery just above the wrist on the thumb side. The middle finger serves as the "feeler." By reference to a stopwatch or a watch with a second hand, the rate or frequency of the pulse may be counted. Simultaneously, the regularity or irregularity may be noted. From the pressure with which the blood strikes against the fingers the force of the pulse may be relatively estimated as strong or weak, and from the extent of the expansion of the artery at each beat, the volume as big or small. By pressing down upon the blood vessel with the finger nearest the heart until the pulse, as felt by the middle finger, is obliterated, the tension inside the vessel may be roughly gauged, as normal, high, or low. By lightly rolling the blood vessel under the fingers, the condition of the arterial wall, either normally soft and elastic or abnormally solid and fixed, may be assessed.

Each quality of the pulse has its meaning, although interpretation is not as easy as reading a book. Thus, the average pulse rate of normal individuals is usually given as 70 beats/min. A rapid pulse, for example, 90 beats/min, may accompany excitement, fear, elation, fever, hyperthyroidism, heart disease, and so on. A slow pulse may indicate a failing heart, as in a case of myocardial degeneration, or a forceful heart, as often is seen in a well-trained athlete. An experienced doctor can differentiate between the two because of the small volume of the pulse in the former case and the big volume in the latter. On the other hand, a strong, big pulse does not always mean good health; it may be a sign of a disease such as hypertension.

For one without much clinical experience it is safer to look with caution upon a case of either too high pulse rate (above 90 beats/min while at rest) or too low (below 50 beats/min), especially when accompanied with irregularity in rhythm or force. A thorough medical examination should be made before taking tests of physical fitness. On the other hand, it has been repeatedly observed that some cardiac irregularities, such as premature beats and drop beats, may be physiological in origin and may disappear on taking exercise regularly.

The measurement of arterial blood pressure is an important procedure and is usually performed on the arm with the subject in a resting, recumbent state. Physical activity performed within 10 or 15 min of the measurement may cause abnormally high readings. Average normal values for young male adults are about 120 mm Hg systolic (that is, during the contraction of the heart) and 70 mm Hg diastolic (that is, during the relaxation of the heart); it is usually written 120/70 mm Hg. The pressures rise with age, so that at 60 years they may have become 150/80 mm Hg. The limits are 10 to 15 mm Hg lower for females.

The blood pressure reflects the functional condition not only of the heart but also of several other organs, namely, the blood vessels, the kidneys, the endocrine glands, the psyche, even the quality and quantity of the blood. Thus, within limits, a normal pressure indicates a generally healthy condition. A very low blood pressure may mean some abnormality in the heart or general weakness, whereas a high blood pressure may be the symptom of a diseased condition in some of the endocrine organs, the kidneys, or the nervous system. Abnormal values, either on the low or on the high side, always warrant a thorough investigation before demanding tests are conducted.

The abdomen is always interesting and important, and its general appearance may indicate significant information. A well-rounded, muscular abdominal wall is part of a generally "fit" physique, whereas an opulent, pendulous abdomen is an evident sign of poor physical condition. In any case, palpation may give additional information of consequence, such as the presence of a tumor. However, not all palpable masses are due to disease; some may be fairly harmless. For example, chronic constipation may give rise to hardened fecal masses, known medically as scybala, which are easily eliminated with a purgative.

Hernia (rupture) may or may not in itself be incapacitating; however, when present it should always be cause for caution because exercise, even if only moderately severe, may aggravate the condition and precipitate some dangerous complication such as irreducibility or incarceration (retention). A doctor should always be consulted as to the feasibility of physical tests.

The extremities—arms and legs—deserve attention not only from the standpoint of motion but also of balance. Movability of some parts may be reduced by a chronic inflammation in or around the joints concerned. Severe infection or injury such as that resulting from accidents may cause deformities that hinder free movement. Angulation of the elbow is a common example; it may be unnoticed under ordinary circumstances but, when finer adjustments are required, it may be troublesome because of the variety of movements involved at the joint. The same is true of the hip joint where a slight abnormality may escape casual observation. Although the arms are more prone to acquire abnormalities arising from accidents, the legs suffer more often from developmental defects. Whatever the etiology, abnormalities of the extremities must be looked for and recorded because they may provide an explanation for some irregularity in the results of certain tests. In fact, some procedures may be impossible in the presence of certain defects, for example, chin-ups in a case of fixation of the elbow, or the broad jump in a case of clubfoot. In older people an anatomical defect involving the bony structure, be it at the extremities or any part of the skeleton, demands special attention and thorough investigation. It may be the result of a dangerous condition common in the aged, known as osteoporosis, in which the bones are rarified and relatively brittle. The jolt accompanying a jump may be sufficient to cause multiple fractures in such a case.

Laboratory Examinations

In a medical examination, laboratory tests are desirable in many, and necessary in some, cases to eliminate doubt and confirm some ambiguous point. In most instances simple procedures such as qualitative tests on the urine may suffice, although more sophisticated examinations are sometimes necessary, especially in the very young and the very old.

Proteinuria or albuminuria, the presence of protein in the urine, must always be treated with concern and should dictate the need for further investigation regarding the function of the kidneys. Microscopic examination of the urine and chemical analysis of the blood are usually necessary to exclude serious diseases of the kidneys such as subacute nephritis, which may contraindicate physical exertion, or chronic nephritis, in which exercise could be undertaken with precaution. The finding of protein in the urine in itself may be of little or no significance because it may be functional, such as that due to strong excitement (emotional proteinuria), or accidental, such as that due to admixture of menstrual blood. In many otherwise normal individuals proteinuria may be detected after heavy exertion, such as a game of basketball or football. The condition is known as exercise proteinuria.

Glycosuria, the presence of sugar in the urine, may be transient or persistent. In the former case it is usually without significance, and may be brought about by some temporary, physiological cause, for example, ingestion of a large amount of sugar (ingestive or alimentary glycosuria). If persistent, the glycosuric condition is likely to be due to diabetes mellitus. Although this disease is not a contraindication to exercise in itself, in certain stages severe physical stress is not advisable. In case of doubt, a specialist should be consulted.

Measurement of the vital capacity is an easy and useful procedure. Although it is by no means an estimate of the capacity of the lungs as the name suggests, it shows one aspect of breathing ability. Because vital capacity is influenced by many interacting factors, it is more useful as an indicator of changes in the same person, for example, as the result of training or of a disease process, than as an indication of superiority or inferiority in the comparison of individuals. A considerable increase in vital capacity is a reliable sign of progress in ventilatory ability or respiratory function. A high value, for example, over 5 liters, provides evidence of being well trained, whereas a low value usually accompanies poor health or feeble physique. Very low results, for example, below 3 liters, may be due to a pathological process, such as obstruction, fibrosis, or other changes in the bronchi, the lungs, the pleura, or the chest cavity. In a suspicious case the forced expiratory volume should be determined, since it is a better indicator of bronchial obstruction. If this condition is indicated or suggested, the advice of a specialist should be sought because it may be the symptom of some serious affection, for example, bronchial carcinoma (cancer of the wind pipes).

In the examination of the blood the estimation of hemoglobin content is the simplest and the most frequently performed analysis. It is an indicator of the all around "fitness" or "health" of the individual from the standpoint of nutrition. Hemoglobin concentration in healthy subjects lies between 13 and 16 gram percent (g%). Values below 12 g% denote anemia, which may be a result of improper diet, for example, a diet low in meat or iron content, or of some serious disease such as malaria or pernicious anemia. Whatever the cause, the anemic condition will result in a poor score in physical tests, especially as far as stamina is concerned. A hemoglobin concentration below 10 g% should be regarded as a serious condition and a hematologist should be consulted.

Since the discovery of the significance of blood lipids in connection with degenerative changes in the cardiovascular system and the rise in the incidence of heart diseases, estimation of the blood cholesterol has assumed particular importance. Blood cholesterol should be determined as a routine in obese subjects and in persons more than 40 years old because these people are

especially endangered. A result higher than 300 mg% of total blood cholesterol may be evidence of some dangerous condition, for example, an atheroma-
tous affection of the blood vessels or coronary heart disease. It should be
looked upon as a danger sign, and a physical test should not be taken without the consent of a physician.

High blood cholesterol may also indicate the need for an electrocardio-
graphic examination of the heart, which usually requires the services of a
cardiologist. With modern, highly efficient instrumentation, recording an
electrocardiogram (ECG or EKG) may be relatively easy; however, the interpretation of the records is always difficult. In principle, a number of "waves"
on the ECG is studied, and from them the functional condition of various
parts of the heart is deciphered. Thus the P wave shows the activity of the
atria and the QRS complex that of the ventricles. From alterations in the
form, height, duration, rhythm, and sequence of the waves, the specialist
visualizes alterations in the work of the heart muscle. Some changes are functional and harmless; some are pathological and dangerous. The cardiologist
must decide whether an exercise test is safe and permissible.

Some other special laboratory tests are performed when particular
information is required. Thus roentgenography of certain bones will tell the
skeletal age of the subject; heart volume estimation, also by means of x-rays,
will give information on the size of the heart chambers and the covering
membranes; blood grouping will disclose the nature and composition of the
antibodies in the blood as well as give some information regarding the
hereditary history of the individual.

Few examinations give highly specific information in themselves. In
general, an accurate interpretation must be based upon a number of tests and
investigations. Of prime importance is the experience of the physician making
the decision.

REFERENCES

Best, C. H., and N. B. Taylor: *The Physiological Basis of Medical Practice*, 8th ed.
    Baltimore, Williams & Wilkins, 1966.

Campbell, E. J. M., C. J. Dickinson, and J. D. H. Slater (eds.): *Clinical Physiology*,
    3rd ed. Philadelphia, F. A. Davis, 1968.

Davson, H., and M. G. Eggleton (eds.): *Starling and Lovatt Evans Principles of
    Human Physiology*, 14th ed. Philadelphia, Lea & Febiger, 1968.

Guyton, A. C.: *Textbook of Medical Physiology*, 4th ed. Philadelphia, W. B.
    Saunders, 1971.

Kampmeier, R. H.: *Physical Examination in Health and Disease*, 3rd ed.
    Philadelphia, F. A. Davis, 1964.

Keele, C. A., and E. Neil (revs.): *Samson Wright's Applied Physiology*, 11th ed.
    London, Oxford University Press, 1965.

Physique and Body Composition

Part **III**

SECTION EDITOR:
J. WARTENWEILER
Zürich, Switzerland

Anthropologic Measurements and Performance

11

J. WARTENWEILER
A. HESS
B. WÜEST
Swiss Federal
Institute of Technology
Zürich, Switzerland

It is well known that a relationship exists between body form and physical fitness. Every sport has different requirements, especially with regard to force input, speed, and endurance. Consequently, the development of the various body systems—muscle, motor, cardiovascular, nervous, and so on—are differentially influenced by the various sports practiced. Changes in body constitution can take place, however, only within certain limits. For example, based on tests involving identical twins Verschuer (1954) concluded that weight, shoulder width, chest circumference, and upper arm circumference were affected by environmental influences, whereas length measurements of the bones were not subject to significant changes.

In order to meet the requirements for championship performance, the athlete should have certain body proportions. A jumper theoretically should have the longest possible legs; a gymnast profits from having short legs and a well-developed chest; a long distance runner is more or less thin; and the hammer thrower has more weight and a higher percentage of fat. In this sense, sport can be a selective factor and can influence appearance.

The method for determining growth phenomena and body form is known as anthropometrics. The use of anthropometrics permits one to ascertain the relationships between body form and performance. To show environmental factors the standards developed by the International Committee for the Standardization of Physical Fitness Tests (ICSPFT) recommend that all lateral measurements be taken on the right side. In genetic studies, however, preference is often given to the left side. These special cases are marked with (left) in this chapter.

Structure and Composition of the Human Body

The structure of the human body is mainly determined by its skeleton and musculature. The combination of bone tissue, musculature, and fat layers constitutes what is referred to as body composition. Taken together the structure and composition of the body determine the body type.

Structure of the Body

The space dimensions of the human body can be measured in terms of length, width, depth, circumferences, and skinfolds by means of anthropometrics (see Table 11-1). Body weight can also be evaluated three dimensionally.

Table 11-1 Basic Body Measurements (As Recommended by ICSPFT Standards)

I. BODY WEIGHT	IV. CIRCUMFERENCE
	Chest circumference at xiphoidal level
II. LENGTH	at the end of normal expiration
Total body length	(at maximal inspiration)
Sitting height	(at maximal expiration)
Trunk length	Upper arm circumference
Total upper extremity length	Thigh circumference
Upper arm length	
Total lower extremity length	V. SKINFOLDS
Thigh length	Skinfold over triceps
	Skinfold over biceps
III. WIDTH	Subscapular skinfold
Biacromial diameter	Suprailiac skinfold
Biiliocristal diameter	Skinfold thigh medial
Biepicondylar diameter humerus	Skinfold thigh lateral
Biepicondylar diameter femur	

Morphological Indices

A human body varies in its proportions, both with respect to absolute measurements as well as with respect to relative measurement or morphological indices. There are persons with relatively long legs and a short trunk, and there are persons with exactly the opposite proportions. There are slender types and sturdy types. If hip and shoulder width are being compared, then women in general are broad hipped, whereas men are broad shouldered. Relatively great circumferences of arms and legs indicate muscular or adipose types.

All body proportions are subject to change during adolescence. For example, children have, not only absolutely but also relative to their body length, shorter arms and legs than adults.

Table 11-2 Basic Morphological Indices

I. LENGTH
Total upper extremity length in percent of total body length
Total lower extremity length in percent of total body length
Upper arm length in percent of total body length
Thigh length in percent of total body length
Total upper extremity length in percent of total lower extremity length

II. WIDTH
Biacromial diameter in percent of total body length
Biiliocristal diameter in percent of total body length
Biiliocristal diameter in percent of biacromial diameter
Biepicondylar diameter humerus in percent of upper arm length or total body length
Biepicondylar diameter femur in percent of thigh length or total body length

III. CIRCUMFERENCE
Chest circumference in percent of the total body length
Upper arm circumference in percent of the upper arm length or total body length
Thigh circumference in percent of the thigh length or the total body length

Ponderal Index

A general impression of body stoutness can be derived from the ponderal index. Weight is the result of the three-dimensional expansion of the body. If weight and body length are compared, it is necessary to compare the total body length with the cube root of the weight. A thorough explanation of this index was given by Hirata and Kaku (1968). The ponderal index is determined by the following ratio:

$$\sqrt[3]{\text{Weight, kg}}/\text{Total body length, cm} \times 1000$$

Tables of Growth and Comparison of Sport Types (Constitutions)

It is advisable to be very cautious when analyzing the results of measurements. The particular method of measuring that was used to obtain the results should be taken into account. There are, for example, several ways to measure the total lower extremity length: (1) trochanterion height, (2) iliospinal height, (3) iliocristal height, and (4) subischial length (in subtracting sitting height from standing height). The reservations mentioned above should be kept in mind while studying Figures 11-1 through 11-43.

The figures depicting growth (Figures 11-1 through 11-21) were derived from a longitudinal study completed in Zurich involving children 1–15 years of age.* The measurement results involving sport types (Figures 11-22 through 11-43) were taken from the investigations conducted by Correnti (1964) and Tanner and coworkers (1964) in Rome during 1960 using Olympic

* The authors would like to thank Prof. Dr. A. Prader, Director of the Children's Hospital of the University of Zürich for his permission to publish preliminary results of the growth study.

[Text continues on page 235.]

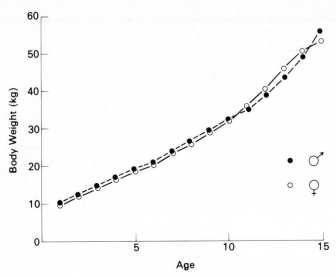

Figure 11-1. Body weight and age.*

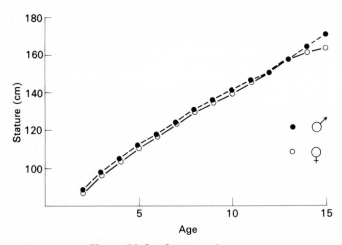

Figure 11-2. Stature and age.

* The data for Figures 11-1 through 11-21 are courtesy of Prof. Dr. A. Prader, Director of the Children's Hospital of the University of Zürich.

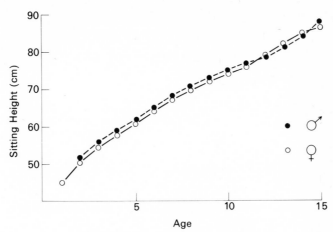

Figure 11-3. Sitting height and age.

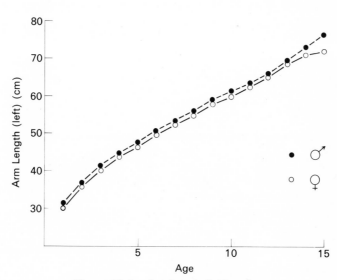

Figure 11-4. Arm length (left) and age.

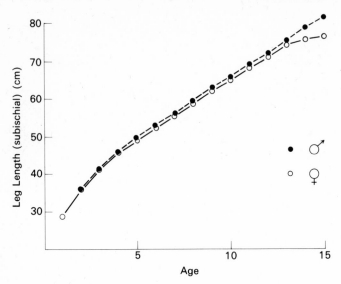

Figure 11-5. Leg length (subischial) and age.

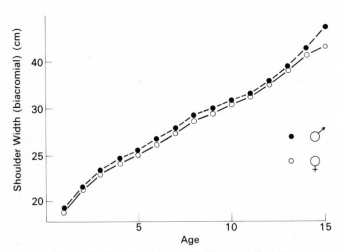

Figure 11-6. Shoulder width (biacromial) and age.

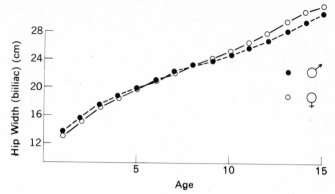

Figure 11-7. Hip width (biiliac) and age.

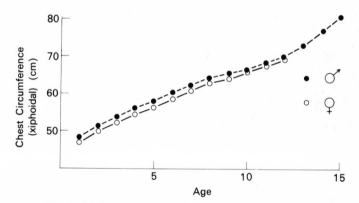

Figure 11-8. Chest circumference (xiphoidal) and age.

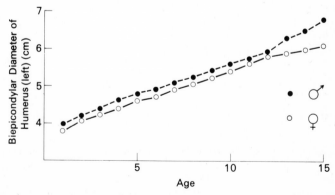

Figure 11-9. The biepicondylar diameter of the humerus (left) and age.

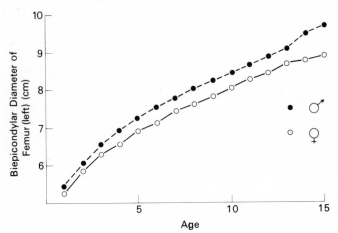

Figure 11-10. The biepicondylar diameter of the femur (left) and age.

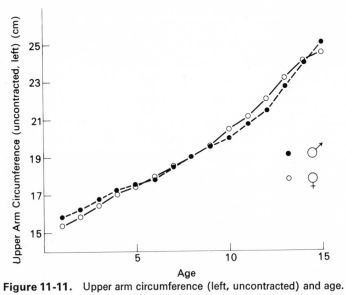

Figure 11-11. Upper arm circumference (left, uncontracted) and age.

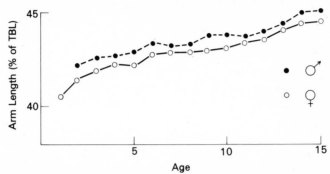

Figure 11-12. Arm length as a percentage of total body length (TBL) and age.

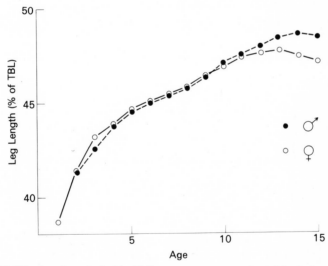

Figure 11-13. Leg length (subischial) as a percentage of total body length (TBL) and age.

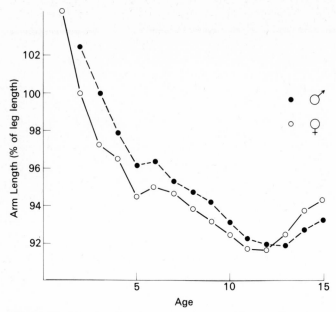

Figure 11-14. Arm length as a percentage of leg length and age.

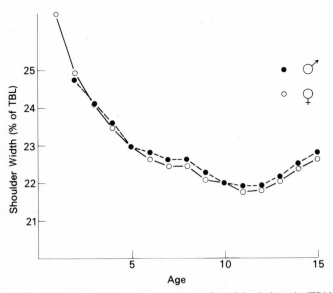

Figure 11-15. Shoulder width as a percentage of total body length (TBL) and age.

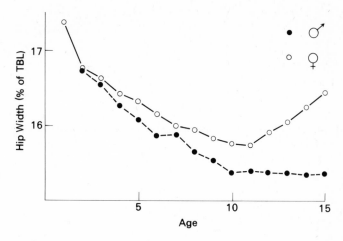

Figure 11-16.   Hip width as a percentage of total body length (TBL) and age.

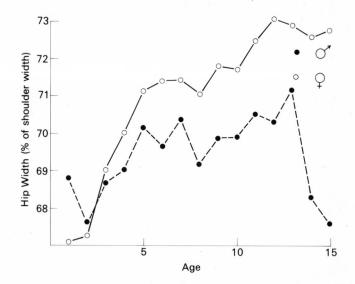

Figure 11-17.   Hip width as a percentage of shoulder width and age.

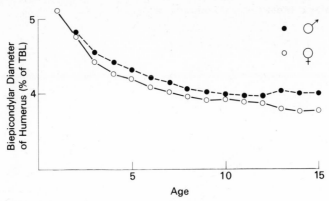

Figure 11-18. Biepicondylar diameter of the humerus as a percentage of total body length (TBL) and age.

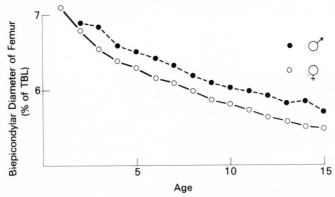

Figure 11-19. Biepicondylar diameter of the femur as a percentage of total body length (TBL) and age.

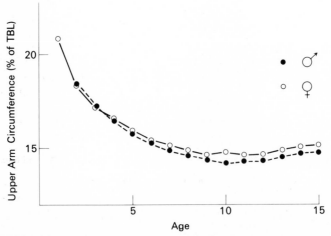

Figure 11-20. Upper arm circumference as a percentage of total body length (TBL) and age.

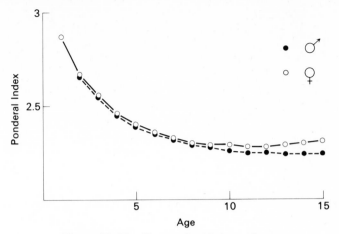

Figure 11-21. The ponderal index and age.

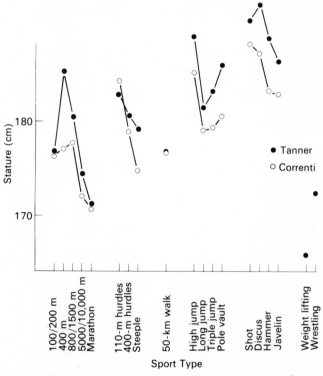

Figure 11-22. Differences in stature and sport type.*

* The data for Figures 11-22 through 11·46 come from V. Correnti: *Olympionici 1960.* Roma, 1964; and J. Tanner, R. H. Whitehouse, and S. Darmann: *The Physique of the Olympic Athlete.* London, George Allen, 1964.

223

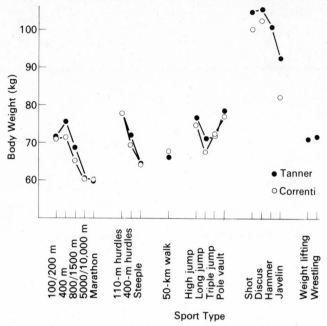

Figure 11-23. Differences in body weight and sport type.

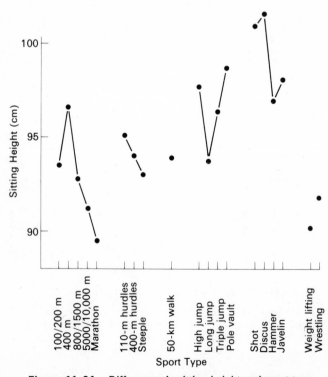

Figure 11-24. Differences in sitting height and sport type.

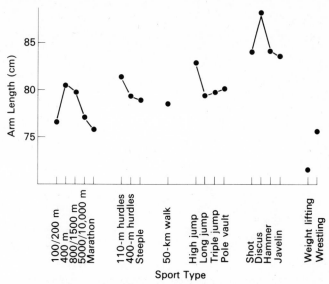

Figure 11-25. Differences in arm length (left) and sport type.

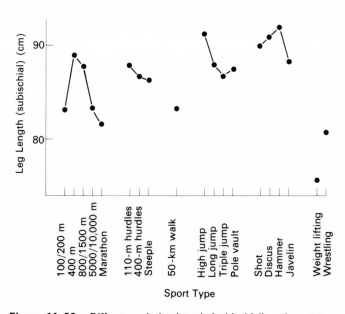

Figure 11-26. Differences in leg length (subischial) and sport type.

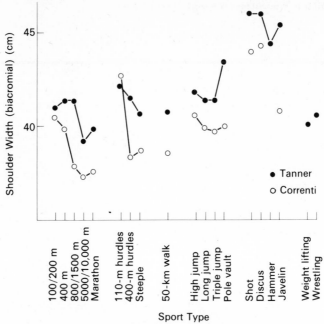

Figure 11-27. Differences in shoulder width (biacromial) and sport type.

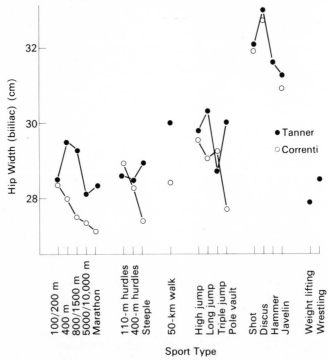

Figure 11-28. Differences in hip width (biiliac) and sport type.

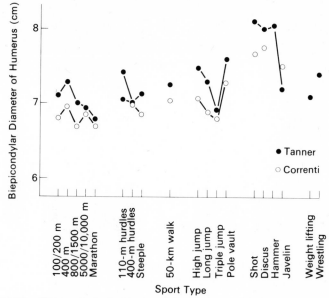

Figure 11-29. Differences in the biepicondylar diameter of the humerus and sport type.

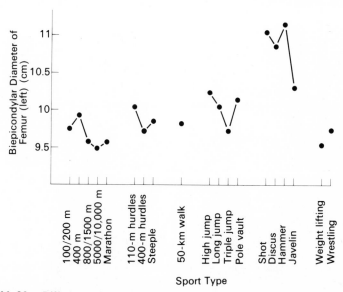

Figure 11-30. Differences in the biepicondylar diameter of the femur and sport type.

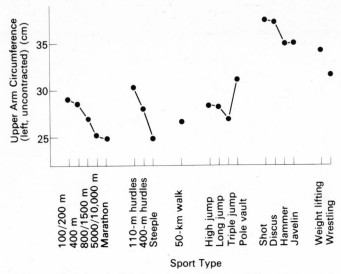

Figure 11-31.   Differences in upper arm circumference (left, uncontracted) and sport type.

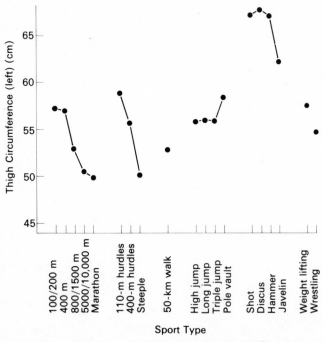

Figure 11-32.   Differences in thigh circumference (left) and sport type.

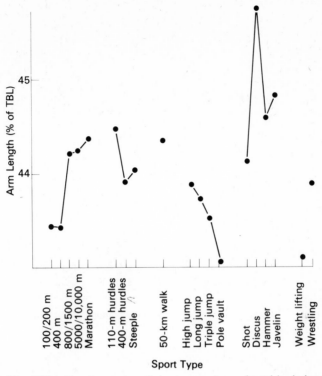

Figure 11-33. Differences in arm length as a percentage of total body length (TBL) and sport type.

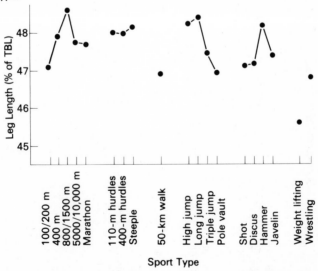

Figure 11-34. Differences in leg length as a percentage of total body length (TBL) and sport type.

229

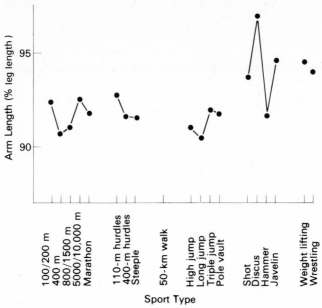

Figure 11-35. Differences in arm length as a percentage of leg length and sport type (Tanner).

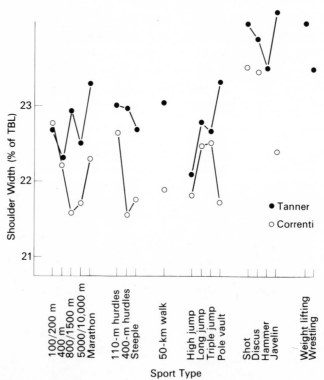

Figure 11-36. Differences in shoulder width as a percentage of total body length (TBL) and sport type.

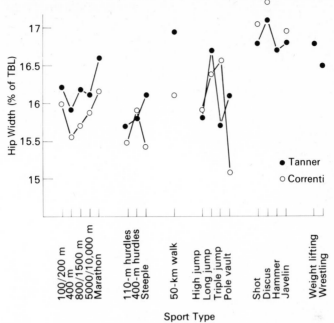

Figure 11-37. Differences in hip width as a percentage of total body length (TBL) and sport type.

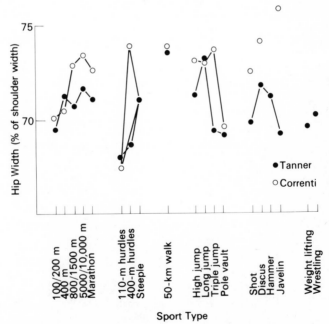

Figure 11-38. Differences in hip width as a percentage of shoulder width and sport type.

231

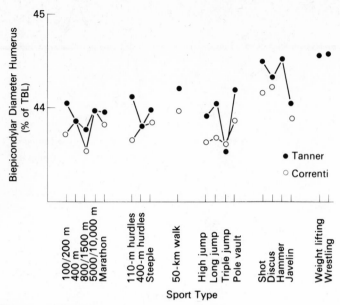

Figure 11-39. Differences in the biepicondylar diameter of the humerus as a percentage of total body length (TBL) and sport type.

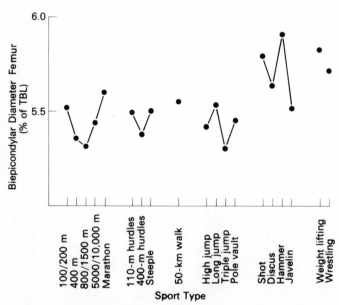

Figure 11-40. Differences in the biepicondylar diameter of the femur as a percentage of total body length (TBL) and sport type (Tanner).

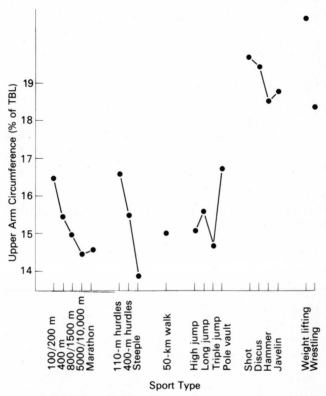

Figure 11-41. Differences in upper arm circumference as a percentage of total body length (TBL) and sport type (Tanner).

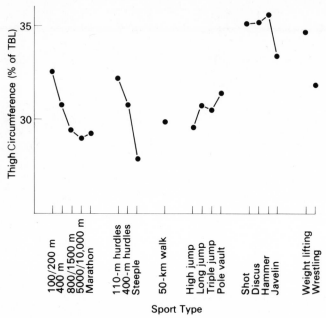

Figure 11-42. Differences in thigh circumference as a percentage of total body length (TBL) and sport type (Tanner).

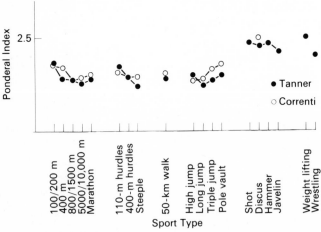

Figure 11-43. Differences in the ponderal index and sport type.

athletes. When these two studies are compared, it is readily apparent how greatly data obtained from similar investigations can differ. The differences may be attributable to differences in measurement technique. It seems that the high values of body lengths and sitting heights obtained by Tanner were due to the method of gentle stretching that he used in which he lifted the head before measuring. In addition, Tanner measured arm length by means of photographs. The width measurements of Correnti (shoulder and hip width) also generally have lower values than those of Tanner et al.

Table 11-3 Number of Athletes of Various Sport Types at the 1960 Olympic Games Who Were Subjects in Studies Conducted by Correnti (1964) and by Tanner et al. (1964)

Event	100 m 200 m	400 m	800 m 1500 m	5000 m 10,000 m	Mara-thon	110-m Hurdles	400-m Hurdles	Steeple Chase	50-km Walk
Number of individuals (Tanner)	12	11	16	19	9	3	5	4	6
Number of individuals (Correnti)	25	19	12	20	23	5	7	4	27

Event	High Jump	Long Jump	Triple Jump	Pole Vault	Shot	Discus	Ham-mer	Javelin	Weight Lifting	Wrestling
Number of individuals (Tanner)	8	2	3	2	6	2	2	2	15	32
Number of individuals (Correnti)	12	5	4	3	8	6	—	3	—	—

Composition of the Body

The human body consists of different kinds of tissue, such as bone, muscle, and skin/fat layers. Tissue indices are used to describe the body composition that consists of these kinds of tissue. The indices are based on simple anthropological measurements. To determine the tissue indices both upper and lower extremities can be used. For tissue indices based on measurements at the upper extremity the following data are required: (1) upper arm circumference, (2) epicondylar diameter of the humerus, (3) skinfolds over triceps and biceps, (4) total upper extremity length, and (5) body weight. To simplify matters it is assumed that the cross section of the upper arm is circular and that either half of both measured skinfolds represents the average skin/fat layer. Figure 11-44 shows a cross section of tissue area at the upper arm.

The bone diaphysis diameter appears consistently proportional to the

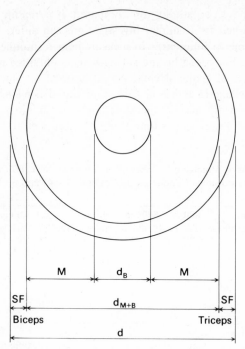

$$SF = \text{Skin/fat thickness} = \frac{\text{skinfold}}{2}$$

$$M = \text{Muscle}$$

$$d = \text{Diameter of the upper arm} = \frac{\text{circumference}}{\pi}$$

$$d_B = \text{Diameter of the bone}$$

$$d_{M+B} = \text{Diameter of the muscle} + \text{Bone} = d - (SF_{\text{biceps}} + SF_{\text{triceps}})$$

Figure 11-44.   Schematic cross section in the middle of the upper arm.

epiphysis breadth. The constant α* of this proportionality amounts to 3.1 (± 0.07) for the humerus of the male.

Calculation of the Bone (B), Muscle (M),
and Skin/Fat (SF) Area

$$\text{Surface } B = \left(\frac{d_B}{2}\right)^2 \cdot \pi = \frac{d_{\text{epiphysis}}^2}{4\alpha^2} \cdot \pi \qquad \text{in cm}^2$$

$$\text{Surface } M = (d_{M+B}^2 - d_B^2) \cdot \frac{\pi}{4} \qquad \text{in cm}^2$$

$$\text{Surface } SF = (d^2 - d_{M+B}^2) \cdot \frac{\pi}{4} \qquad \text{in cm}^2$$

* The constant α was calculated by Wüest from the specifications that Tanner gave for the athletes at the Olympic Games in 1960. These specifications were tested on students in Zürich and were found to be correct.

Tissue volumina were obtained by multiplying tissue surface areas by total arm lengths. (It would have been better if measurements of the upper arm had been taken. Specifications on upper arm lengths are, however, very rarely documented. We have therefore chosen the total arm length.)

Calculation of the Bone, Muscle, and Skin/Fat Volumina

Volume B = Surface area B × Total upper extremity length in dm³
Volume M = Surface area M × Total upper extremity length in dm³
Volume SF = Surface area SF × Total upper extremity length in dm³

It is possible to determine tissue weight by multiplying the tissue volume by the specific weight of that particular tissue.

Calculation of the Bone, Muscle, and Skin/Fat Weight

Weight B = Volume$_B$ × 1.4	in kg
Weight M = Volume$_M$ × 1	in kg
Weight SF = Volume$_{SF}$ × 0.9	in kg

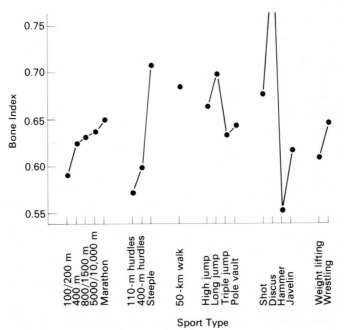

Figure 11-45. Differences in the bone index and sport type.

The tissue index is expressed by considering the tissue weight as a percentage of the body weight. Tissue indices refer to the constitution of the body.

Calculation of the Bone,
Muscle, and Skin/Fat Indices

$$\text{Index } B = \frac{\text{Weight}_B \times 100}{\text{Body weight}}$$

$$\text{Index } M = \frac{\text{Weight}_M \times 100}{\text{Body weight}}$$

$$\text{Index } SF = \frac{\text{Weight}_{SF} \times 100}{\text{Body weight}}$$

While fat layers have a body distribution which differs from type to type, tissue indices should not only be determined at the level of the upper arm, but also at other body levels, such as the thigh. The method used is always the same as the one for the upper arm. As constant α, which designates the relation of the epicondylar width to the diaphysis diameter, we propose to take the value 3 uniformly for the upper arm, lower arm, thigh, and calf.

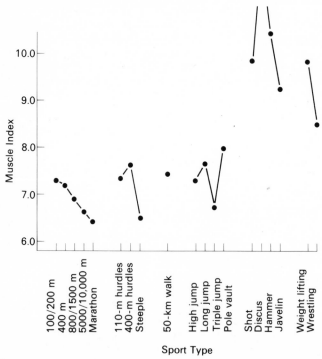

Figure 11-46.   Differences in the muscle index and sport type.

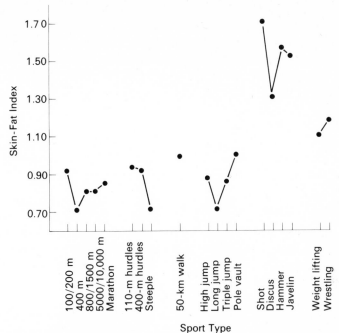

Figure 11-47.   Differences in the skin-fat index and sport type.

Figures 11-45 through 11-47 show bone, muscle, and skin/fat proportions of competitors in the 1960 Olympic Games at Rome and were calculated from the measurements taken by Tanner. Even though the tested groups were relatively small, there are definite differences among the various sports. The muscle index of runners and jumpers is low. As a rule, runners have a lower index if the distance is longer. High indices are found for throwers, weight lifters, and wrestlers. The skinfold index is also low for runners and jumpers, whereas weight lifters and wrestlers show average values and throwers have the highest values. The bone indices displayed such a wide range of differences that we have not attempted to interpret the results yet.

REFERENCES

Budliger, H.: Longitudinal growth study at the childrens' hospital of the University of Zürich. In preparation.

Correnti, V.: *Olympionici 1960.* Roma, 1964.

Grimm, H.: *Einführung in die Anthropologie.* Jena, Fischer Verlag, 1961.

Hiràta, K., and K. Kaku: *The Evaluating Method of Physique and Physical Fitness and its Practical Application.* Hirata Institute of Health, Gifu City, 1968.

International Committee for Standardization of Physical Fitness Tests—Standards (See Part VII, pp. 449–533.)

Martin, R., and K. Saller: *Lehrbuch der Anthropologie*, Vols. I–IV. Stuttgart, Fischer Verlag, 1957, 1959, 1960, 1966.

Saller, K.: *Leitfaden der Anthropologie*. Stuttgart, Fischer Verlag, 1964.

Tanner, J., R. H. Whitehouse, and S. Darmann: *The Physique of the Olympic Athlete*. London, George Allen, 1964.

Verschuer, O.: *Wirksame Faktoren im Leben des Menschen*. Wiesbaden, Franz Steiner Verlag, 1954.

Analysis of Body Compartments

12

LADISLAV P. NOVAK
Southern Methodist University
Dallas, Texas

The development of indirect methods for the analysis of body composition provided scientists with opportunities to compartmentalize the human body in several ways, depending on the purpose of the study. This *in vivo* approach is new in its concept and has practical implications for scientific studies investigating the effect of physical activity on the body composition of man.

From an historical point of view, Matiegka, the Czech anthropologist, tried 50 years ago to point out the broad avenues of somatometric evaluation of man's physique for various purposes. One of these was the appropriate choice of athletic events according to his evaluation. Matiegka (1921) proposed the following four compartments into which the body weight (W) could be divided: O = weight of skeleton (ossa, bone), D = skin (derma) plus subcutaneous adipose tissue, M = muscles, and R = remainder. Anthropometric measurements provided the necessary information for estimating the first three components. The weights of bone, skin and subcutaneous tissue, and muscles were estimated independently; that is, they were separate components of body weight.

The anthropometric approach to the appraisal of human physique has been used by various scientists. Subsequent measurements of limb or chest circumferences and diameters of bones are helpful, but extremely limited, indicators of "robusticity" or the gracile structure of a man. All these measurements belong to "surface anthropometry" and do not indicate the changes of various tissues inside a man which occur, for example, under a regimen of habitual exercise. Modern biology is interested in the identification of body compartments under the skin, that is, in the study of "inner man" (Brožek, 1963).

Introduction of skinfold calipers into the measurement of subcutaneous

241

fat plus use of the following formula for lean tissues of limbs helped in estimating the amount of lean tissues found under the skin:

$$d^1 = \frac{C}{\pi} - S$$

where d^1 = corrected diameter of limb, C = circumference of limb, π = 3.14159, and S = skinfold measured at site where circumference was taken. Determination of lean tissues of upper and lower extremities is described in detail in Part VII, Section 4, Article 78.0.

Roentgenograms and Ultrasonic Measurements of Subcutaneous Fat

Subcutaneous fat that is deposited directly under the skin can be seen and measured on radiographs. Garn (1957) and Brožek et al. (1958) provided details of methodologies for soft-tissue roentgenograms. The x-ray measurements are helpful in the determination of deposits of subcutaneous fat where the skinfolds cannot be measured and provide additional information about the muscle and bone. Recently, visualization of organs or tissues by ultrasound proved to be rather successful. The observations are not made from shadow pictures but are based on cross sections built up from echo formation over the period when a scanning system is used.

Analyses

Direct Analysis. Before any discussion of indirect biochemical or biophysical methods for analysis of body composition can be attempted, it is necessary to consider the available data from direct analyses of human bodies. Table 12-1 shows the results of chemical analyses of three male

Table 12-1 Results of Chemical Analyses of Three Male Cadavers

Cadaver	Age years	Height cm	Weight kg	Water %	Fat %	Protein %	Ash %	Water %: Fat-Free Weight
1	35	183.0	70.6	68.2	12.5	14.5	4.8	77.9
2	25	179.0	71.8	62.0	15.0	16.6	6.4	72.9
3	46	168.5	53.8	56.0	19.6	18.8	5.6	69.6
Average	35.3	176.8	65.4	62.6	15.3	16.4	5.7	73.9

cadavers obtained by Mitchell et al. (1945), Widdowson et al. (1951), and Forbes et al. (1953). The first two cadavers apparently represent normal bodies, but the third one is subject to question.

It is evident that some variation exists in the amount of water and total fat present in these few cadavers as well as in the relative amount of water in the fat-free body weight. These few examples do, however, point toward cautious acceptance of so-called constants for the hydration of the fat-free body for which evidence has also been obtained in numerous animal studies.

Four-Compartmental Analysis. From the physiological point of view, the human body could be subdivided into two components: one that is metabolically very active and another that is practically inert. The first component consists of cells and has been termed "active tissue mass" by Rubner (1902). It represents a large part of the body weight. In a muscular man it could exceed 50% of body weight, whereas in an obese individual it could account for only 30% of body weight. The other component of the body includes body fat, extracellular water, and mineral elements in the skeleton. In the normal, healthy individual the most variable part of this relatively inert component of the body is body fat. Thus, the human body can be considered as a four-compartmental system:

$$\text{weight} = \text{fat} + \text{extracellular water} + \text{cells} + \text{minerals}$$

This four-compartmental subdivision of the human body into fat, extracellular water, cells, and bone minerals seems to be warranted from the metabolic point of view and coincides reasonably with presently available methodology for the determination of body composition *in vivo*. However, four-compartmental analysis requires profound methodology which is available in only a few laboratories.

Two-Compartmental Analysis. Historically, the first approach of densitometry, described by Behnke et al. (1942), Brožek et al. (1949), and Goldman and Buskirk (1961), utilized concepts of body volume and body density which permitted division of the body into two compartments, that is, fat and fat-free, according to the equation

$$M = M_1 + M_2$$

where M = total body mass; M_1 = fat; and M_2 = fat-free mass.

If the densities of the compartments are known, the density of the total body can be determined as follows

$$D = \frac{M_1 + M_2}{(M_1/d_1) + (M_2/d_2)}$$

if

$$M_1 + M_2 = 1$$

then

$$D = \frac{1}{(M_1/d_1) + (M_2/d_2)}$$

Solving for M_1 yields

$$M_1 = \frac{1}{D} \times \frac{d_1 \times d_2}{(d_2 - d_1)} - \frac{d_1}{(d_2 - d_1)}$$

if M_2 is desired

$$M_2 = \frac{1}{D} \times \frac{d_1 \times d_2}{(d_1 - d_2)} - \frac{d_2}{(d_1 - d_2)}$$

The density of human fat extracted by ether from adipose tissue has a density of 0.9007 g/ml at 37°C according to Fidanza et al. (1953). The density of fat-free body was reported by Behnke et al. (1942) as 1.100 g/ml. If these densities of the two compartments are used, body fat can be calculated. It should be emphasized at this point that few laboratories have underwater weighing apparatus. The construction of a simple system is not expensive, but the methodology is not suitable for small children, elderly subjects, or subjects who are afraid to be submerged in water.

Reference Man. The practical application of body composition analysis needs to be verified first against theoretical computations. Total body fat is the most variable compartment of the body and is readily determined by indirect methods in two-compartmental analysis. From a practical point of view the following question can be raised: How much body fat should a young man have for a given height?

The answer to that question came from the classic research of Keys and Brožek (1953) and of Brožek et al. (1963). They proposed a "reference man" who is clinically healthy, who is 25 years of age, and whose weight equals the average in the United States for given height according to standard height-weight tables. Such a reference body has a density of 1.064 g/ml at 37°C and 15.3% fat. These figures help, in practice, to appraise the ratio of leanness to fatness of various individuals. Those with lower densities will gravitate to relative fatness, whereas those with higher densities than that of the reference man will be relatively lean.

Total Body Fat*

Apparatus. Any type of water-filled tank or swimming pool may be used if the water is still. The underwater weighing system may be a suspension or platform type; the suspension system is the most prevalent. With the suspension system, the subject is lowered under water by means of a hoist while sitting in a chair or a canvas sling or while supine on a stretcher. With the platform, the subject sits in a chair anchored to a scale platform and immerses himself by leaning forward until he is under water.

Scale. The scale used for underwater weighing should be properly

---

* Refer to Part VII, Section 4, Article 79.0.

damped so that maximal oscillations due to water turbulence and pendulum action of the chair will not exceed 20 g stability. The scale should have a maximal capacity of at least 15 kg calibrated and should be adjusted to read to the nearest 0.10 g.

Thermometer. The thermometer should be secured in the water tank and available for accurate readings.

Weights. Lead weights are necessary to maintain the subject's fully submerged position.

Residual Volume Equipment. Equipment for determination of residual volume by helium dilution, nitrogen washout, oxygen rebreathing, hydrogen rebreathing, plethysmography, and so forth.

Spirometer. A reliable spirometer may be used to determine the subject's vital capacity (VC) if the residual volume (RV) is to be estimated ($RV = 30\% \, VC$). Residual volume may be estimated from standard tables, but this is a less desirable method.

Description. The total body volume is determined by the hydrostatic weighing technique, using the Archimedean principle, whereby the volume of the body is determined from its displacement in water.

Scoring

$$\text{Body density} = D_B = \frac{\text{Weight}_A/(\text{Weight}_A - \text{Weight}_W)}{\text{Density}_W}$$

where A = air and W = water.

Since a certain amount of air is in the lungs and respiratory passages during submersion of the subject, a correction factor for the air of the gross body volume must be applied. Thus the complete body density formula becomes

$$\text{Body density} = D_B = \frac{\text{Weight}_A/(\text{Weight}_A - \text{Weight}_W)}{\text{Density}_W} - RV_A$$

where RV_A = residual volume of air remaining in the lungs at the end of maximal expiration.

Calculation

1. Water temperature.
2. Water density at temperature observed.
3. Weight in air.
4. Submerged weight.
5. Weight of submerged apparatus.
6. Total gas volume = $RV + V_{gi}$ (volume of gastrointestinal gas, in milliliters).
7. Weight of gas volume = milliliters of gas × water.
8. Corrected submerged weight = $(4 + 7) - 5$.*

* Numerals refer to statements in the list.

9. Difference in air-to-water weight $= 3 - 8$.
10. Body volume $= 9 \div 2$.
11. Body density $= 3 \div 10$.

Estimation of Body Fat From Body Density. When the densities of the two proportional masses in the two-compartmental analysis are known, then the total density can be calculated.

$$M_1 = \frac{1}{D} \times \frac{d_1 \times d_2}{(d_2 - d_1)} - \frac{d_1}{(d_2 - d_1)}$$

where $M_1 =$ the fat expressed as a function of total body mass; $d_1 =$ the density of the fat; and $d_2 =$ the density of the fat-free body.

When the known densities of human fat and fat-free body are substituted in the above formula, the equation for calculating fat content of an individual is

$$\text{Fat} = \frac{4.570}{\text{Density}} - 4.142$$

This equation has been proposed by Keys and Brožek (1953) and is recommended for its uniformity. It is also applicable for the estimation of fat in individuals free of large, recent fluctuations of fat.

General Guide and Regulations. The principle of the estimation of body fat from calculations based on measurements of body density depends on the following assumptions:

1. That the separate densities of the body components are additive.
2. That the densities of the constituents of the body are relatively constant from person to person.
3. That an individual differs from a "standard reference man" only in the amount of adipose tissue he possesses.

The difference between the body weight in air and the body weight completely immersed in water is the weight of the displaced volume of water. If the water density is known, the volume displaced or the body volume can be calculated. The density of the whole body (D_B) is determined as follows:

$$D_B = \frac{M_{BA}}{V}$$

The density of the water (D_W) can be determined from standard tables if the temperature is known and the water is adequately mixed and free of air bubbles.

It is necessary to maintain a water temperature at mean body temperature value (35–36°C) since extremes in water temperature could induce changes in mean body temperature (that is, produce shivering).

The residual volume may be determined in the following ways:

1. Simultaneously with density determination, for greater accuracy.
2. Prior to or following the weighing procedure without appreciable loss of accuracy.
3. By estimation from known lung volumes.
   (a) 20% of the total lung capacity.
   (b) 30% of the vital capacity.

If the residual volume is assumed, the effect of age, sex, and posture must be considered. The volume of gas in the gastrointestinal tract (V_{gi}) has been estimated most accurately at 100 ml (body temperature and pressure saturated with water vapor) in the postabsorptive state. In addition to errors arising from variations in the foregoing measurements, gas bubbles adhering to the skin and the hair on the body surface must be removed. If the subject is not weighed in the nude, air may be trapped in the bathing suit or bathing cap (in the long hair of female subjects) and will produce an error in the estimation of the density.

Density should be determined while the subject is in a postabsorptive state to reduce the amount of gastrointestinal gas to a minimum. The test should be fully explained in order to alleviate any apprehension and, if possible, several trial runs should be made. Prior to weighing, the residual volume should be determined (or the vital capacity) with the subject in the same position in which he will be weighed.

The subject's body weight on land is determined and recorded, as well as the weight of submerged apparatus (that is, chair, cot, added weights, and so forth). The subject then assumes his position in the apparatus and is partially lowered into the water. The body is scrubbed to dislodge gas bubbles in the skin and hair. A nose clip is applied and tested for leaks. The subject performs a maximal expiration (as in performing the residual volume) and flexes at the neck until the top of the head is barely submerged. In this position the scale is read to the nearest 10 g. After the reading, the subject is touched on the head and surfaces simply by raising the head.

The test is repeated until the *heaviest* measured weight is obtained on at least three different trials. The water temperature (centigrade) is recorded after each weighing. The barometric pressure is recorded at the beginning and at the end of each session. The weight of the submerged apparatus is again recorded after each subject's weighing is completed.

Total Body Water Measurements*

Total amount of water in the body can be estimated with ease even under field conditions. It requires oral administration of a certain amount of deuterium oxide and collection of two urine samples, the first during a short

* Refer to Part VII, Section 4, Article 80.0.

equilibration period and the second approximately 1 hr after equilibration. Sealed samples of urine can be carried or shipped to the laboratory and analyzed by mass spectrometer as proposed by Solomon et al. (1950). Samples of urine give identical results of total body water with plasma samples. If plasma is available, several other methods can be used for the estimation of total body water, namely, the falling drop method of Schloerb et al. (1950), infrared absorption as proposed by Turner et al. (1960) using Beckman IR 5 spectrophotometer, freezing point elevation as described by Reaser and Burch (1958) using Fiske Deuterium Cryoscope, and gas chromatography as proposed by Arnett and Duggleby (1963).

Apparatus. Mass spectrometer and reduction train. Deuterium oxide, D_2O (99.8%), paper cups, plastic bottles, pipettes, graduated cylinders.

Description. Total body water can be determined by the dilution principle based on the following formula for scoring.

Scoring

$$V_F = \frac{C_1 V_1 - C_E V_E}{C_F}$$

where V_F = final volume of body water into which test substance has diffused at equilibrium; C_1 = concentration of test substance administered; V_1 = volume of test substance administered; C_E = concentration of test substance lost during equilibration time; V_E = volume of test substance lost during equilibration time; and C_F = final concentration of test substance after equilibration has been achieved.

It has been well documented that the loss of test substance during equilibration time is less than 0.25%; it can therefore be omitted from calculations. Thus, the formula is reduced to

$$V_F = \frac{C_1 V_1}{C_F}$$

Calculation. The subject, a female weighing 55.0 kg, is given 30 g of D_2O orally (99.8% in purity, density 1.11 g/ml). During the 2 hr of the equilibration period, 200 ml of urine were collected at a concentration of 0.0900 mole/100 ml excess. Samples of urine collected over 3 and 4 hr had an average concentration of 0.0992 mole/100 ml excess. With the dilution principle, total body water is calculated as follows:

$$TBW = \frac{\left(\frac{99.8\%}{100} \times \frac{30 \text{ g } D_2O}{1.11 \text{ g/ml}}\right) - \left(200 \times \frac{0.0900\%}{100}\right)}{\frac{0.0992\%}{100}}$$

$$TBW = \frac{26.972 \text{ ml} - 0.180 \text{ ml}}{\frac{0.0992\%}{100}} = 27{,}009 \text{ ml or } 27.01 \text{ liters}$$

$$TBW = 49.11\%.$$

Fat-Free Mass and Fat from Total Body Water. The fat-free mass contains not only the cellular mass but also the extracellular supporting structures such as extracellular water, collagen, and bone mineral. The cellular mass has high oxygen consumption whereas the extracellular supporting structures represent low oxidizing tissues. Therefore, fat-free mass represents heterogeneous components of the body. The derivation of fat-free mass from total body water is valid only in the normal state, where the relationship of body water to dry lean body tissues remains constant. In pathologic states, when either extracellular or intracellular water accumulates, this relationship does not hold. However, a correction factor for the excess of the extracellular water has been proposed by Keys and Brožek (1953). Fat-free mass can be calculated from the determination of total body water (*TBW*) under the assumption that it has a "constant" amount of water, namely, 73.2%, and that body fat is practically anhydrous. Then,

$$LBM, \% = \frac{TBW\%}{0.732} \quad \text{or} \quad LBM, \text{kg} = \frac{TBW_L}{0.732}$$

where *LBM* is lean body mass, $TBW\%$ is total body water expressed in percent of body weight (*BW*), TBW_L is total body water expressed in liters, and 0.732 is a constant of hydration for fat-free mass (*FFM*) based on analyses of small laboratory rodents according to Pace and Rathbun (1945).

Fat, % = 100 − LBM% or Fat, kg = BW, kg − FFM, kg

Further calculations:

Total body solids, kg = Body weight, kg − Total body water, kg

Fat-free solids, kg = Total body solids, kg − Total body fat, kg

General Guide and Regulations. The principle of dilution of total body water is based on the following assumptions:

1. The ideal test substance should be diffusible into all the fluid compartments of the body within a short time.
2. The ideal test substance should reach a stable and uniform equilibrium after a short time.
3. The ideal test substance should not be selectively stored, secreted, or metabolized.
4. The ideal test substance should be completely exchangeable with body water.

Usually 1 g D_2O/kg of body weight is given orally to the subject after his bladder is emptied. Two hours are required for D_2O to equilibrate with body water. After 2 hr have passed, the subject empties his bladder into the toilet. Samples of urine are collected into plastic bottles at 3 and 4 hr after the time that D_2O was administered. The volume of each urine sample is measured, noted, and aliquots are taken of each sample into 5-ml plastic vials. The urine samples are sealed and sent to the mass spectrometer laboratory. Urine samples do not have to be frozen.

Both samples containing D_2O are analyzed by mass spectrometer for the ratio of hydrogen 2 to hydrogen 1 ($^2H:^1H$) and should provide identical results. If the results of both samples disagree more than 5%, equilibrium was not achieved and the 4-hr urine sample should provide the true volume distribution.

In cases of abnormal hydration, the time for equilibration of D_2O with body water has to be extended at least to 4 hr. The subject should not drink fluids excessively, if at all, during the period of urine collections. The primary inherent error of this method is in the exchange of deuterium atoms with labile hydrogen atoms of organic molecules. This exchange occurs rapidly and therefore represents only a small loss of deuterium. The loss has been estimated to have a water equivalent between 0.5% and 2.0% of body weight. Thus, for the average man who has 45 liters of body water, the D_2O method will overestimate his body water by 700–1000 ml. This figure will set the limits on the accuracy of body water measurements. Thus, corrected volume can be obtained by an average decrease of 1%.

Instructions for Total Body Water Determination. Ask the subject to empty his bladder before administration of the dose. Give subject 25 ml of D_2O orally in a plastic or paper cup. He must empty the cup totally. Fill the cup with tap water and ask the subject to drink this water also, making sure that no residual drops of water are left in the cup. Explain to the subject that he is not to drink additional water or any liquid from the time the dose is given until the final collection of urine (4 hr later).

At 2 hr after the dose has been given, ask the subject to empty his bladder into the toilet (about 0.25% of the dose will be lost in this equilibration urine, which will cause a negligible error in the total calculation of total body water). At 3 hr after the dose has been given, ask the subject for the first sample of urine (mark this bottle with the name of the subject and as No. 1). Measure the total volume of urine, record it, place an aliquot into 5-ml vial, and seal. At 4 hr after the dose has been given, ask the subject for the second sample of urine (mark this bottle with the name of the subject and as No. 2). Measure the total volume of urine, record it, place an aliquot into a 5-ml vial, and seal. Store samples in a cool place. Samples are reduced to a gaseous state and analyzed for the ratio of $^2H:^1H$ on the mass spectrometer.

Total Body Potassium*

Since potassium (K) is present mainly inside the cells, the measurement of the amount of potassium in the body offers possibilities for estimation of

* Refer to Part VII, Section 4, Article 81.0.

fat-free mass and the body cell mass. Though potassium content of the body can be determined from the measurement of total exchangeable potassium by the isotopic dilution method using ^{42}K as a tracer, whole-body counting of naturally emitted γ-rays in ^{40}K will always be preferred in normal subjects for measurement of total body potassium.

The direct estimation of total body potassium was introduced by Sievert (1951) and was developed at Los Alamos by Anderson (1957). The two methods of estimating potassium in the body are reasonably accurate, though the ^{42}K method provides lower values than the ^{40}K method by about 5–10% according to Anderson (1965). Whole-body counters are available in the main cities of most countries, and the location can be found in the *Directory of Whole-Body Radioactivity Monitors* published by the International Atomic Energy Agency, Vienna, 1964.

Apparatus. Steel room, whole-body counter with sodium iodide (NaI), plastic or liquid scintillating detectors. Phantom made of plastic containers and filled with known amount of potassium as potassium chloride (KCl). Sugar phantom, hospital cart.

Description. Total body potassium can be determined by the measurement of naturally occurring radioactivity of the body due to the ^{40}K content. This ^{40}K emits γ-rays of maximal energy 1.46 million electron volts (Mev) and is in a constant ratio of 0.0119% to the two stable potassium isotopes: ^{39}K, 93.08%; and ^{41}K, 6.91%. These γ-rays are detected and counted by sensitive detectors surrounding the subject.

Scoring

$$TBK = \frac{\text{Subject cps} \times \text{Efficiency counter (day)}}{\text{Weight/height correction factor cps/g K}}$$

where TBK = total body potassium in grams; Subject cps = counts per second of subject and counts per second of appropriate sugar phantom; Efficiency counter = 0.3619 cps/g of K phantom (known amount of K) divided by the daily counts per second per gram of K; and Weight/height correction factor = counts per second per gram of K based on the regression line obtained from calibration of the counter with ^{42}K.

Remark: The sugar phantom is used to stimulate body thickness and to correct for the internal absorption of γ-rays within the body.

Calculation

1. Weight in kilograms and height in centimeters of the subject.
2. Counts per second of the subject.
3. Counts per second of appropriate sugar phantom.
4. Counts per second of adult K phantom.
5. Net subject cps = 2 − 3.*

* Numerals refer to statements in the list.

6. Efficiency of daily counting = $0.3619/[(4 - 3) + 850]$, where 850 equals grams of K in a phantom.
7. Subject efficiency correction derived from weight/height.
8. Total body K = $(5 \times 6) + 7$.

Estimation of Fat-Free Mass From Total Body Potassium. In the adult human the K concentration of the fat-free body mass, as determined by chemical analysis, averages 68.1 milliequivalents per kilogram (mEq/kg) of fat-free body mass (range, 66.6–72.3 mEq). Thus,

$$\text{Fat-free mass, kg} = \frac{\text{Total body K, mEq}}{68.1}$$

$$\text{Fat, kg} = \text{Body weight, kg} - \text{Fat-free mass, kg}$$

However, the K concentration in the fat-free mass of newborns seems to be between 48 and 50 mEq/kg; at 1 year of age, approximately 58 mEq/kg; at 10 years of age, 60 mEq/kg; and at 15 years of age, 68.1 mEq/kg (Forbes, 1962; Oberhausen and Onstead, 1965).

Estimation of Cell Mass from Total Body Potassium. The body cell mass is a pure culture of living cells. It consists of the cellular components of the skeletal, cardiac, and smooth muscles; viscera (liver, kidney, spleen, lungs, heart); intestinal tract; blood; glands; reproductive organs (uterus, ovaries, testes); and the cells of the brain. If one assumes that these cellular tissues have an average potassium to nitrogen ratio of 3 mEq/g and that their total net weight (excluding extracellular water) is equal to their nitrogen content multiplied by the coefficient 25, then the weight of body cell mass can be calculated as proposed by Moore et al. (1963):

$$\text{Body cell mass, g} = \frac{\text{Total body K, mEq} - \text{Extracellular K, mEq}}{3} \times 25$$

Since the correction for extracellular potassium causes negligible error in the calculations of body cell mass, it can be omitted and the equation becomes

$$\text{Body cell mass, g} = \text{Total body K, mEq} \times 8.33$$

General Guide and Regulations. Before calculations of total body potassium can be achieved, the whole-body counter has to be calibrated. This is usually done by giving an oral dose of ^{42}K to subjects of various weights. ^{42}K has maximal energy (1.52 Mev) similar to that of ^{40}K, and it has a conveniently short half-life (12.5 hr).

First, a fasting subject is counted for ^{40}K before the administration of ^{42}K. The subject then receives 5 microcurie (μcurie) of ^{42}K and is counted at 1 hr, 6 hr, 24 hr, and 48 hr. Urine is collected between each whole-body counting period, and the bottles of urine are counted in order to determine the amount of tracer lost; thus subject counts can be corrected for urinary loss of ^{42}K.

A phantom containing a known amount of KCl is then substituted for the subject, counted in the whole-body counter, and compared to a calibrated quantity of ^{42}K in the same phantom. From these data the subject's potassium can be calculated as follows:

$$TBK, \text{g} = \text{cps } ^{40}K \text{ (man)} \times \frac{\text{g K (phantom)}}{\text{cps } ^{40}K \text{ (phantom)}} \times \frac{\text{cps } ^{42}K \text{ (phantom)}}{\text{cps } ^{42}K \text{ (man)}}$$

The relationship of counts per second per gram of K to the ratio of weight/height is determined from the regression equation, which includes various ranges of weight and height.

$$\log(\text{cps/g K}) = -0.30122(\text{weight/height}) + 0.65499$$

which, expressed arithmetically, is

$$\text{cps/g K} = -0.23317(\text{weight/height}) + 0.42640$$

Table 12-2 Example of Total Body Potassium Determination
(Male: weight = 71.0 kg, height = 169.0 cm, age = 40 years.)

Source	Time of Counting	Counts per Second Average	Net
Room background	600	92	0
Phantom (850 g K)	600	398	306
Subject	600	140	48

$$TBK, \text{g} = \text{Subject net cps} \times \frac{\text{Counter efficiency}}{\text{Correction for weight/height}}$$

$$TBK, \text{g} = \frac{48 \times (0.3619/0.3597)}{0.337} = 143 \text{ g or } 2.0 \text{ g/kg}$$

$$\frac{143 \times 1000}{39.1} = 3646 \text{ mEq or } 51.3 \text{ mEq/kg.}$$

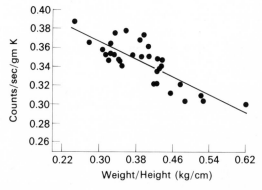

Figure 12-1. Relationship of counts per second per gram K to ratio of weight (kg) to height (cm).

This regression equation also can be expressed on an arithmetic graph (see Figure 12-1). The difference in correlation coefficients of log cps/g K and cps/g K is negligible, $r = 0.822$ and $r = 0.815$, respectively.

Table 12-2 gives an example of this calculation.

REFERENCES

Anderson, E. C.: Scintillation counters: the Los Alamos human counter. *Brit. J. Radiol. Suppl.* **7**:27–32 (1957).

Anderson, E. C.: Determination of body potassium by 4π gamma counting. In G. R. Meneely and S. M. Linde (eds.): *Radioactivity in Man*. Springfield, Ill. Charles C Thomas, pp. 211–231, 1965.

Arnett, E. M., and P. M. Duggleby: A rapid and simple method of deuterium determination. *Anal. Chem.*, **35**:1420–1424 (1963).

Behnke, A. R., Jr., B. G. Feen, and W. C. Welham: The specific gravity of healthy men: body weight ÷ volume as an index of obesity. *J. Amer. Med. Assoc.*, **118**:495–498 (1942).

Brožek, J.: Quantitative description of body composition: anthropology's fourth dimension. *Curr. Anthropol.* **4**:3–39 (1963).

Brožek, J., F. Grande, J. T. Anderson, and A. Keys: Densitometric analysis of body composition: revision of some quantitative assumptions. *Ann. N.Y. Acad. Sci.*, **110**:113–140 (1963).

Brožek, J., A. Henschel, and A. Keys: Effect of submersion in water on the volume of residual air in man. *J. Appl. Physiol.*, **2**:240–246 (1949).

Brožek, J., H. Mori, and A. Keys: Estimation of total body fat from roentgeno-grams. *Science*, **128**:901 (1958).

Fidanza, F., A. Keys, and J. T. Anderson: Density of human body fat in man and other animals. *J. Appl. Physiol.*, **6**:252–256 (1953).

Forbes, G. B.: Methods for determining composition of the human body: with a note on the effect of diet on body composition. *Pediatrics*, **29**:477–494 (1962).

Forbes, R. M., A. R. Cooper, and H. H. Mitchell: The composition of the adult human body as determined by chemical analysis. *J. Biol. Chem.*, **203**:359–366 (1953).

Garn, S. M.: Roentgenogrammetric determinations of body composition. *Hum. Biol.*, **29**:337–353 (1957).

Goldman, R. F., and E. R. Buskirk: Body volume measurement by underwater weighing: description of a method. In *Techniques for Measuring Body Composition*. Washington D.C., National Academy of Science, pp. 90–107, 1961.

Keys, A., and J. Brožek: Body fat in adult man. *Physiol. Rev.*, **33**:245–325 (1953).

Matiegka, J.: The testing of physical efficiency. *Am. J. Phys. Anthropol.* **4**:223–230 (1921).

Mitchell, H. H., T. S. Hamilton, F. R. Steggerda, and H. W. Bean: The chemical composition of the adult human body and its bearing on the biochemistry of growth. *J. Biol. Chem.*, **158**:625–637 (1945).

Moore, F. D., K. H. Olesen, J. D. McMurrey, H. V. Parker, M. R. Ball, and C. M. Boyden: *The Body Cell Mass and Its Supporting Environment: Body Composition in Health and Disease*. Philadelphia, W. B. Saunders, 1963.

Oberhausen, E., and C. O. Onstead: Relationship of potassium content of man with age and sex: results of 10,000 measurements of normal persons; factors influencing potassium content. In G. R. Meneely and S. M. Linde (eds.): *Radioactivity in Man*. Springfield, Ill. Charles C Thomas, pp. 179–185, 1965.

Pace, N., and E. N. Rathbun: Studies on body composition. III. The body water and chemically combined nitrogen content in relation to fat content. *J. Biol. Chem.*, **158**:685–691 (1945).

Reaser, P. B., and G. E. Burch: Determination of deuterium oxide in water by measurement of freezing point. *Science*, **128**:415–416 (1958).

Rubner, M.: *Die Gesetze des Energieverbrauchs bei der Ernährung*. Leipzig, Franz Deuticke, 1902.

Schloerb, P. R., B. J. Friis-Hansen, I. S. Edelman, A. K. Solomon, and F. D. Moore: The measurement of total body water in the human subject by deuterium oxide dilution: with a consideration of the dynamics of deuterium distribution. *J. Clin. Invest.* **29**:1296–1310 (1950).

Sievert, R. M.: Measurements of radiation from the human body. *Ark. Fyst*, **3**:337–346 (1951).

Solomon, A. K., I. S. Edelman, and S. Soloway: The use of the mass spectrometer to measure deuterium in body fluids. *J. Clin. Invest.*, **29**:1311–1319 (1950).

Turner, M. D., W. A. Neely, and J. D. Hardy: Rapid determination of deuterium oxide in biological fluids. *J. Appl. Physiol.*, **15**:309–310 (1960).

Widdowson, E. M., R. M. McCance, and C. M. Spray: The chemical composition of the human body. *Clin. Sci.*, **10**:113–125 (1951).

Physique, Body Composition, and Performance

13

LADISLAV P. NOVAK
Southern Methodist University
Dallas, Texas

Body composition analysis of the human body is a suitable tool for characterization of individuals who habitually exercise as compared to those individuals who lead a sedentary life. Physical activity can have a profound influence on the human body. By determination of specific gravity of football players, Behnke et al. (1942) pointed out that individuals with excessive weight for their age might be erroneously regarded as obese, according to standard height–weight tables. Brožek (1954) documented that active men more than 50 years of age, who were matched for age and height with inactive men, were found to have lower fat content and higher fat-free mass. Other investigators such as Pascale et al. (1955), Buskirk and Taylor (1957), and Behnke and Taylor (1959) utilized biochemical and biophysical methods to document the influence of intensive physical training on the body composition of soldiers, students, and athletes. Changes in body composition of Olympic gymnasts were studied by Pařízková (1962) as they prepared for the Olympic Games.

The reverse trends in body composition with increase in body fat after 15 weeks of relaxation were characterized by lower body densities. The body fat, fat-free mass, and cell mass seem to be affected differently by various physical activities, depending on the caloric expenditure necessary for each particular athletic event, as Novak et al. (1968) described in a study of various groups of highly trained collegiate athletes.

This presentation is concerned with differences in body composition of senior high school boys or adults who participated habitually in various physical activities as compared to those individuals, matched for age and weight or height, whose mode of life could be classified as "inactive."

256

Body Density and Physical Activity

Eighteen boys were selected randomly from a group of 43 boys who were members of high school basketball and football teams. The control group of 20 boys was selected randomly from 91 senior high school boys and matched for age and weight. Body density was determined by the underwater weighing method as described by Keys and Brožek (1953). Skinfolds were measured by Lange calipers with constant pressure of 10 g/mm² and corrected diameters were calculated as described in the standards of the International Committee for Standardization of Physical Fitness Tests (ICSPFT).

Table 13-1 provides information about heights, weights, and body density of the active and inactive groups of boys. The active boys were slightly, but not significantly, taller than the inactive boys. The weights of both groups were practically the same. When body densities of both groups were compared, however, the active boys seemed to have higher body density —1.0827 g/ml as compared to 1.0648 g/ml measured in the group of inactive boys. This difference of 0.0179 g/ml between the means was highly significant.

Table 13-1 Heights, Weights, and Body Density of Active and Inactive Boys

	Active			Inactive			
	Number	Mean	SD[1]	Number	Mean	SD	t
Height, cm	18	175.5	6.79	20	172.1	8.22	1.38
Weight, kg	18	67.3	10.1	20	66.7	10.6	0.16
Body density, g/ml	18	1.0827	0.0122	20	1.0648	0.0164	3.81***

SOURCE: L. P. Novak: Physical activity and body composition of adolescent boys. *J. Amer. Med. Assoc.*, **197**:891–893 (1966).
[1] SD = Standard deviation.
*** Significant at 0.001 level.

When the fat fraction of the body was calculated from the known densities, the active boys had only 7.2% of fat, whereas the average amount of fat for the inactive group of boys was twice as high, namely, 14.9%.

The results of body density were substantiated further by anthropometric appraisal of leanness-fatness. Table 13-2 shows the results of three skinfolds and two corrected diameters for both active and inactive boys. The means of all three skinfolds, which were significantly lower in the active group of boys, indicated less subcutaneous fat tissues at the sites sampled, that is, the upper arm, calf, and under the shoulder blade. Because approximately 50% of body fat is deposited subcutaneously, these results of lower skinfold measurements substantiate well the findings about lower total body fat and higher body density found in the group of active boys.

The corrected diameters, which relatively measure lean tissues of the extremities, indicated significantly larger musculature at least in the upper

Table 13-2 Skinfolds and Corrected Diameters of Active and Inactive Boys

Factors	Active			Inactive			
	Number	Mean	SD[1]	Number	Mean	SD	t
Skinfolds							
Upper arm, mm	18	8.3	2.29	20	13.0	6.59	2.94**
Subscapular, mm	18	8.4	2.81	20	11.6	6.17	2.10*
Calf, mm	18	9.9	2.29	20	14.2	7.16	2.53*
Correct diameters							
Upper arm, cm	18	8.0	0.86	20	7.6	0.68	1.74**
Calf, cm	18	10.8	0.67	20	10.4	0.83	1.39

SOURCE: L. P. Novak: Physical activity and body composition of adolescent boys. *J. Amer. Med. Assoc.*, **197**:891–893 (1966).
[1] SD = Standard deviation.
* Significant at 0.05 level.
** Significant at 0.01 level.

arm, whereas corrected diameter of the calf of active boys did not differ significantly from that of inactive boys.

Conclusion

From the results of this study it can be said that habitual participation of adolescent boys in sports (basketball and football) affected their body composition in such a way that they had significantly less body fat as estimated by densitometry and skinfolds when compared with inactive adolescent boys of the same age.

Total Body Water and Physical Activity

Habitual physical activity affects cardiovascular performance and also, by the various metabolic demands on the body, profoundly modifies and influences body composition. Collegiate and professional athletes, in particular, must exert themselves in their daily training programs to the maximum in order to sustain a certain degree of physical and physiological fitness; they are working under a constant caloric expenditure which is either equal to or surpassing their caloric intake, depending on the caloric load each particular activity requires for top performance. This demand for each performance modifies, in turn, the body composition of each athlete.

The purpose of this investigation was to study five groups of highly trained collegiate athletes whose physical activities necessitated varied caloric demands. A matter of further interest was the influence of long-term participation in various physical activities on the body composition and, in particular, on the total body water of the athlete.

Subjects and Methods

The subjects for this study were 7 swimmers, 9 track-and-field men, 7 gymnasts, 10 baseball players, and 16 football players who were members of the University of Minnesota Intercollegiate Athletic teams. All athletes were tested within 2 weeks after the end of the competitive season and presumably at the peak of their physical condition.

Total body water was determined by the dilution principle as described in the methods of the International Committee for Standardization of Physical Fitness Tests (ICSPFT). About 25 ml of D_2O was given to the subjects orally. Samples of urine after equilibration time were analyzed by mass spectrometer in duplicate, and the total body water was calculated according to the proposal of Schloerb et al. (1950). Fat-free mass was calculated from the results of total body water according to the formula proposed by Pace and Rathbun (1945). Body fat was obtained by subtracting fat-free mass from body weight. Total body solids or dry body weight was calculated by subtracting total body water from body weight. Fat-free solids were determined by subtracting body fat from total body solids.

Results

Table 13-3 presents means and standard deviations (SD) of ages, heights, and weights of the five groups of athletes. The results indicate that there was no significant difference in the age or height of the athletes. However, the weight of the football players was found to be significantly different from the mean weights of the other four groups of athletes.

Table 13-3 Ages, Heights, and Weights of Athletes

Athletic Group	Number	Means ± SD		
		Age, years	Height, cm	Weight, kg
Swimmers	7	20.6 ± 0.92	182.9 ± 5.02	78.9 ± 7.22
Track-and-field men	9	21.3 ± 1.08	180.6 ± 6.62	71.6 ± 12.73
Gymnasts	7	20.3 ± 0.86	178.5 ± 5.35	69.2 ± 5.37
Baseball players	10	20.8 ± 0.92	182.7 ± 6.65	83.3 ± 11.41
Football players	16	20.3 ± 0.92	184.9 ± 4.70	96.4 ± 10.84

SOURCE: L. P. Novak, R. E. Hyatt, and J. F. Alexander: Body composition and physiologic function of athletes. *J. Amer. Med. Assoc.*, **205**:764–770 (1968).

Table 13-4 presents means and standard deviations of total body water, body fat, and fat-free mass. The absolute mean values of total body water of football players (60.46 liters) and of swimmers (55.23 liters) differ significantly from the means for the other three groups. However, when total body water was expressed in percentage of body weight, the baseball and football players had the lowest mean values, namely, 62.82% and 63.08%, respectively. On the other hand, relative values of total body water of swimmers, track-and-field men, and gymnasts reached similar percentages, that is, 69.58%, 70.52%, and 69.82%, respectively, and were significantly different from the values for the other two groups.

Table 13-4 Total Body Water, Body Fat, and Fat-Free Mass of Athletes

Athletic Group	Number	Total Body Water		Body Fat		Fat-Free Mass	
		L	%	Kg	%	Kg	%
Swimmers	7	55.23	69.58	3.92	4.95	74.97	95.05
		± 5.91	± 3.25	± 3.61	± 4.48	± 7.48	± 4.48
Track-and-field men	9	50.04	70.52	3.29	3.66	68.36	96.34
		± 5.64	± 5.18	± 7.14	± 7.08	± 7.86	± 7.08
Gymnasts	7	48.23	69.82	3.33	4.63	65.88	95.37
		± 2.46	± 2.45	± 2.63	± 3.35	± 3.37	± 3.35
Baseball players	10	51.30	62.82	12.24	14.18	70.08	85.82
		± 4.63	± 4.92	± 6.69	± 6.72	± 6.33	± 6.72
Football players	16	60.46	63.08	13.84	13.83	82.58	86.17
		± 4.51	± 4.90	± 8.05	± 6.70	± 6.17	± 6.70

SOURCE: L. P. Novak, R. E. Hyatt, and J. F. Alexander: Body composition and physiologic function of athletes. *J. Amer. Med. Assoc.*, **205**:764–770 (1968).

Interestingly, the high level of hydration of the swimmers, track-and-field men, and gymnasts signifies values close to the assumed hydration of fat-free mass which ought to be 73.2%. These three groups of athletes were extremely lean, which points out clearly the metabolic demands of the three activities, which do not seem to allow any accumulation of body fat.

Table 13-5 shows means and standard deviations (SD) of total body solids and fat-free solids of athletes. The mean absolute values of total body solids were distributed according to the weight of athletes. The football and base-ball players had significantly higher mean values than those of the other three groups of athletes. However, even in percentage of body weight, the football and baseball players had significantly higher amounts of body solids, more than 37% as compared to 30% found in the swimmers, track men, and gymnasts. The interpretation of these figures indicates that the first two groups included athletes with large amounts of fat. This was well demonstrated when means of fat-free solids were taken into consideration. In absolute terms there were no significant differences among the means of the various groups. However, a slightly clearer picture appeared when the means

Table 13-5 Total Body Solids and Fat-Free Solids of Athletes

Athletic Group	Number	Total Body Solids		Fat-Free Solids	
		Kg	%	Kg	%
Swimmers	7	24.01 ± 3.55	30.41 ± 3.28	20.09 ± 2.00	25.46 ± 1.20
Track-and-field men	9	21.61 ± 8.31	29.47 ± 5.18	18.32 ± 2.06	25.82 ± 1.90
Gymnasts	7	20.99 ± 3.25	30.18 ± 2.45	17.65 ± 0.90	25.55 ± 0.90
Baseball players	10	31.02 ± 7.73	37.18 ± 4.92	18.78 ± 1.69	23.00 ± 1.80
Football players	16	35.96 ± 8.45	37.07 ± 4.95	32.13 ± 1.65	23.08 ± 1.80

SOURCE: L. P. Novak, R. E. Hyatt, and J. F. Alexander: Body composition and physiologic function of athletes. *J. Amer. Med. Assoc.*, **205**:764–770 (1968).

of fat-free solids expressed in percentage of body weight were studied. In these terms, the baseball and football players had relatively less fat-free solids (23%), whereas swimmers, track-and-field men, and gymnasts registered a higher percentage (25%). This difference, however, did not reach statistical significance.

Conclusions

From the results of this study it can be concluded that habitual participation in various physical activities molds the body composition. Since total body water is primarily confined to lean tissues, estimates of total body water also provide information about fat-free mass or fat-free solids. Total body water showed that swimmers, track-and-field men, and gymnasts had significantly higher percentages when compared with baseball and football players. Similarly, the fat-free mass and fat-free solids of the first three groups mentioned were greater than those of the latter two groups.

Total Body Potassium and Physical Activity

In 1902 Rubner called attention to "active tissue mass" as the fundamental base line for determinations of body heat production. Measurements of actively metabolizing tissues of the body had to wait several decades for the development of methods that would allow estimation of cellular mass. The new concept of "body cell mass" proposed by Moore et al. (1963) encompasses the totality of cellular material of the body. It includes the cellular population of all viscera and skeletal muscles as well as the few cells of tendon, dermis, skeleton, fascia, cartilage, collagen, elastin, and adipose tissue. Body cell mass can be estimated well from the measurements of total body potassium content because 98% of the potassium is inside the cells. Because of the availability of a sensitive instrument, the whole-body counter, a small percentage of the potassium which naturally is radioactive can be detected with accuracy and, thus, the amount of total body potassium of an individual can be determined.

This investigation was concerned with comparisons of total body potassium, body cell mass, and maximal oxygen consumption of active middle-aged women versus sedentary women.

Subjects and Methods

The subjects for the study were 13 women who participated in a voluntary YWCA swimming contest, covering 30–50 miles intermittently during a period of 3 months. The control group of 13 women matched for age were not participating in any physical activities aside from their household or office duties.

Total body potassium was determined by whole-body counting of ^{40}K, naturally radioactive potassium which emits γ-rays of 1.46 Mev and which represents 0.0119% of the stable potassium pool consisting of ^{39}K (93.08%) and ^{41}K (6.91%). Two 5-min counts were averaged for each subject, corrected to counts per second, and corrected for background. Further correction was made for the efficiency of the counter by using a ratio of height/weight.

The body cell mass was calculated from total body potassium according to the formula proposed by Moore et al. (1963) and the fat-free mass according to the formula of Forbes and Hursh (1963). Maximal oxygen consumption was determined with a bicycle ergometer, which was pedaled at 50 cycles/sec to a metronome eliciting audio and visual stimuli. The methodology of ICSPFT for obtaining maximal oxygen consumption was followed.

Results

Table 13-6 presents means and standard deviations (SD) of heights, weights, and total body potassium of both groups. Though the active group of women was taller by 4.5 cm and heavier by 4.4 kg, no statistical difference between the means was obtained. Total body potassium in absolute values, however, was greater by 440 mEq. This difference between the means of the two groups was highly significant in favor of the active women. When total body potassium was expressed in milliequivalents per kilogram of body weight, the difference between the mean 45.9 mEq/kg of the active group and the mean 42.1 mEq/kg of the inactive group was also statistically significant.

Table 13-6 Heights, Weights, and Total Body Potassium of Active and Inactive Women

| | | | | | Means ± SD | |
Group	Age, years	Number	Height, cm	Weight, kg	Total Body mEq	Potassium mEq/kg
Active	41.0 ± 10.5	13	166.6 ± 6.0	63.5 ± 7.6	2905*** ± 411.5	45.9* ± 5.3
Inactive	42.8 ± 7.7	13	162.1 ± 7.7	59.1 ± 9.4	2465 ± 281.8	42.1 ± 3.8

* Significant at 0.05 level.
*** Significant at 0.001 level.

Table 13-7 presents data on body composition with means and standard deviations (SD). It is evident that sustained swimming had an effect on the body composition of active women in reducing, to a degree, the amount of fat both in absolute and relative values, even though the active women had higher weight. The fat-free mass reached statistical significance in favor of the active group when their absolute value of 47.3 kg was compared to 41.6 kg for the inactive women. Also, the slightly higher percentage of fat-free mass in active women, namely, 74.9% as compared to 71.1%, indicated that they had leaner bodies, but the difference did not reach statistical significance.

Table 13-7 Fat, Fat-Free Mass, and Body Cell Mass of Active and Inactive Women

| | | Means ± SD | | | | | |
| | | Body Fat | | Fat-Free Mass | | Body Cell Mass | |
Group	Number	Kg	%	Kg	%	Kg	%
Active	13	16.2±6.7	25.1±8.6	47.3**±6.0	74.9±8.6	24.2***±8.4	38.2*±4.4
Inactive	13	17.5±7.0	28.9±7.4	41.6±4.9	71.1±7.4	20.5±2.4	35.1±3.1

* Significant at 0.05 level.
** Significant at 0.01 level.
*** Significant at 0.001 level.

When body cell mass expressed in absolute and relative values was taken into consideration, the means of the active group, 24.2 kg and 38.2%, were both significantly higher when compared to 20.5 kg and 35.1% for the inactive group of women.

Table 13-8 presents means and standard deviations (SD) of maximal oxygen consumption elicited on a bicycle ergometer. The active women achieved significantly higher maximal oxygen consumption in absolute terms or, when expressed per square meter of surface, per kilogram of body weight or per kilogram of cellular mass. Moreover, these differences were obtained under a significantly greater workload. When these results are compared to the tables of Åstrand (1960) for the evaluation of aerobic capacity based on five scales for women, it is satisfying to note that the active women would fall in the average classification of aerobic capacity according to their age (range, 32–40 ml/kg), whereas the inactive group would qualify for inclusion in the lowest group of aerobic capacity according to their age (range, ≤ 25 ml/kg). These data indicate that a reasonably good degree of cardiovascular fitness can be maintained in middle-aged women with intermittent swimming three or four times a week. On the other hand, sedentary life seems to diminish the cardiovascular potential.

Table 13-8 Maximal Oxygen Consumption of Active and Inactive Women

| | | | | Means ± SD | | | |
| | | | | Maximal Oxygen, ml/min | | | |
Group	Number	Rate, cycles/min	Workload, kpm	Total	Surface Area, m²	Body weight, kg	Cell Mass, kg
Active	13	50	669**	2064***	1206***	32.6***	85.7***
			± 99	± 330	± 170	± 4.9	± 11.4
Inactive	13	50	542	1472	907	25.1	71.6
			± 130	± 280	± 147	± 4.1	± 10.2

** Significant at 0.01 level.
*** Significant at 0.001 level.

Conclusions

According to the results of this study, it seems appropriate to say that habitual swimming had a profound effect on body composition and cardiovascular performance of middle-aged women. Compared to inactive females matched for age, the active women had significantly higher total body potassium, fat-free mass, body cell mass, and maximal oxygen consumption than the inactive women.

REFERENCES

Astrand, I.: Aerobic work capacity in men and women with special reference to age. *Acta Physiol. Scand.*, 49 Suppl., **169**:1–92 (1960).

Behnke, A. R. and W. A. Taylor: Some aspects of recent findings pertaining to the body composition of athletes, obese individuals and patients. United States Naval Radiological Defense Laboratory, Report No. USNRDL-TR 339, San Francisco, 1959.

Behnke, A. R., Jr., B. G. Feen, and W. C. Welham: The specific gravity of healthy men: body weight ÷ volume as an index of obesity. *J. Amer. Med. Assoc.*, **118**:495–498 (1942).

Brožek, J.: Physical activity and body composition. *Arh. Hig. Rada. Toksikol.*, **5**:193–212 (1954).

Buskirk, E., and H. L. Taylor: Maximal oxygen intake and its relation to body composition, with special reference to chronic physical activity and obesity. *J. Appl. Physiol.*, **11**:72–78 (1957).

Forbes, G. B., and J. B. Hursh: Age and sex trends in lean body mass calculated from K40 measurements: with a note on the theoretical basis for the procedure. *Ann. N.Y. Acad. Sci.*, **110**:255–263 (1963).

Keys, A., and J. Brožek: Body fat in adult man. *Physiol. Rev.*, **33**:245–325 (1953).

Moore, F. D., K. H. Olesen, J. D. McMurrey, H. V. Parker, M. R. Ball, and C. M. Boyden: *The Body Cell Mass and Its Supporting Environment: Body Composition in Health and Disease.* Philadelphia, W. B. Saunders, 1963.

Novak, L. P.: Physical activity and body composition of adolescent boys. *J. Amer. Med. Assoc.*, **197**:891–893 (1966).

Novak, L. P., R. E. Hyatt, and J. F. Alexander: Body composition and physiologic function of athletes. *J. Amer. Med. Assoc.*, **205**:764–770 (1968).

Pace, N., and E. N. Rathbun: Studies on body composition. III. The body water and chemically combined nitrogen content in relation to fat content. *J. Biol. Chem.*, **158**:685–691 (1945).

Pařízková, J.: Izměněnia aktivnoj massy i reservnovo zhira u gimnastov pri trenirovke rozlitchnoy intensivnosti. *Teor. Prakt. Fizitcheskoy Kultury Sporta*, **25**:37–40 (1962).

Pascale, L. R., I. L. Faller, and E. E. Bond: Report of changes in body composition of soldiers during paratrooper training. United States Army Medical Nutrition Laboratory Project No. 6-60-11-019, Report No. 156, Denver, 1955, pp. 1–14.

Rubner, M.: *Die Gesetze des Energieverbrauchs bei der Ernährung.* Leipzig, Franz Deuticke, 1902.

Schloerb, P. R., B. J. Friis-Hansen, I. S. Edelman, A. K. Solomon, and F. D. Moore: The measurement of total body water in the human subject by deuterium oxide dilution: with a consideration of the dynamics of deuterium distribution. *J. Clin. Invest.*, **29**:1296–1310 (1950).

Body Type and Performance

14

MARCEL HEBBELINCK
Vrije Universiteit Brussel
Brussels, Belgium

WILLIAM D. ROSS
Simon Fraser University
Burnaby, Canada

Body Type Classification

Competitive sport, particularly at the championship level, appears to have definite physique requisites. Kohlraush (1929), Cureton (1947, 1951), Correnti and Zauli (1964), Tanner (1964), Azuma (1964), Tittel (1965), Hirata (1966), Ziemilska (1970), Carter (1970), and others have demonstrated the importance of size and shape parameters in identifying those who excel at certain sports.

From a purely geometric point of view, if shape and composition are similar for any given linear measurement, all lengths, widths, circumferences and thicknesses would be a linear function; all areas would be a function raised to the second power and all volumes a function raised to the third power. These observations are not recent. In fact, about three hundred years ago Galileo commented on size relationships in animal forms and in 1729 Swift immortalized his perceptions in *Gulliver's Travels*. Thompson (1917), Huxley (1932), Brody (1945), and Hill (1950) have also elaborated and speculated on size, shape, and performance relationships.

In recent years, with a biological rationale and experimental evidence that indicates strength or muscular force is directly related to area of cross section of muscle tissue, it follows that, dimensionally, force is a function of the square of any criterion linear dimension (L), such as stature. As discussed by Georgian (1964), von Döbeln (1956), and Astrand and Rodahl (1970), the basic quantities of length, mass, and time and their derivatives may be expressed in physiological terms, where length has the dimension L, mass L^3

and time L. These relationships furnish theoretical models to observe growth, training, and performance phenomena.

When reviewing weight lifting records, Karpovich and Sinning (1971) found the theoretical relationship between strength (L^2) and body weight (L^3), (that is, where strength is some function raised to the power 0.6667) was reflected in the calculated formula $\log W = 1.5123 + 0.6748 \log BW$, when ($W$) was weight lifted and (BW) was body weight. The weight lifting champions, we assume, had relatively the same shape and composition, similar skill, and their training approached optimal levels. Ekblom (1969) used longitudinal stature curves and theoretical relationships with size dimensions L, L^2, and L^3 to observe departure from the expected geometrical increase with growth in order to evaluate training effects and infer hormonal activity.

The implicit assumption in using a theoretical size relationship for comparative purposes is that the human design is similar when viewed cross sectionally or longitudinally. However, although the mean conformation may be relatively stable, there are vast individual differences at every age. Scientists have been aware of individual physique differences for centuries. Martin and Saller (1957) present a table listing 38 physique classification systems starting with Hippocrates. These systems, based on a variety of individual and group measurements or rating techniques, were evolved to identify different body types or classify structural dominance.

Essentially what these studies have in common is the attempt to provide classifications of body form or some convenient way to give a "gestalt" or overall impression of the body type in order to relate this to other human characteristics and expressions. The aim in many of these systems has been to dissociate "size" from "shape" or to do conceptually what Hirata (1968) does when he projects photographs so that the length of the image from the top of the head to the soles of the feet is the same for all subjects. Sheldon et al. (1940, 1954), influenced by the work of the Italians de Giovanni (1904) and Viola (1932) and the German Kretschmer (1922), evolved an elaborate and ingenious system of physique analysis that included a taxonomy which gave a lexicon of physique terminology to the public domain. Strictly speaking, a somatotype, by Sheldonian definition is "... a quantification of the three primary components determining the morphological structure of the individual expressed as a series of three numerals, the first referring to endomorphy, the second to mesomorphy and the third to ectomorphy."

In popular parlance endomorphy, or the first component, may be interpreted as relative fatness; mesomorphy, or the second component, as the level of musculoskeletal development for an individual's height or relative lean body mass; and ectomorphy, or the third component, as the relative linearity, ponderosity, or "stretched-outness." A subject's physique may be dominant in a single component, and such a subject could be classified as an endomorph, mesomorph, or ectomorph. If there is a secondary dominance the physique might be classified as an endomorphic-mesomorph or endo-mesomorph, which indicates primary dominance of mesomorphy with a secondary dominance of endomorphy. Physiques having no single dominance may be described as having "balanced" components such as balanced mesomorphy and ectomorphy.

Sheldon's original terminology, concepts, and methodology have been widely adapted as discussed by Carter (1970, 1971), who points out the importance in making comparisons of taking into account the methods of rating because there are often pronounced differences among methods.

Classification Problems in the Sport Sciences

A basic dilemma exists in the sport sciences. From a biogenetic point of view, the ideal system of physique classification is one that identifies the basic morphological pattern or genotype. The Sheldonian concept of the somatotype as a "trajectory or pathway along which a subject is destined to travel under average conditions of nutrition and in the absence of major illness" is both attractive and useful. Parnell (1954, 1958), Damon et al. (1962), and Peterson (1967) have prescribed methodology that attempts to minimize the effect of age on the body type classification. Viewed strictly from an environmentalist point of view rather than genetically, "the present mor-phological characteristics" are of overriding importance. According to Carter and Heath (1971), citing fourteen supportive studies, the overwhelming evidence is in the direction of plasticity and inconstancy of physique values. For them, and perhaps for kinesiologists, physical educators, and coaches, the ideal system of physique classification should reflect growth and training changes. Indeed, unlike the criterion of "constancy" found in the Sheldonian systems, the more sensitive the physique rating system is to changing shape and composition the greater its applicability to fitness and performance studies.

The system of physique rating advocated by Heath and Carter (1967) provides for ratings of three components on open-ended scales and may be used for both sexes. Their criterion is essentially an arbitrary photoscopic rating of the outer configuration which may be derived anthropometrically by their procedures as adapted and indicated in the tables and figures shown in this chapter.

Similar to other modified somatotype methods (Hooten, 1951; Parnell, 1954), the Heath-Carter third component is related to the reciprocal of the ponderal index (*RPI*) or the quotient obtained when height in inches is divided by the cube root of weight in pounds. Actually any ratios of height and weight adjusted to the same dimension might have been used. Although

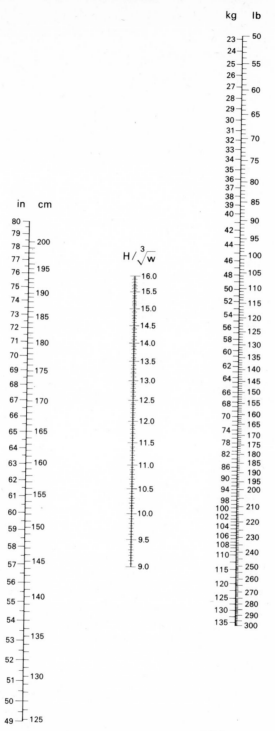

Figure 14-1. Nomogram of *RPI* ($H/\sqrt[3]{W}$) for children and adults.

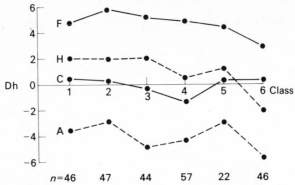

Figure 14-2. Deviation from height for each of six grade levels of girls from a single school in Belgian performance and talent project using an adult model as prototype. Bone widths and girths relative to height. *F*, Femur width; *C*, calf girth uncorrected for fat; *H*, humerus width; *A*, flexed and tensed arm girth uncorrected for fat. Deviations according to Heath-Carter somatotype scales.

a nomogram as shown in Figure 14-1 or a computer table* may be used to convert metric measures to the *RPI* which is in English units, it might have been simpler to use a metric index such as that proposed by McCloy (1936) and Hirata (1968) where the cube root of weight in kilograms is divided by stature in centimeters and the quotient is multiplied by 10^3. Nevertheless, the same argument for the dimensional reasonableness of Hirata's *F*-index, as he terms it, is appropriate for the *RPI* adopted by Sheldon and many of the modifiers of his methodology.

In obtaining the second component by anthropometric procedure, Heath and Carter essentially use the same approach as that used in the M.4 deviation chart method devised by Parnell (1958). This approach involved determining deviations of girths and bone widths from stature values. Since girths, widths, and stature are in the same dimension, the procedure does not violate geometric principles. Parnell, faithful to the genetic point of view, makes an age correction to adjust for the fat tissue reflected in the girth measurement, which is estimated from the sum of the skinfold measures. Heath and Carter, disregarding age, simply subtract triceps and medial calf skinfold thicknesses from arm and calf girths, respectively. Although the corrections in both procedures are rational, they may not be optimal.

Another as yet not fully appreciated point of concern is the differential growth rates of bone and muscle tissue, relative to height in children. When an adult model is used as a prototype, bone widths in the upper and lower

---

* When height (*H*) is in centimeters and weight (*W*) is in kilograms, the *RPI* or height in inches divided by cube root of weight in pounds can be obtained by multiplying H_{cm} by 0.3937 $(2.205\ W_{kg})^{-1/3}$.

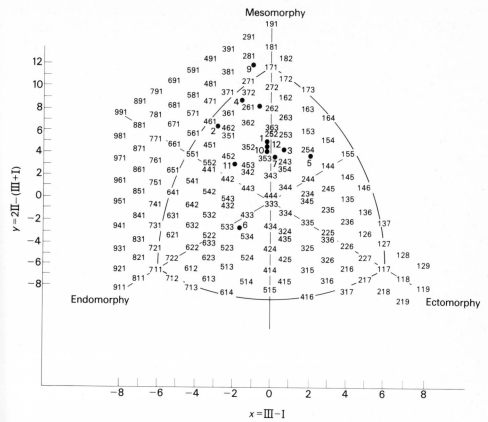

Figure 14-3. Mean somatotype of male champion athletes (Carter, 1970) assembled and plotted on the somatochart. 1. Cureton's champion swimmers; 2. San Diego State football players; 3. Cureton's track-and-field champions; 4. 1960 Olympic track-and-field athletes (throwers); 5. Olympic distance runners; 6. United States "nonathletes;" 7. University of Iowa basketball players; 8. British Empire Games wrestlers; 9. British Empire Games weightlifters; 10. British Empire Games boxers; 11. San Diego State golfers; 12. San Diego State rowers.

extremities tend to have positive deviations whereas the respective girths tend to have negative deviations. This phenomenon is illustrated in Figure 14-2, which shows the deviations from height for each of six grade levels of girls from a single school taken from the Belgian national study on performance and talent (Hebbelinck and Cliquet, 1970). The mean of four deviations from height values on the Heath-Carter scales, in effect, serves only as a general musculoskeletal robustness indicator. In other words, the same mesomorphic estimate in children and adults disregards the differing contribution of bone and muscle in its derivation. This apparent preponderance of bone to muscle relative to height in children may, in part, explain the lower relative maximal aerobic power in children. As discussed by Astrand and Rodahl (1970), this was calculated by Asmussen and Heeböll-Nielsen (1956) to be proportional to $h^{2.896}$ rather than theoretically L^2, as one would expect from a dimensional analysis and conversion of quantities into physiological equivalents as previously discussed.

In both Parnell and the Heath-Carter procedures, the first component or relative fatness-leaness is indicated by the sum of the three skinfold

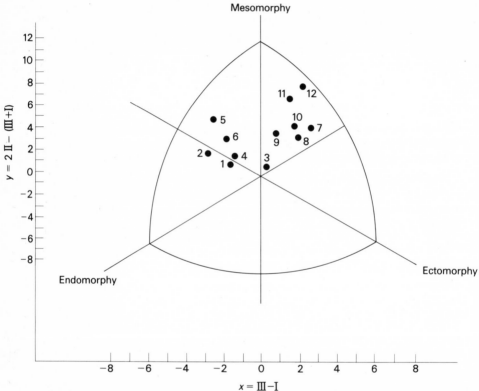

Figure 14-4. Mean somatotype of female champion athletes (Carter, 1970), early and late maturing 12-year-old boys (Borms, 1972), young skiers with first component corrected and uncorrected for height (Ross and Day, 1972), and a champion gymnast compared to Mexico Olympic gymnasts (Carter and Hebbelinck, 1972). 1. United States professional golfers (F); 2. San Diego amateur golfers (F); 3. San Diego track and field (F); 4. U.S.S.R. basketball players (F); 5. U.S.S.R. gymnasts (F); 6. New Zealand physical education majors (F); 7. Young skiers uncorrected first component; 8. Young skiers height-corrected first component; 9. Early maturing 12-year-old boys; 10. Late maturing 12-year-old boys; 11. A champion gymnast (example in text); 12. Mexico Olympic gymnasts.

measures. Parnell adjusts for age, whereas Heath-Carter make no correction because, by intent, they are concerned only with the "present morphological conformation." Dimensionally, a skinfold thickness, being the linear distance between the pressure plates of skinfold calipers has the dimension of (L). Theoretically, if shape and composition were constant throughout the entire age and size range, it would be appropriate to make an adjustment for size. The simplest procedure would be to select some arbitrary height standard for adult men and women such as 170.18 cm (5 ft 7 in.) and to adjust the skinfold sums proportionally to this value. In a sample of young skiers aged 8–14 studied by Ross and Day (1972) and illustrated in Figure 14-4, this height correction had the effect of increasing the value of the first component estimate by half a unit; however, this did not appreciably change the component dominances for individuals in this particular sample. In adult samples, innumerable cross-sectional studies using anthropometric variables to predict fat criteria have shown height not to be highly related, and therefore in adults a height correction is probably unjustified.

Subject to some conceptual limitations, the Heath-Carter system of somatotyping by anthropometric procedure is attractive for a number of reasons: (1) it represents a phenotype or present morphological configuration; (2) it has an open-ended scale to accommodate extreme types; (3) it yields a reasonably close estimate of photoscopic ratings as demonstrated by Heath and Carter (1967); and (4) it has been used extensively on samples of sports men and women as reviewed by Carter (1970) and illustrated with ancillary data in Figures 14-3 and 14-4.

Demonstration of Classification Procedures

To demonstrate the procedures we selected a world class gymnast whose basic anthropometric data is shown in Figure 14-5. The form is designed for computer use and contains data spaces for the complete analysis according to Heath-Carter (1967). The first eight spaces for Items 1, 2, and 3 are for subject identification, followed by Item 4 for date of observation and Item 5 for the subject's date of birth expressed as decimal fractions of a year (Appendix A, page 537). The skinfolds are obtained with Harpenden calipers using a repeated series on the right side with recorded values derived by the procedure described in the form footnote.

Right and left epicondylar humerus and femur widths are obtained by using spreading calipers or a vernier scale modified bone caliper as described by Carter (1967); the largest of each width obtained is recorded. Flexed and contracted arm and standing calf girths at the greatest circumferences are obtained, and the largest measurement of each also is recorded. As shown in Items 15 and 16, the procedure makes an adjustment for fat in the arm and calf girths by subtraction of triceps and medial calf skinfolds, which are converted to centimeters from values obtained for Items 8 and 11 which are expressed in millimeters. A simplified anthropometric procedure for cross-sectional studies would be to obtain height and weight, take one measure of each skinfold, and measure only the right side for humerus and femur widths and for flexed-contracted arm and standing calf girth.

To obtain the first component, the sum of the triceps, subscapular, and

ANTHROPOMETRIC DATA FORM (Heath - Carter somatotype)

NO.
01. Subject _World class gymnast_   1 | 0 | 0 | 4 |
              (LAST NAME)   (GIVEN NAMES)

02. Project _Aalst gymnastic show 1971_   4 | 0 | 3 |

03. Identity _Card 1, male 1, anthropometrist 1_   6 | 1 | 1 | 1 |

04. Date of observations ___ | 2 | 8 | day | 1 | 1 | mo | 7 | 1 | year ___   9 | 7 | 1·9 | 0 | 7 |

05. Date of birth ___ | 1 | 9 | day | 0 | 2 | mo | 4 | 4 | year ___   14 | 4 | 4·1 | 3 | 4 |

06. Body weight | 0 | 6 | / | 0 | kg - correction of | · | kg ___   19 | 0 | 6 | 1·0 |

07. Height (cm) _____   23 | 1 | 6 | 6·9 |

08. Triceps skinfold (mm) ___ | 0 | 5·0 | | 0 | 5·0 | | · | 27 | 0 | 5·0 |

09. Subscapular skinfold (mm) ___ | 0 | 5·9 | | 0 | 5·9 | | · | 30 | 0 | 3·9 |

10. Suprailiac skinfold (mm) ___ | 0 | 3·7 | | 0 | 3·7 | | · | 33 | 0 | 3·7 |

11. Medial calf skinfold (mm) ___ | 0 | 3·5 | | 0 | 3·5 | | · | 36 | 0 | 3·5 |

12. Epicondylar humerus width (cm) ___ R | 0 | 7·0 | 9 | L | 0 | 7·0 | 9 | 39 | 0 | 7·0 | 9 |

13. Epicondylar femur width (cm) ___ R | 0 | 9·9 | 6 | L | 0 | 9·8 | 5 | 43 | 0 | 9·9 | 6 |

14. Flexed and tensed arm girth (cm) ___ L | 3 | 1·2 | R | 3 | 2·2 | 47 | 3 | 2·2 |

15. Standing calf girth (cm) ___ L | 3 | 2·2 | R | 3 | 2·6 | 50 | 3 | 2·6 |

16. Arm girth corrected for fat ___ no. 14 - (no. 8/10) ___   53 | 3 | 1·7 |

17. Calf girth corrected for fat ___ no. 15 - (no. 11/10) ___   56 | 3 | 2·2 |

18. Sum of three skinfolds ___ no. 8, 9, 10 ___   59 | 0 | 1 | 4·6 |

19. 1st component (endomorphy) ___   63 | 0 | 1·0 |

20. 2nd component (mesomorphy) ___   66 | 0 | 5·5 |

21. 3rd component (ectomorphy) ___   69 | 0 | 2·5 |

22. 1st component when corrected ___ no. 18 (170.18/no. 7) ___   72 | 0 | 1·0 |

NOTE: Series 8 to 11 is repeated. If difference between first and second measure of any item is less than 5% of first measure, record mean value of the two measures. If difference is greater than 5% take a third measure and record mean of closest pair. Items 12 to 15, record largest of left and right sides.

Figure 14-5. Anthropometric data form (Heath-Carter somatotype).

suprailiac skinfolds is read directly from Table 14-1. If a height correction is used, however, the sum of the skinfolds must be multiplied by an arbitrary height standard (170.18 cm), divided by obtained height, and the result used to enter the table to predict the first component. Since no correction was necessary in our example, the sum of the three skinfolds of 13.1 mm was used to enter the table to yield a first component rating of 1.0.

Table 14-1 Heath-Carter Somatotype
First Component (Endomorphy)

Sum of Skinfolds, mm	Rating
7.0–10.9	$\frac{1}{2}$
11.0–14.9	1
15.0–18.9	$1\frac{1}{2}$
19.0–22.9	2
23.0–26.9	$2\frac{1}{2}$
27.0–31.2	3
31.3–35.8	$3\frac{1}{2}$
35.9–40.7	4
40.8–46.2	$4\frac{1}{2}$
46.3–52.2	5
52.3–58.7	$5\frac{1}{2}$
58.8–65.7	6
65.8–73.2	$6\frac{1}{2}$
73.3–81.2	7
81.3–89.7	$7\frac{1}{2}$
89.8–98.9	8
99.0–108.9	$8\frac{1}{2}$
109.0–119.7	9
119.8–131.2	$9\frac{1}{2}$
131.3–143.7	10
143.8–157.2	$10\frac{1}{2}$
157.3–171.9	11
172.0–187.9	$11\frac{1}{2}$
188.0–204.0	12

The second component is obtained from Table 14-2 by finding the average deviations or average number of rows above or below the height row that the recorded epicondylar widths (Items 12, humerus, and 13, femur) and recorded girths corrected for fat (Items 18, arm, and 17, calf) are. Deviations above the height row are positive and below the row are negative. If the algebraic sum of the deviations is zero, or if there were no deviations from the height row, the subject is rated a 4 in the second component. The formula for the rating (which is $4 + \frac{1}{8}D$) is the algebraic sum of the positive and negative deviations from the height row. The subject's obtained height value of 166.9 cm was closest to the row 67.0 and 170.2. The algebraic sum of the deviations as shown by the underlined values in the table was 11. This

Table 14-2 Heath-Carter Somatotype Second Component (Mesomorphy)

Height, in.	Height, cm	Humerus Width	Femur Width	F. Biceps-Tri	Calf-M.C.
110.5	280.7	10.59	15.10	48.3	56.5
109.0	276.9	10.44	14.90	47.6	55.7
107.5	273.0	10.30	14.69	46.9	55.0
106.0	269.2	10.15	14.48	46.3	54.2
104.5	265.4	10.01	14.27	45.6	53.4
103.0	261.6	9.86	14.06	44.9	52.6
101.5	257.8	9.71	13.86	44.3	51.9
100.0	254.0	9.57	13.65	43.6	51.1
98.5	250.2	9.42	13.44	43.0	50.3
97.0	246.4	9.28	13.23	42.3	49.5
95.5	242.6	9.13	13.03	41.6	48.7
94.0	238.8	8.99	12.82	41.0	48.0
92.5	234.9	8.84	12.61	40.3	47.2
91.0	231.1	8.69	12.40	39.6	46.4
89.5	227.3	8.55	12.19	39.0	45.6
88.0	223.5	8.40	11.99	38.3	44.9
86.5	219.7	8.26	11.78	37.6	44.1
85.0	215.9	8.11	11.57	37.0	43.3
83.5	212.1	7.97	11.36	36.3	42.5
82.0	208.3	7.82	11.15	35.6	41.7
80.5	204.5	7.67	10.95	35.0	41.0
79.0	200.7	7.53	10.74	34.3	40.2
77.5	196.8	7.38	10.53	33.7	39.4
76.0	193.0	7.24	10.32	33.0	38.6
74.5	189.2	<u>7.09</u> *7.09*	10.12	32.3	37.9
73.0	185.4	6.95	<u>9.91</u> *9.96*	<u>31.7</u> *31.7*	37.1
71.5	181.6	6.80	9.70	31.0	36.3
70.0	177.8	6.65 *+5*	9.49 *+4*	30.3 *+4*	35.5
68.5	174.0	6.51	9.28	29.7	34.7
67.0	<u>170.2</u> *166.9*	6.36........	9.08........	29.0........	34.0
65.5	166.4	6.22	8.87	28.3	33.2
64.0	162.6	6.07	8.66	27.7	<u>32.4</u> *32.6*
62.5	158.7	5.93	8.45	27.0	31.6
61.0	154.9	5.78	8.24	26.3	30.9 <u>*−2*</u>
59.5	151.1	5.63	8.04	25.7	30.1
58.0	147.3	5.49	7.83	25.0	29.3
56.5	143.5	5.34	7.62	24.4	28.5
55.0	139.7	5.20	7.41	23.7	27.7
53.5	135.9	5.05	7.21	23.0	27.0
52.0	132.1	4.91	7.00	22.4	26.2
50.5	128.3	4.76	6.79	21.7	25.4
49.0	124.5	4.61	6.58	21.0	24.6
47.5	120.6	4.47	6.37	20.4	23.9
46.0	116.8	4.32	6.17	19.7	23.1
44.5	113.0	4.18	5.96	19.0	22.3
43.0	109.2	4.03	5.75	18.4	21.5
41.5	105.4	3.89	5.54	17.7	20.7
40.0	101.6	3.74	5.33	17.0	20.0
38.5	97.8	3.59	5.13	16.4	19.2
37.0	94.0	3.45	4.92	15.7	18.4
35.5	90.2	3.30	4.71	15.1	17.6
34.0	86.4	3.16	4.50	14.4	16.9
32.5	82.5	3.01	4.30	13.7	16.1
31.0	78.7	2.87	4.09	13.1	15.3

yielded a mesomorphy rating of $4 + (\frac{1}{8} \times 11) = 5\frac{3}{8}$ which was expressed to the nearest half unit as $5\frac{1}{2}$ by interpolation from the actual height value.

The third component rating is obtained from Table 14-3 by using the calculated *RPI* as previously discussed. This was 12.82 for the subject under consideration, which yielded a third component or ectomorphy rating of $2\frac{1}{2}$. Thus, the overall Heath-Carter anthropometric somatotype rating of the gymnast was $1-5\frac{1}{2}-2\frac{1}{2}$. According to the Sheldonian schema he is designated as an ectomorphic mesomorph or ectomesomorph. He was primarily a mesomorph with a secondary dominance in ectomorphy and was similar to the Mexican Olympic gymnasts who, according to Carter and Hebbelinck (1972), had a mean somatotype 1.4–5.9–2.4.

Table 14-3 Heath-Carter Somatotype Third Component (Ectomorphy)

$H/\sqrt[3]{W}$	Rating
up to 11.99	$\frac{1}{2}$
12.00–12.32	1
12.33–12.53	$1\frac{1}{2}$
12.54–12.74	2
12.75–12.95	$2\frac{1}{2}$
12.96–13.15	3
13.16–13.36	$3\frac{1}{2}$
13.37–13.56	4
13.57–13.77	$4\frac{1}{2}$
13.78–13.98	5
13.99–14.19	$5\frac{1}{2}$
14.20–14.39	6
14.40–14.59	$6\frac{1}{2}$
14.60–14.80	7
14.81–15.01	$7\frac{1}{2}$
15.02–15.22	8
15.23–15.42	$8\frac{1}{2}$
15.43–15.63	9

The subject may be located by X, Y coordinates on the modified Heath-Carter somatochart shown in Figure 14-3, where $X = III - I$, and $Y = 2II - (I + III)$ or, as illustrated from our subject's somatotype of $1-5\frac{1}{2}-2\frac{1}{2}$, $X = 2\frac{1}{2} - 1 = 1\frac{1}{2}$ and $Y = 2(5\frac{1}{2}) - (1 + 2\frac{1}{2}) = 7\frac{1}{2}$.

Relationship Between Body Type and Performance

The Heath-Carter somatotype procedure provides useful information. However, at best it is a gross physique classification technique best suited to nonparametric analysis. It has special value in physical fitness studies because it distinguishes extreme types and considerable comparative data are available. Except for cases where the only estimation of structure is available from a photograph, somatotype ratings should not be used parametrically. The correlation of a single component with a performance criterion is not always meaningful, since it is the relative dominance of the components that is of prime concern. For example, in a recent study by Borms (1972) correlation techniques revealed only trivial relationships between maturity and each of the components for 12-year-old boys from the performance and talent project (Hebbelinck and Cliquet, 1970). However, when extreme groups of early and late maturers were examined nonparametrically, 18% of the early maturers were endomorphic whereas only 1% of the late maturers had this dominance. Other physique rating systems usually based on reference group or within group normative data may be designed for general or specific purposes. The essential methodology is to decide on physique parameters and provide appropriate comparative scales.

The selection of physique factors is primarily conceptual. As summarized by Oliver (1960), the traditional point of view of the French school has been to recognize four basic body types: a vertical type (cérébral or longiligne), middle type (respiratoire or medioligne), and a horizontal type (breviligne) that is usually subclassified into muscular short type (musculaire) and visceral short type (digestive). A morphogram based on five measures presented on a sigma scale may be used to aid in verbal description of body types.

One of the earliest systems that is still noted in basic textbooks is that of the French physician Manouvrier (1902) who used simple proportions of sitting height to stature and leg length to sitting height to define body types as marscoskèle, brachyskèle, and mesoskèle.

Probably the most universal descriptive physique classification is that of the German psychiatrist Kretschmer (1922) whose basic terminology of leptosome (asthenic), pyknic, and athletic types and constitutional observations still permeate current clinical thinking.

One of the first comprehensive systems of physique rating was that evolved by Viola (1932) which provided for a technique of measurement using lengths and transverse and sagittal diameters to estimate trunk, thorax, and abdominal volumes. These measurements in association with lengths of upper and lower extremities were related to reference values. For reference, Viola used a theoretical average man whose values he arrived at statistically, in much the same way as Quételet (1870) had done to distinguish brevi-, longi-, and normotypes.

Another quantitative approach was that used by Lindegard (1953), who selected physique factors a priori and used a norming procedure. Primarily on the basis of 181 cooperating male subjects from a longitudinal project in Sweden, he selected four factors that were identified as length, relative sturdiness, relative muscle, and fat. Alternate ways of deducing these four factors from anthropometric and dynamometric measures were presented along with a sigma scale for each factor for determining relative dominance. The use of such a standard deviation scaling procedure, besides having the advantage of ascribing relative dominance, may also have the advantage of relating directly to any other physique, maturity, or performance parameters.

The Medford Boys' Growth Study (Clarke, 1971) makes extensive use of such a technique utilizing Hull scores. A convenient procedure is to use modified Hull scores or standard scores with the mean set at 50 and standard deviation at 14. This procedure is employed in the Belgian national study which involves large numbers of subjects from randomly selected schools and a comprehensive array of physique, performance, social and genetic parameters (Hebbelinck and Cliquet, 1970).

In the use of reference groups for physique analysis, one of the most extensive samples is that used by Hirata (1968) who developed three indices: F, stout-lean index $(\sqrt[3]{Wt/h})10^3$; b, relative chest circumference index $(C/h)10^2$; and t, relative sitting height index $(T/h)10^2$ which he interprets by use of a chart based on a pseudo ellipse. A polar coordinate chart is also proposed as a means of observing physique status for cross sectional and longitudinal studies.

Behnke (1961b, 1963) based a physique rating system on the observation that the sum of eleven circumferences (C) was related to the square root of the ratio of body weight (W) to height (h) by a constant (K) which was approximately the same value in dissimilar groups. By obtaining proportional constants (k) for each circumference (c) for a "reference man" it is possible to derive a profile to show percent deviation of c/k values from the composite ratio C/K. A similar approach is described for the prediction of lean body weight from the sum of measurements of four diameters (biacromial, biiliac, wrists, and knees).

Milicer (1970) reports extensive use of standard deviations or z scores in Polish studies of physique and performance. Based largely on the work of Perkal (1953), the basic stratagem is to establish a reference group, obtain relevant anthropometric data, transpose raw scores into z scores and form subsets of highly correlated variables (for example, girths, breadths, lengths). For any given individual or group of subjects represented by the mean z score for each variable, x values are obtained by finding the mean z scores for each subset and an m value is obtained by finding the mean of all the z scores irrespective of the subset. The m score is interpreted as an index of size. Thus, Perkal indices or the differences between x scores and m scores indicate the relative size of each subset to the overall size estimate. Perkal indices for each z score, or the difference between the z score and x value, indicate the relative size of the variable with respect to some reference sample.

Summary

When shape and composition are similar, there are dimensional relationships that provide theoretical models to study structural and functional phenomena with respect to performance, growth, training, diet, or other concerns related to physical performance.

Human material, however, exhibits differences in shape and composition. These differences invite classification, and many systems have been evolved for artistic, medical, and scientific purposes.

Contemporarily the age-old dilemma about the relative contribution of endowment or environment as the basis of human destiny exists. From a biogenetic or constitutional point of view, the basic genotype is of great concern; hence, the preference for a system of physique classification relatively unaffected by age or environmental effects. From a functional point of view, which is perhaps of greatest concern in physical fitness assessment, a phenotypical representation of physique is preferred.

For this reason and because extensive information is now, and shortly shall be, available on Heath-Carter somatotypes of sportsmen and sportswomen, this methodology which is modified in format but not substance is presented in detail.

As yet, the problems of using an anthropometric procedure to estimate the Heath-Carter somatotype in children are not resolved. Our concern is reflected in our comments on the dimensional rationale for a height correction for the first component. Although mesomorphy may serve as a musculo-skeletal robustness indicator, bone widths and circumferences may have differing growth patterns with respect to height and these differences will be obscured when the mean deviation from a height standard is used to estimate the second component.

The scope of this paper precluded a review of other often ingenious and useful physique rating systems except to mention the pioneering work of Manouvrier and his objectification of physique ratings; Viola and his anthropometric system using a theoretical average man; the French school and its consistent conceptualization; the basic contribution of Kretschmer to clinical thinking; the approach used by Lindegard involving factors and standard deviation scales that have particular relevance in relating somatic and motoric variables in longitudinal and cross-sectional studies; the norming procedure of Hirata; the body composition approach by Behnke; and the stratagem of Perkal in viewing proportional physique differences by z score indices.

In conclusion, it is apparent that the study of physique and performance, taking into consideration the complications of growth and training, requires a plethora of techniques. There is, as yet, no single comprehensive integrated procedure for the analysis of size, shape, proportion, and composition. This chapter is therefore an overview of partial solutions and approaches to the overall problem of physique and performance, which is a major concern for an area of research interest that, for the want of a better term, we identify as kinanthropometry.

Acknowledgment: Some of the data in this chapter are from the project "Performance and Talent," sponsored and supported by the Belgian Ministry of Education and Culture (Administration of Physical Education and Sports), The Ministry of Health and Family (Center of Studies on Population and Family), The University of Brussels (Physical Education Research Laboratory), the University of Ghent (Anthrop-biological Research Unit), and the Belgian Fund for Fundamental Research (F.K.F.O. Research Program 935). The participant investigator was sponsored by a Simon Fraser University President's research grant.

REFERENCES

Asmussen, E., and K. Heeböll-Nielsen: A dimensional analysis of physical performance and growth in boys. *J. Appl. Physiol.*, **7**:593–603 (1955).

Asmussen, E., and K. Heeböll-Nielsen: Analyse des rapports de grandeur des performances physiques et de la croissance des garcons. *FIEP—bulletin*, **26**:1–12 (1956).

Astrand, P. O., and K. Rodahl: *Textbook of Work Physiology*. New York, McGraw-Hill, 1970.

Azuma, T. (ed.): Olympic medical archives. Organizing Committee for the Games of the XVIII Olympiad. Tokyo, 1964.

Behnke, A. R.: Anthropometric fractionation of body weight. *J. Appl. Physiol.*, **16**:949–954 (1961a).

Behnke, A. R.: Quantitative assessment of body build. *J. Appl. Physiol.*, **16**:960–968 (1961b).

Behnke, A. R.: Anthropometric estimation of body size, shape and fat content. *Postgrad. Med. J.*, **34**:190–198 (1963).

Borms, J.: Relaties tussen biologische leeftijd, lichaamsstruktuur, somatotype, lichaamsrijping en lichamelijke prestatiegeschiktheid. Doctoral Dissertation, University of Brussels, Vrije Universiteit Brussel, 1972.

Brody, S.: *Bioenergetics and Growth*. New York, Hafner, 1945.

Carter, J. E. L.: The somatotypes of athletes—a review. *Hum. Biol.*, **42**:535–569 (1970).

Carter, J. E. L. and B. H. Heath: Somatotype methodology and kinesiological research. *Kinesiol. Rev.*, **1**:10–19 (1971).

Carter, J. E. L. and M. Hebbelinck: Physical anthropology of the athletes. In A. L. de Garay, L. Levine, and J. E. L. Carter (eds). *Genetical and Anthropological Studies of 1265 Athletes of the XIX Olympic Games Mexico City 1968*. New York, Academic Press, in press.

Clarke, H. H.: *Physical and Motor Tests in the Medford Boys' Growth Study*. Englewood Cliffs, N.J., Prentice-Hall, 1971.

Correnti, V., and B. Zauli: *Olympionici, 1960*. Roma, Tipolitografia Marves, 1964.

Cureton, T. K.: *Physical Fitness Appraisal and Guidance*. St. Louis, Mo., C. V. Mosby, 1947.

Cureton, T. K.: *Physical Fitness of Champion Athletes*. Urbana, University of Illinois Press, 1951.

Damon, A., H. K. Bleibtreu, O. Elliot, and E. Giles: Predicting somatotype from body measurements. *Amer. J. Phys. Anthropol.*, 20:461–472 (1962).

De Giovanni, A.: *Morfologia del corpo umano 1, 2, 3*. Milano, Ulrico Hoepli, 1904.

Ekblom, B.: Effect of physical training in adolescent boys. *J. Appl. Physiol.*, 27:350–355 (1969).

Georgian, J. C.: The temperature scale. *Nature*, 281:695 (1964).

Heath, B. H., and J. E. L. Carter: A comparison of somatotype methodology. *Amer. J. Phys. Anthropol.*, 24:87–99 (1966).

Heath, B. H., and J. E. L. Carter: A modified somatotype method. *Amer. J. Anthropol.*, 21:57–74 (1967).

Hebbelinck, M., and R. L. Cliquet: Performance and talent. *Gymnasion*, 7:7–15 (1970).

Hill, A. V.: The dimension of animals and their muscular dynamics. *Proc. Royal Inst. Gt. Brit.*, 34:450 (1950).

Hirata, K. I.: Physique and age of Tokyo Olympic champions. *J. Sport Med. and Phys. Fitness*, 6:207–222 (1966).

Hirata, K. I. and K. Kaku: *The Evaluating Method of Physique and Physical Fitness and its Practical Application*. Gifu City, Hirata Institute of Health, 1968.

Hooton, E. A.: *Handbook of Body Types in the United States Army*. Cambridge, Mass., Department of Anthropology, Harvard University, 1951.

Huxley, J.: *Problems in Relative Growth*. New York, Dial Press, 1932.

Karpovich, P. V. and W. E. Sinning: *Physiology of Muscular Activity*. Philadelphia, Saunders, 1971.

Kohlraush, N.: Zusammenhänge von Körperform und Leistung. *Arbeitsphysiol.*, 1:187–204 (1929).

Kretschmer, E.: *Körperbau und Charakter*. Berlin, Springer, 1922 and 1961.

Lindegard, B.: Variations in human body-build, a somatometric and X-ray cephalometric investigation in Scandanavian adults. *Acta Psych. et Neurol.*, Suppl. 86 (1953).

Lindegard, B.: *Body-Build, Body-Function and Personality*. Lund, Gleerup, 1956.

McCloy, C. J.: *Appraising Physical Status: Selection of the Measurements*. Iowa City, State University of Iowa, 1936.

Manouvrier, L.: Etude sur les rapports anthropométriques et sur les principales proportions du corps. *Mém. Soc. Anthropol.*, 2:3–19 (1902).

Martin, R. and K. Saller: *Lehrbuch der Anthropologie*. Stuttgart, Gustav Fisher, 1957.

Milicer, H.: Anthropological problems in physical education and sports. Physical education and sport. Suppl. 1. *Wych. /Z sport*. 4:41–56 (1970).

Oliver, G.: *Pratique Anthropologique*. Paris, Vigot Frères, 1960.

Parnell, R. W.: Somatotyping by physical anthropometry. *Amer. J. Phys. Anthropol.*, 12:209–239 (1954).

Parnell, R. W.: *Behaviour and Physique*. London, Edward Arnold, 1958.

Perkal, J.: Owskaznikach antropologicznych. *Prezegl. Antropol. Poznan*, 19

(1953). Cited in: Milicer, H. (1970), see also Perkal, J. and F. Szczotka: Eine neue methode der Analyse eines Kollektivs von Merkmalen. *Biom. Z.*, **2**:108–116 (1960).

Petersen, G.: *Atlas for Somatotyping Children*. Springfield, Ill., Charles C Thomas, 1967.

Quételet, A.: *Anthropométrie ou Mesure des Differentes Facultés de l'Homme*. Bruxelles, Muguardt, 1870.

Ross, W. D., and J. A. P. Day: Physique and performance in young skiers. *J. Sport Med. and Phys. Fitness* **21**:30–37 (1972).

Sheldon, W. H., S. S. Stevens, and W. B. Tucker: *The Varieties of Human Physique*. New York, Harper Bros., 1940.

Sheldon, W. H., C. W. Dupertuis, and E. McDermott: *Atlas of Men*. New York, Harper Bros., 1954.

Tanner, J. M.: *The Physique of the Olympic Athlete*. London, George Allen and Unwin, 1964.

Thompson, D. W.: *On Growth and Form*. Cambridge, Cambridge University Press, 1917.

Tittel, K.: Zur Biotypologie und funktionellen Anatomie des Leistungssportlers. *Nova Acta Leopoldina*, **30** (172):1–255 (1965).

Viola, G.: La constituzione individuale dottrina. Metodo tipi morfologia, vols 1 et 2. Bologna, Lucindo Capelli, 1932 et 1933.

von Döbeln, W.: Human standard and maximal metabolic rate in relation to fat free body mass. *Acta Physiol. Scand.*, Suppl. 126 (1956).

Ziemilska, A.: Body build of Polish Olympic athletes. Physical Education and Sport. Suppl. 1. *Wych. Fiz. i. Sport*, **4**:65–69 (1970).

Applied Physiology

Part IV

SECTION EDITOR:
BRUNO BALKE
The University of Wisconsin

The Physiological Factors

15

M. Ikai
University of Tokyo
Tokyo, Japan

One of the main purposes of physiological measurement is the collection of information on the essential factors that contribute to integrated organic functioning at all levels of energy expenditure. However, only important physiological factors should be selected for this limited purpose. It is not an easy matter to identify those factors which specifically influence physiological performance because of their inseparable association with the total process of functional adaptations geared to maintain or restore homeostasis. The following formula may be used to express the contribution of essential factors to performance.

$$P = K \int E(M)$$

where P is performance, K is a cybernetic factor, E is a sum of energy, and M is motivation.

The cybernetic factor denotes the individual's skill or mechanical efficiency in carrying out a particular task and therefore directly affects the energy requirements for the task. If differences in the cybernetic factor exist, different patterns of performance will be revealed in individuals even though they possess a similar capacity for energy expenditure. From a physiological point of view, every attempt should be made to minimize the effects of cybernetic factors when measuring the factors of energetics.

Each of the factors contained in the formula for performance can be measured, although sophistication of technique and degree of accuracy vary considerably. Performance can be measured in any one, or combination, of four ways; namely, (1) by ascertaining the mechanical power developed on a staircase or on a bicycle ergometer, (2) by obtaining the duration of running on a treadmill at defined grades and speeds, (3) through measuring the time required to run a given distance, and (4) by establishing the distance run in a given period of time. Energy expenditure can be determined readily by measuring the oxygen consumption during exercise.

287

The measurement of the cybernetic factor is relatively complex and involves assessment of the mechanical efficiency of the body together with establishing the pattern of grading, spacing, and timing of the nervous discharges from the motor center to the acting muscles. In performance testing, motivation can exert a profound effect upon the level of physiological reactions. Although its complexity makes this factor difficult to assess accurately, researchers have assumed that motivation is at a high level when the heart rate and the lactic acid concentration in the blood have reached maximal values during exercise.

Energy Metabolism and Work Capacity

Maintenance of human life and the ability to do physical work are ensured by the energy-yielding splitting of elemental compounds. The complex cycling of these biochemical processes requires a supply of oxygen commensurate with the intensity of the energy demands. The energy used is only partly converted into mechanical work and actual performance. Although internal and external factors of resistance and friction may use up another part of the total energy expenditure, a much greater part shows up in generated heat.

The total energy used is comprised of the metabolic rate at rest and the extra energy required for performing any given physical task. The ratio of the metabolic rates at work and at rest is used as an index of the intensity of exercise. It has become customary to use the symbol "Met" as an expression of the unit value for the resting metabolic rate.

The basal metabolic rate (BMR) represents the energy expenditure of the organism under completely relaxed resting conditions unaffected by extra internal loads, such as digestion, excess temperature regulation, or psychomotoric tenseness. Actually, the BMR consists of the energy requirements of the cardiac and respiratory muscles and other vital organic functions at absolute rest and of the energy required to maintain the body temperature within the relatively normal range. The relationship between the energy required to do a certain amount of mechanical work and the actual metabolic energy release, minus the resting metabolic rate, serves as a clue for understanding a person's work efficiency.

The level or intensity of energy output per unit of time is directly related to the mechanical work performed. It is measured by determining the oxygen consumption over a given period of time. Because the work performed per unit of time constitutes mechanical power, the measured oxygen consumption represents the equivalent metabolic power. The maximum workload that can be performed under aerobic conditions, that is, requiring the maximum amount of oxygen that can be supplied to the working tissue, constitutes the maximum aerobic power. The range of potential energy release up to maximum aerobic power defines the aerobic work capacity. If a certain metabolic power is applied for such a duration that exhaustion occurs in available energy-providing substrates, the metabolic capacity for this power setting is defined.

The relation between the intensity (power) of, and the capacity for, energy expenditure is not always clear, especially not at the level of maximum oxygen intake. The latter is actually limited by the attainment of maximum oxygen transport functions encompassing mainly the circulatory and respiratory systems. Thus, maximum aerobic power is dependent on the "capacity"—or ability—of these systems to make the coordinated adjustments necessary for maximum oxygen transport. Because the attainment of maximum oxygen transport is used as the physiological criterion, the relationship between the intensity (power) and capacity of energy for work is expressed by the following formula:

$$C = \int_{t_0}^{t_a} I\, dt$$

where C is capacity, t_a is time of start, t_0 is time to exhaustion, dt is change in time, and I is intensity.

Aerobic Power

Aerobic power is, according to Wilkie (1960), developed 3 or 4 min after the start of intensive exercise and may continue for a period of approximately 15–30 min through optimally coordinated circulatory and respiratory adjustments resulting in maximum delivery of oxygen to the active tissues. A close relationship exists between maximum aerobic power and metabolic capacity. Metabolic capacity is an index of work capacity and is represented by the amount of energy-yielding substances maximally available from the body stores under aerobic conditions for a period of 2–3 hr. However, the maximum oxygen intake is not the only index of metabolic capacity. Many other physiological factors including high cardiac output, glycogen storage, and efficient water balance within the body are also related to metabolic capacity.

Maximum Oxygen Intake and Body Size

Maximum oxygen intake is usually dependent upon body size; the larger the amount of body tissues, the greater is the oxygen requirement for work. A useful index for the comparison of work capacity among populations with different body sizes is the ratio between maximum oxygen intake and body weight. In studies employing this index the highest values have been observed in marathon runners, cross-country skiers, and other athletes involved in endurance events.

Maximum Oxygen Intake and Active Tissues

Recently much attention has been paid to the index of maximum oxygen intake per unit weight of lean body mass. It is realized that adipose tissue, although constituting a large proportion of the body weight, is nevertheless fairly inert metabolically so that its exclusion may be important in the evaluation of the oxygen transportation capacity.

Maximum Oxygen Intake and Limiting Factors

The following factors suggested by Astrand and Rodahl (1970) limit maximum aerobic power: (1) the oxygen content of the inspired air, (2) pulmonary ventilation, (3) diffusion of oxygen from alveolar space to hemoglobin, (4) hemoglobin content, (5) blood volume, (6) ability of the heart to pump blood, (7) distribution of blood flow, (8) ability of muscle tissues to receive the blood, (9) diffusion from capillaries to the working cells, (10) venous blood return, (11) efficiency of the mitochondria in transferring aerobic energy to the ATP-ADP machinery, (12) access to fuel, (13) neuromuscular system, and (14) motivation.

Cardiac Output

The maximum capacity of the heart can be evaluated only by measuring the cardiac output during physical exertion. However, the direct measurement of cardiac output, although very valuable in cardiac diagnosis and prognosis, is virtually impossible because the heart is quite inaccessible for the determination of stroke volume. The most direct method may be by calculation of changes in cardiac volume from the cardiac silhouette on roentgenographic plates.

Physiological measurements have been conducted by indirect methods based on the Fick principle. Blood flow can be determined if a substance is removed from, or added to, the blood during its flow. Applied to the lungs, the Fick principle is used to calculate the volume of blood flow in a given time from the amount of oxygen taken up and from the difference of the oxygen content in the arterial and mixed venous blood.

During exercise cardiac output increases with the intensity of work and in a linear relationship to the amount of oxygen intake. The highest volume of cardiac output is closely related to the maximum oxygen intake. Another indirect way of estimating cardiac output, that is, the product of heart rate and stroke volume, is the use of the product of pulse pressure and heart rate, as suggested by Erlanger and Hooker (1904). Other indirect methods of assessing cardiac output involve rebreathing procedures with acetylene, carbon dioxide, nitrous oxide, and so forth.

Oxygen Pulse

During muscular work not only do body cells take more oxygen out of the arterial blood but also the amount of blood ejected from the heart with each beat is augmented. The combined effect of these two factors results in an increased delivery of oxygen to the tissues. The amount of oxygen taken out of the blood per pulse beat is called the oxygen pulse and is calculated by dividing the oxygen intake by the heart rate over a given period of time. During exercise the oxygen pulse increases and in most cases reaches its maximum value of 11–17 ml at a pulse of 130–140 beats/min. With further acceleration of the heart, the oxygen pulse tends to decrease.

Heart Size

The size of the heart can be observed by means of roentgenograms, and its volume can be calculated by the application of an empirical formula. A high correlation has been established in healthy younger persons between heart volume and various other parameters, such as blood volume, total amount of hemoglobin, and stroke volume. The difference between the athlete's heart and the dilated heart of a patient is represented by the disproportion between heart size, maximum aerobic power, and other physiological parameters such as total hemoglobin.

Total Hemoglobin

Total hemoglobin is closely correlated with maximum oxygen intake because it determines the potential capacity of the blood to carry oxygen. The maximum oxygen content in the arterial blood depends, in addition to the hemoglobin content, on factors affecting the oxygen saturation.

Diffusing Capacity

The diffusing capacity of the lungs is defined as the quantity of oxygen transferred each minute for each millimeter of mercury difference in partial pressure of oxygen on the two sides of the alveolar membrane. It has been observed that diffusing capacity increases in trained athletes, suggesting that a larger surface area develops that facilitates better transference of oxygen in the lungs.

Rate of Oxygen Removal

The efficiency of respiration is represented by the ratio of oxygen intake ($\dot{V}_{O_2}$) to lung ventilation ($\dot{V}_E$) per minute. This ratio is called the "rate of oxygen removal" and refers to the volume of oxygen absorbed into the blood from 1 liter of air. After a period of training this ratio will increase considerably. It will noticeably decrease, however, when an individual approaches exhaustion as a result of strenuous exercising.

Heart Rate

In many types of exercise, the increase in heart rate is linearly related to the increase in work intensity. The maximum heart rate is of more concern than the resting rate in the study of physical fitness. As age increases the maximum heart rate decreases. Although it is obvious that there is a considerable individual variation within each age group, the average maximum heart rate for a given age group is used in the assessment of maximum aerobic power from the extrapolation of the heart rate at submaximal work intensities with known oxygen requirements.

Arterial Blood Pressure

During exercises of any type, the amount of blood supplied to the muscles and the amount of blood flow through the lungs must be increased to meet the increased demand for oxygen. Arterial blood pressure will be raised by increased contractile forces of the heart muscle. Systolic pressure rises with increases in heart rate in both athletes and nonathletes. The trained subjects do not show as large an increase for a given heart rate, possibly because of the marked decrease in peripheral resistance during exercise resulting from vasodilation, a phenomenon which is usually accompanied by a decrease in diastolic pressure.

Pulse Pressure

The pulse pressure is the arithmetic difference between the systolic and diastolic pressures. Because, during exercise, the diastolic pressure changes little and the systolic pressure increases considerably, the pulse pressure

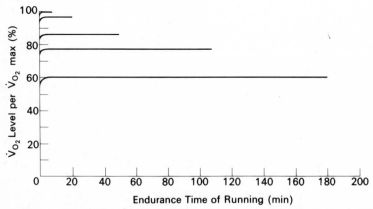

Figure 15-1. Power-endurance: Ordinate shows the percentage of a subject's maximum aerobic power, and abscissa shows the duration he can maintain the respective levels of power.

usually increases. The pulse pressure is an index of the effective pumping force of the heart and suggests an increase in stroke volume.

Anaerobic Power

Oxygen Debt

Total work capacity is a sum of the capacities for aerobic and anaerobic work. Anaerobic energy is provided not only by glycogenolysis or glycolysis but also by the breakdown of ATP and creatine phosphate. Anaerobic power can be maintained for only a short period of time. It is known that the resynthesis of phosphagen after work requires a supply of oxygen. Therefore, the measurement of oxygen intake during the recovery period serves as an assessment of the anaerobic power of the subject, that is, of his "oxygen debt capacity." The maximum oxygen debt is usually attained within 40–60 sec after the start of an exercise requiring maximum effort. The maximum value of this measurement is called the "maximum oxygen debt."

Lactic Acid in the Blood

During and after exercise in which the oxygen demand exceeds the oxygen supply, lactic acid accumulates in the muscle and diffuses from there into the blood. The lactic acid accumulation becomes a useful indication of the severity of the exercise. A maximum concentration of lactic acid is usually found a few minutes after termination of acute maximum exercise. It may take up to 60 min or even longer before the resting level is attained again.

Mechanical Power

Mechanical power of an anaerobic nature is an index of physical performance capacity. Margaria et al. (1966) introduced a test in which power could be measured: The subject runs at top speed up a staircase, two steps at a time. A constant speed is attained in about 1–2 sec and remains constant until the fifth second before declining. The exercise is a convenient ergometric procedure, because it appears that the energy requirement for speed maintenance in running a given distance depends upon the mechanical work per second. The mechanical power output is expressed in kgm/kg·sec.

Another method for measuring mechanical power of anaerobic nature has been introduced by Ikai et al. (1967) using a bicycle ergometer. The subject is invited to work on the ergometer with a certain load for a predetermined period of time. The number of revolutions of the wheel is recorded by a photoelectric circuit and the mechanical work is calculated. The value is expressed in kgm/sec.

Metabolic Capacity

As was mentioned earlier, metabolic capacity is understood as the amount of energy-yielding substances maximally available from the body stores under conditions of high aerobic energy demands for periods of approximately 2–3 hr. Because maximum oxygen intake has been observed to be closely related to endurance performance on the treadmill or bicycle ergometer as well as in distance running or swimming, metabolic capacity is usually estimated from the measurement of maximum oxygen intake in individuals. There are many individual differences, however, in the work time maintained at a certain level of oxygen intake. For example, elite distance runners or cross-country skiers can work at 80% of their aerobic power for up to 2 hr. However, it may be too difficult to keep a steady state at 50% of maximum for many working days in a row (Figure 15-1).

REFERENCES

Assmussen, E., and K. Heeböll-Nielsen: A dimensional analysis of physical performance and growth in boys. *J. Appl. Physiol.*, **7**:593–603 (1955).

Astrand, P. O., and K. Rodahl: *Textbook of Work Physiology.* New York, McGraw-Hill Book Co., 1970.

Erlanger, J., and D. R. Hooker: An experimental study of blood pressure and of pulse-pressure in man. *Johns Hopkins Hosp. Rep.*, **12**:145–378 (1904).

Hill, A. V.: *Muscular Activity.* Baltimore, Williams and Wilkins Co., 1926.

Ikai, M.: Trainability of muscular endurance as related to age. *Proc. X ICHPER Congr.*, Vancouver, Canada, 29–35, 1967.

Karpovich, P. V., and W. E. Sinning: Physiology of Muscular Activity. Philadelphia, W. B. Saunders, 1971.

Margaria, R., P. Aghemo, and E. Rovelli: Measurement of muscular power (anaerobic) in man. *J. Appl. Physiol.*, **21**:1662–1664 (1966).

Wilkie, D. R.: Man as a source of mechanical power. *Ergonomics*, **3**:1–8 (1960).

The Measurement of Physiological Factors

16

BRUNO BALKE
The University of Wisconsin
Madison, Wisconsin

In the process of human evolution man has developed as a multifactorial entity of living matter designed and prepared to withstand a variety of environmental forces threatening the preservation of his existence. In this entity a multitude of organs and organ systems are working together in ever-changing responses to intrinsic and extrinsic physical, sensory, mental, or psychological stimuli. They are coordinated by the most intricate and complex command and computer system, the human brain and nervous system.

Although it may appear absurd to search for a single element or factor which keeps the millions of body cells alive and functioning there is, in fact, such an element: *oxygen*. The human organism depends on a continuous and adequate flow of oxygen to all body cells, most importantly to the organs controlling the life processes. Any restriction of oxygen flow to tissues in urgent need of it will result in quick deterioration of efficient functioning of this particular organic tissue. The most familiar examples are "strokes" and "infarcts," the former caused by obstructions to the blood supply of the brain, the latter caused by occlusion of a coronary artery branch supplying the heart muscle with oxygenated blood. Depending on the size of such occlusions, the resulting damage to the tissue can vary from light to most severe. Major damage to the brain or heart can cause sudden death.

These introductory remarks were meant to prepare the ground for a better understanding of the fact that in the search for physiological criteria of human performance capacity so much emphasis is placed on the determination and discussion of oxygen demands and consumption under situations of physical, environmental, and psychological stress.

295

Crude Signs of Life

Even the crudest means of detecting signs of human life utilize simple methods for appraising the existence or intensity of circulatory or respiratory activity. The first and simplest measurement of the existing level of life intensity is obtained by palpation of readily accessible arteries, most usually of the radial artery. For the inexperienced observer, detectable pulsation would mean life; the lack of pulsation would indicate imminent danger for life, or death. To the experienced observer, the frequency, intensity, and regularity of the arterial pulsation serve as indicators of normal, intensified, or reduced blood circulation.

Another crude sign of life is the existence of rhythmic breathing. From the frequency, the depth, and the time course of inhalation and exhalation the experienced observer can size up pulmonary ventilation as normal or abnormal for given situations.

There are instances, however, in which the apparent nonexistence of these crude signs of life must not be indicative of death. During the course of cold exposure, for example, an undercooling of the body can occur that results in a state of hypothermia in which circulatory and respiratory functions have practically ceased. In such case, a check of reflex activities may be useful for judging the severity of the life-endangering condition. This judgment can be supported by the measurement of the body core temperature, which is usually maintained at a very narrow range. In acute hypothermia a core temperature of 25°C might not be incompatible with restoring life. Normally, however, temperatures only slightly below the usual range, if they coincide with the cessation of circulatory and respiratory functions, can be interpreted as termination of life processes.

Clinical Manifestations of the State of Health

The "crude signs of life" are useful only for a quick appraisal of whether any form of life is still present or irreparably lost. They might serve the purpose of encouraging attempts at resuscitation with some hope or expectation of success. For the simple clinical assessment of normal or pathological nuances of life, similar measurements of circulatory or respiratory parameters are generally in use. For instance, the measurement of heart rate, blood pressure, total blood volume, amount of hemoglobin, size and configuration of the heart, venous pulsation, peripheral edema, all may help to establish the status of clinical conditions of the cardiovascular system. The existence of eupnea or dyspnea, of quick deep breathing, of periodic breathing, of noiseful shortness of breath, of symmetric or unilateral abdominal or thoracic movements during the breathing cycle, any of these observations might be indicative of certain types of respiratory problems.

The measurement of body temperature is a common clinical tool for ascertaining not only the seriousness of infectious diseases but also disturbances in temperature regulation resulting from an imbalance between heat production, heat transfer, and heat loss.

Physiological Energy Exchange—Quantification of Life Intensity

Life is characterized by continuous dissimilation and assimilation of energy in the body cells. The intensity of this energy exchange in the total organism can be determined by direct or indirect calorimetry. The lowest intensity is measured during supine rest in an absolutely relaxed state several hours after the last meal and after any previous physical exertion. The energy expenditure in such a state is known as basal metabolic rate (BMR). It is comprised of the minimum metabolic processes necessary to maintain the body temperature and the continuous work done by the heart and the respiratory muscles. The slightest muscular activity, increased demands on temperature regulation, and food intake result in a rise of the BMR.

The magnitude of the BMR is related to the size, weight, age, and sex of an individual. In earlier attempts to establish norms for the BMR of different species of warm-blooded animals, it was found that the energy expenditure per unit of body weight (kg) increased in inverse proportion to the animal's size. That is, the smaller the animal the greater, relatively, is the body surface area and, therefore, the potential heat transfer. Because the greater part of the BMR is utilized to maintain equilibrium of body temperature, the smaller animal with the relatively greater surface area has to maintain a higher metabolic rate. Since the same law applies to man; a comparison of the BMR among individuals and groups of individuals is possible only on the basis of their surface area. When surface area is taken into consideration, it becomes evident that younger people have a higher BMR than older people and the female population usually has a lower energy expenditure in the basal state than the male population. This interrelationship between BMR, age, sex, and the surface area is shown in Table 16-1 (Rein, 1941).

Table 16-1 Basal Metabolic Rate in Kilocalories per 24 Hours per Square Meter

Age	Male	Female
14	1100	1030
18	980	920
30	930	880
50	900	820
60	860	810

SOURCE: Hermann Rein: *Physiologie des Menschen*, 5th and 6th ed. Berlin, Springer-Verlag, 1941, p. 153.

As an empirical formula for predicting the body surface area the same author used

$$SA = 167.2 \times \sqrt{W_{kg}} \times \sqrt{H_{cm}}$$

where SA = surface area, W_{kg} = weight in kilograms, and H_{cm} = height in centimeters.

The physiological measure of energy expenditure is either the amount of oxygen consumed during a given time ($\dot{V}_{O_2}$) or its caloric equivalent, the kilocalorie (kcal), that is, the energy required to raise the temperature of 1000 ml of water by 1°C. The energy set free is determined either directly or indirectly. In direct calorimetry the radiating body heat is measured as the difference of air or water temperature before entering and after leaving the calorimeter in which the man or animal has been placed.

In the indirect procedure the respiratory gas exchange is determined qualitatively and quantitatively, procuring a measure of the amount of oxygen consumed and of carbon dioxide produced. The relationship between $\dot{V}_{O_2}$ and $\dot{V}_{CO_2}$, the respiratory quotient (RQ), under steady state gas exchange conditions provides an indication of the type of fuel used in the metabolic process.

$$RQ = \dot{V}_{CO_2}/\dot{V}_{O_2}$$

Thus, fat combustion is represented by an RQ of 0.7, whereas the sole utilization of carbohydrates is indicated by an RQ of 1.0. The type of substrate utilized alters somewhat the calorific value of oxygen consumed: at an RQ of 0.7 the caloric value of 1 liter of oxygen is 4.7 kcal, whereas at an RQ of 1.0 it is 5.05 kcal. For a quick estimation of caloric energy expenditure from measured values of oxygen consumed during exercise, the value of 5 kcal for 1 liter of $\dot{V}_{O_2}$ can be used as a conversion factor without overestimating the actual energy expenditure by more than 2–3%.

For practical purposes it is more applicable to relate exercise metabolic rate to a unit of resting energy expenditure (the Met) that differs slightly from the BMR in having less stringent requirements. The only need in measuring the Met is for a relaxed period of about 10–20 min in a sitting or supine position before the gas collection begins. In addition, the energy expenditure during exercise is much less related to the surface area—as previously mentioned for the BMR—than to the body mass. Therefore, oxygen requirements during exercise are more practically compared with those during the resting state which, on the average, amount to about 3.5 ml/kg of body weight per minute. This figure has been defined as the absolute value for the unit of the resting metabolic rate, namely 1 Met. The expression of energy expenditure during exercise or during any other energy-consuming stress situation in the relative term of Mets permits a quick estimation of the total oxygen requirements if the body weight is known. For example, the metabolic requirement for walking at a speed of 3 miles per hour (mph) is 3 Mets or 10.5 ml/kg·min of oxygen. The total oxygen costs for an individual of 50 kg would amount to 525 ml/min, for a 100 kg man to 1050 ml/min.

Ranges of Oxidative Energy Metabolism

The Met concept is very useful for the appraisal of submaximal or maximal working efforts. There are patients, for instance, who may reach limitations of the oxygen transport system at 2 Mets. The average aerobic work tolerance of many male population groups peaks between 9 and 10 Mets. The expression of maximum aerobic power in Mets may serve as a better criterion of physical fitness than the absolute value of maximum $\dot{V}_{O_2}$. For example, at a maximum $\dot{V}_{O_2}$ of 6 liters/min, a well-conditioned tall football player of 125 kg body weight may perform maximally at a level of 13.5 Mets, whereas a cyclist, a cross-country skier, or a middle-distance runner weighing only 75 kg would perform at a level of about 23 Mets.

Aerobic Metabolism

From a strictly physiological point of view let us assume that adequate oxygen transport is the most important function that enables all the body cells to work in unison toward the common goal of total performance. Because all the components of the intricate system contributing to this function (blood, circulation, and respiration) cannot be triggered on a moment's notice to make such immediate adjustments as are necessary for sudden changes in metabolic demands, mechanisms have been provided in the active cell tissue to release energy on an "anaerobic" basis for a limited period of time. Thus, an oxygen-deficient phase of energy exchange is initially involved in any work situation, even one of minimum intensity. This energy turnover, proceeding on a partly anaerobic basis, disturbs the existing homeostasis and activates a feedback loop by which homeostatic conditions in the tissue are to be restored at a higher metabolic level. If, however, the work demands are so high that they exceed the maximal possible oxygen transport functions, work can only go on until all the energy stores available for anaerobic energy exchanges are exhausted.

The best indication of a disturbed or of a restored homeostasis is the measurement of $\dot{V}_{O_2}$. If the fractionated determination of oxygen intake shows a continuous increase after the beginning of a given activity level, adequate oxygen supply to the active tissue has not been achieved and the metabolic turnover still proceeds on a partly anaerobic basis. Eventually, though, the oxygen transport mechanisms will catch up with the demands, and this will be indicated by the leveling of the oxygen consumption values. The attainment of a "steady state" $\dot{V}_{O_2}$ is considered to be an indication of balanced supply and demand, that is, of prevailing aerobic conditions, unless it marks the attainment of the maximum level of oxygen consumption during overload work with even greater demands. In that case an oxygen debt accumulates forcing termination or a considerable reduction of the exercise performed.

Blood

The blood serves as the actual oxygen carrier in addition to carrying the energy substrates from the site of mobilization to the muscles and removing the metabolic waste products from active tissue. The blood also has an important function in the regulation of body temperature. To fulfill these various purposes effectively, the total volume of blood is as essential as a number of other qualitative properties. Changes in blood volume affect the capacity for aerobic work; acute blood loss results in a lower maximum $\dot{V}_{O_2}$. However, three or four days after spending an amount of blood as is customary in blood donations an overcompensating increase of plasma volume has been observed with a parallel increase in maximum $\dot{V}_{O_2}$. The capacity for aerobic work is also affected by changes in the relation of red blood cells to plasma (hematocrit), by the total number of red cells, by their hemoglobin content, and by properties that determine the buffering capacity of the blood.

Each organ has a range of responsiveness to functional demands with a definite limitation of adaptability. For the oxygen transport function of the blood, the limitation is set by the oxygen-carrying capacity, that is, by the amount of hemoglobin (Hb) attached to the red blood cells. Each gram of Hb can carry maximally 1.34 ml of oxygen. Assuming an average Hb of 15 g in 100 ml of blood, the oxygen-carrying capacity of such blood is 20 ml O_2/100 ml of blood, or 20 volume percent (Vol %). However, the actual content of oxygen carried by the blood is dependent on the oxygen saturation, which, in turn, is dependent upon a series of other factors that determine the diffusing capacity of oxygen in the lung tissue, apparently a strictly respiratory process. A quick glance at the factors that determine oxygen diffusion in the lungs will let us recognize the complex nature of this process.

1. The total area available for the diffusing process. (This is actually an anatomical factor because it entails the size of the lungs and the thorax cavity.)
2. The thickness of the alveolar-capillary membrane which may change with the expansion and collapse of the alveoli. (This is a partly anatomical, partly functional factor.)
3. The difference between the oxygen pressure in the alveolar air and that in the blood passing through the lung capillaries. (This pressure differential is influenced by the efficiency of alveolar ventilation in relation to the perfusion of lung tissue with blood and by the reduced oxygen tension in the venous blood returning to the lungs.)
4. The total blood flow through the lung tissue.

5. The duration of time during which the passing blood is exposed to the alveolar-capillary interphase.
6. A diffusion constant that differs for the various fractions of the respiratory gases.

Thus it becomes clear that the oxygen transport is accomplished not only by functions of the blood but also by those of the pulmonary-respiratory and of the cardiovascular systems.

Pulmonary Ventilation

The measurement of lung functions includes the determination of total lung volume and its components, the residual volume and vital capacity. The residual volume is usually determined by a nitrogen washout procedure. Vital capacity can be obtained either by measuring the three components, tidal volume and inspiratory and expiratory reserve volumes separately, or by measuring the volume of air which is maximally exhaled after a maximal inspiration. Although the magnitude of vital capacity is not a criterion of physical fitness *per se*, it can have an essential bearing on the maximum breathing capacity. At rest, about 20% of vital capacity is used in normal rhythmic breathing pattern. During maximal work about 66–75% of vital capacity might be utilized. Thus, individual A with a vital capacity of 4.5 liters, breathing at a maximum frequency of 50 breaths/min at two thirds of his vital capacity, will maximally breath 150 liters/min; whereas subject B, with a vital capacity of 6 liters, breathing at the same frequency, will achieve a ventilatory volume of 200 liters/min. This difference in pulmonary ventilation could result in a difference of 1–2 liters of potential oxygen intake at the maximum rate of work.

The measure of timed vital capacity is used to obtain information on the patency or obstruction of airways. The measure of maximum voluntary ventilation, formerly maximum breathing capacity, is frequently used as a test of maximal pulmonary function. However, the relatively short maneuver (10–20 sec) of maximal breathing effort at the optimum tidal-volume/frequency relationship is not so useful as an auxiliary indication of physical fitness as is the volume of air an individual might be able to move under conditions of maximum physical exertion.

Only that part of air which reaches the lung alveoli will affect the partial oxygen pressure in the lungs. The air remaining in the anatomical or physiological dead space of the airways does not contribute directly to the gas exchange within the lungs. Generally, the larger the tidal volume and the lower the respiratory frequency for a given total ventilation, the greater is the efficiency of pulmonary ventilation.

The more commonly used criterion of ventilatory efficiency, however, is the ventilation equivalent for oxygen, that is, the volume of air inhaled or exhaled during a given time in relation to the amount of oxygen taken up. To be a true indicator of ventilatory efficiency under varying atmospheric conditions, the ventilation volume is corrected for BTPS conditions but oxygen intake is corrected, as usual, for STPD conditions (where BTPS stands for the volume of gas at body temperature 37°C, ambient atmospheric pressure, and saturated with water vapor; STPD for standard sea level pressure at 0°C and dry gas). Thus, ventilatory efficiency is expressed either as $\dot{V}_{BTPS}:\dot{V}_{O_2}$, both in liters per minute, or as the reciprocal value, namely $\dot{V}_{O_2}:\dot{V}_{BTPS}$ in ml of oxygen intake per 1 liter of ventilation. Although the ventilatory equivalent for oxygen varies with changing atmospheric pressure and changing metabolic demands in any given individual, it may be used as a guiding factor in the evaluation of physical fitness when determined and compared at given metabolic loads.

Respiratory Gas Exchange

According to the concept that life depends on adequate oxygen supply, the determination of oxygen demands and of the actual amounts of oxygen consumed in given life situations is essential.

The measurement of oxygen consumption is a relatively simple laboratory procedure. All that needs to be done is to collect expired air during a given "steady state" metabolic condition, analyze this air for its partial gas content, (carbon dioxide, oxygen, nitrogen), and then measure the collected gas volume. The accurate computation of the amount of oxygen consumed and of carbon dioxide eliminated requires corrective considerations, however, because the collected expired air does not have the same volume as the air inspired. Usually, the expired volume of air is smaller than the inspired volume because less carbon dioxide is produced than oxygen consumed. The gas that does not change its volume during the respiratory cycle is nitrogen because it does not take any part in the metabolic gas exchange. In the ambient air the nitrogen content is 79%; in expired air, however, it might be 79.8%— besides 3.5% carbon dioxide and 16.7% oxygen, for example. Then the equivalent of 100 ml of expired air would be $(100 \times 79.8)/79 = 101$ ml of inspired air, which contained $(101 \times 20.9)/100 = 21.1$ ml of oxygen. The oxygen consumption per 100 ml of air inspired was therefore $21.1 - 16.7 = 4.4$ ml or, for the total ventilatory volume measured, that is, 6 liter/min (STPD) a total $\dot{V}_{O_2}$ of 264 ml/min. The $\dot{V}_{CO_2}$ would be 3.5% of 6 liter/min = 215 ml/min. The value of the respiratory exchange ratio, R, would be $215/264 = 0.815$.

In moderate exercise the difference between the oxygen fraction of the inspired and expired air usually becomes somewhat greater than at rest, that is, more oxygen is extracted from the air per unit of respiratory volume. With severe exercise this trend is reversed, although well-trained athletes may maintain a high utilization rate at very high workloads. This is usually paralleled by a lower pulmonary ventilation for the well trained at comparable intensities of work. In other words, the ventilation equivalent for oxygen of the endurance type athlete is indicative of a greater respiratory efficiency.

Cardiovascular Functions

Oxygen transport is mediated via the blood flowing in a system of tubes that vary in caliber size from the nearly 1-in. wide aorta to only microscopically visible capillaries. The pressure pumping action of the heart maintains the flow of blood on the arterial side. This pulsatile flow, with a relatively high pressure peak during the systolic ejection period, is smoothed out somewhat by the "Windkessel" function of the elastic aorta which expands when, in systole, the left ventricular volume is ejected. The recoil action of the aorta then serves to impart an additional force to the volume of blood entering the arterial tree, as well as to the blood entering the coronary arteries. It is during diastole that the relaxing heart muscle receives the major portion of blood supply. This fact is mentioned because it may explain why the measurement of arterial blood pressure during severe exercise is so important for the determination of critical limitations in the work capacity of the heart itself. At the high heart rates that accompany maximum aerobic work, the diastolic relaxation periods of the heart muscle are getting so short that only a higher aortic pressure could maintain a coronary blood flow adequate for the high myocardial oxygen requirements. Thus, a leveling or, worse, a decrease of arterial blood pressure at this point of effort serves as an essential criterion of approaching cardiac limitation.

In addition to the driving forces of ventricular contraction and aortic recoil two other factors contribute to the circulation of blood during exercise. One is the muscular "milking action" of the contracting muscle, which assists in squeezing the venous blood back toward the heart, an action especially important in areas disposed to favor the gravitational pooling of blood. The other factor is the rhythmically exerted negative pressure in the thorax during the inspiratory phases of pulmonary ventilation, which assists in returning the venous blood to the chest cavity and thus to the heart.

The determination of cardiovascular function includes a variety of measurements most of which require elaborate procedures. The most important measurement would be the cardiac output ($\dot{Q}$), that is, the measurement of the quantity of blood ejected during a given time interval. Two equations relate cardiac output to different components: equation (16-1)

$$\dot{Q} = V_s \times f \qquad (16\text{-}1)$$

where $\dot{Q}$ = cardiac output in liter/min; V_s = stroke volume; and f = heart rate per minute and the Fick principle, equation (16-2), which states that

$$\dot{Q} = \frac{\dot{V}_{O_2}}{\Delta O_2 a - \bar{v}} \qquad (16\text{-}2)$$

where $\dot{V}_{O_2}$ = the oxygen consumption in ml/min and $\Delta O_2 a - \bar{v}$ = the oxygen difference, in vol %, between the arterial and the mixed venous blood.

A combination of both equations shows that

$$\dot{V}_{O_2} = V_s \times f \times \Delta O_2 a - \bar{v}$$

The components of $\dot{V}_{O_2}$ and f are readily measurable. For the determination of $\Delta O_2 a - \bar{v}$ there is only one direct method, but several indirect procedures available. In the direct method the arterial blood is sampled from any artery; however, the sampling of mixed venous blood requires the more elaborate procedure of putting a catheter into the pulmonary artery, usually via a brachial vein, the vena cava, the right atrium, and the right ventricle. Because this procedure requires a rather complex laboratory set-up and is not without risks to the experimental subject, its use as a routine procedure is prohibitive. Also, the subject's maximum aerobic work tolerance does not seem to be fully achievable under the conditions of a catheter passing through two heart valves.

For the indirect determination of differences between the content of a given indicator in arterial and mixed venous blood two basically different methods can be employed. The first is the injection of indicator substances into the bloodstream followed by arterial sampling of blood for the determination of these substances. This indicator dilution principle is based on the following assumption: The amount of a substance S, when uniformly mixed in a volume V, will be diluted to a concentration C such that

$$S = C \times V \qquad (16\text{-}3)$$

If S and C are known

$$V = \frac{S}{C} \qquad (16\text{-}4)$$

For measuring flow ($\dot{Q}$), the volume per unit time (V/t) must be determined, that is

$$\dot{Q} = \frac{V}{t} \qquad (16\text{-}5)$$

By substituting the expression from equation (16-4) for V in equation (16-5), equation (16-6) is obtained.

$$\dot{Q} = \frac{S}{C \times t} \qquad (16\text{-}6)$$

In practice, a known amount of dye such as Evans blue, indocyanine green, or albumen labeled with I^{131} is injected into a vein. This injection should be made quickly and as close to the heart as possible so that complete mixing in the right heart is accomplished fast. The arterial blood is then sampled continuously and the concentration of dye is analyzed and plotted.

Because of the problem in obtaining the concentration of an indicator substance in the mixed venous blood as required for the application of the direct Fick principle mentioned previously, other indirect methods use respiratory, that is, pulmonary gas exchange, procedures. It can be assumed that the concentration of carbon dioxide, for example, at the end of exhalation is representative of the alveolar carbon dioxide concentration which, in turn, is assumed to be in equilibrium with the arterial blood. Then, by collecting the volume of a deep exhalation in a small bag and rebreathing this air several times, the carbon dioxide concentration at the end of another exhalation is assumed to be in equilibrium with the venous blood. In similar respiratory techniques for estimating the concentration differences of a certain gas between arterial and mixed venous blood, acetylene, gaseous nitrogen, and nitrous oxide have been utilized.

All these techniques for determining cardiac output can be useful tools in the hands of experienced and skilled investigators under special laboratory conditions. Within the usual laboratory procedures for determining maximum aerobic work tolerance, their applicability is rather restricted. Therefore, several attempts have been made to estimate at least relative changes of cardiac output during exercise from the changes of heart rates and blood pressures, assuming that changes in systolic pressure, in mean pressure, or in pulse pressure, may reflect appropriate changes in stroke volume.

Although in tests of functional adaptations to exercise the absolute values of arterial blood pressure are rather meaningless as quantitative indicators of work intensity in contrast with heart rates, which do correlate with work, they may be very useful as relative indicators of adequate or inadequate myocardial function. This is especially important in the functional evaluation of individuals handicapped by incipient or manifested heart disease.

Electrocardiogram

Here might be the appropriate place to mention briefly the role of the electrocardiogram (ECG) in the evaluation of physical fitness. It must be made clear that the ECG is not a measure of cardiac function, but it is an important tool for detecting abnormalities in the conduction of the cardiac action potentials, usually indicative of some type of heart disease. Since beyond the age of 35 many apparently healthy men may be silently afflicted with atherosclerotic disease of coronary arteries and other major vessels, the ECG recorded during rest and exercise might give the only warning of existing high risk. A resting ECG recorded in young and healthy people can be valuable for future comparison. Routine physical fitness testing by non-medical personnel is contraindicated in the presence of abnormal ECG tracings recorded during rest or exercise. In the hands of the knowledgeable investigator, however, the gradual ECG changes during a progressive-type exercise test may offer a chance to render clear advice with regard to the amount of work the patient is allowed to perform during daily work or in recreational activities.

Similar to the use of the value $\dot{V}_{BTPS}/\dot{V}_{O_2}$ as an indicator of ventilatory efficiency, the value $\dot{V}_{O_2}/HR$, the "oxygen pulse," is frequently calculated to serve as an expression of cardiac or circulatory efficiency. Since $\dot{V}_{O_2} = f \times V_s \times \Delta O_2 a - \bar{v}$, the oxygen pulse equals the product of $V_s \times \Delta O_2 a - \bar{v}$. Neither the stroke volume nor the arteriovenous oxygen difference, however, can be determined without elaborate techniques; therefore, it will remain a wide open question whether a change of the "oxygen pulse" represents a change mainly in V_s or in the $\Delta O_2 a - \bar{v}$. Under optimal conditions, V_s can increase only by a factor of 2 during maximum aerobic exercise, whereas $\Delta O_2 a - \bar{v}$ might increase by a factor of 4 under that condition. Thus, the oxygen pulse is hardly a measure of "cardiac efficiency" but rather a crude expression of the respiratory activity at the muscle tissue level.

During the last few years great strides forward have been made in the biochemistry of muscular activity, especially concerning the oxidative and nonoxidative, that is, the aerobic and anaerobic, mechanisms of energy release by the muscle tissue. It has been suggested that the availability of oxidative enzymes and the quantity and quality of mitochondria might be the limiting factors in aerobic work tolerance rather than the oxygen transport functions of blood, respiration, and circulation. This is an understandable revolutionary trend which tends to deemphasize old established principles in the face of new disclosures. However, the result of the discussion might be that the maximum oxygen intake in relation to respiratory and circulatory factors will remain the preferred measurement for the practical determination of maximum aerobic power.

Important progress has also been made in research on the limiting factors of prolonged physical work. Work capacity for submaximal work depends on the intensity and duration of the energy demands. The choice of fuel— carbohydrate fat, or, in rare cases, protein, may depend among other things on the training state of the individual. Until more data become available and also relatively simple methods for determining metabolic work capacity become established, the maximum aerobic power will remain a useful indicator of the capacity for long-duration work. A higher level of maximum aerobic work tolerance usually permits longer periods of submaximal work at a higher percentage of maximum than found in individuals with less maximum aerobic power.

Another area in which research must make more contributions to understanding physical fitness, detraining, overtraining, fatigue, exhaustion, and reactions to environmental stress concerns the hormonal interactions that may be involved in the regulation of many physiological functions. Are there, for example, limitations in the production of stress hormones necessary for sustained heavy work? Answers to this and related questions will probably result in the development of practical, and therefore more valuable, procedures for measuring physiological factors of physical fitness.

REFERENCE

Rein, H.: *Physiologie des Menschen*, 5th and 6th ed. Berlin, Springer Verlag, 1941.

The Validity of Physiological Determinations

17

C. H. WYNDHAM
University of the Witwatersrand
South Africa

The human body is able to increase many fold the energy it can make available for external work. Thus, a champion track cyclist can increase the work he performs on a bicycle ergometer, for example, from 1 to 400 watts. The immediate source of energy for muscular work is the degradation of adenosine triphosphate (ATP) to adenosine diphosphate (ADP) and the resynthesis of ATP from ADP utilizing the high-energy reservoir in muscle, creatine phosphate (CP). The reserves of ATP and CP in muscle are limited and are soon exhausted during heavy exercise. The main source of energy for the resynthesis of ATP during sustained physical exercise is the oxidation of carbohydrate and free fatty acids.

The breakdown of 1 mole of glycogen to pyruvic acid releases 2 moles of ATP. If there is adequate oxygen, pyruvic acid enters the Krebs cycle and undergoes oxidation and decarboxylation to form acetate, which bonds with Coenzyme A and transfers the acetyl group to oxalacetic acid to form citric acid. This completes the first step in the Krebs cycle. Free fatty acids contribute to the resynthesis of ATP by entering the Krebs cycle in a similar way; 32 moles of ATP are formed for every 2 moles of pyruvic acid that enter the Krebs cycle, a net gain of 36 moles of ATP for every mole of glycogen metabolized. The net gain of ATP from free fatty acid is even greater; 129 moles of ATP are formed for every mole of palmitic acid that is metabolized.

If the delivery of oxygen to working muscle is inadequate, part of the energy for muscular work comes from anaerobic metabolism. Pyruvic acid and free fatty acid cannot enter the Krebs cycle, and pyruvic acid is reduced to lactic acid. The yield of ATP in these circumstances is low, the muscle rapidly exhausts its reserves of CP, and the force of contraction diminishes.

It will be clear from the above that from the point of view of energy release it is important to maintain aerobic conditions during sustained muscular exercise. The ability to do so depends upon the capacities of the various components of the oxygen transport system from atmospheric air to working muscle. The lungs and heart are the two main elements in this transport system.

This chapter is concerned with the validity of the measurement of aerobic metabolism or power at different levels of physical effort and of the measurement of maximum aerobic power or maximum oxygen intake. It will also deal with the validity of the measurement of anaerobic power and capacity.

Measurement of Aerobic Power

The measurement of the energy released by aerobic processes during muscular exercise is one of the most fundamental measurements in exercise physiology. In this section we shall consider, first, how energy is released by the oxidation of foodstuffs and then, with this background, we shall examine the techniques we have available for measuring the energy expenditure of muscular effort. Secondly, we shall examine the intra- and interindividual variability in the measurement of oxygen consumption in different types of exercise and at various levels of effort in order to determine whether these are significant day-to-day variations in oxygen consumption and whether these variations do not "swamp" the differences between individuals in this measurement. We shall consider the relationship between oxygen consumption and such body-size parameters as surface area, body weight, and height in order to assess the validity of comparisons between individuals, or groups, in terms of these body-size parameters. Finally, we shall consider the validity of the use of heart rate or minute pulmonary ventilation for "predicting oxygen consumption."

The Energy Released from the Oxidation of Foodstuffs

If a foodstuff is put into a bomb calorimeter and ignited, all of the organic material is oxidized and heat is released. The heats of combustion of the main foodstuffs are shown in the table below.

Foodstuff	Heat of Combustion, Kcal/g	Available Energy, Kcal/g
Carbohydrate	4.1	4.0
Protein	5.7	4.0
Fat	9.4	9.0

In the human body carbohydrate and fat are oxidized completely to carbon dioxide and water, but the oxidation of protein is never complete. Urea, uric acid, and creatinine, which are derived from protein, are excreted in the urine. The heat of combustion of these unoxidized portions of protein in the urine is about 1.3 kcal/g of protein.

Furthermore, not all of the ingested foodstuffs are absorbed. It was estimated by Atwater that 92% of protein, 95% of fat, and 97% of carbohydrate is absorbed. Applying these "Atwater factors" to the heats of combustion of the three main foodstuffs gives the available energies shown in the table above. It must be understood, however, that these values for available energy are only rough approximations. The digestibility of the coarse corn meal, which is the staple diet in southern Africa, is not 97%.

Tables are available (McCance and Widdowson, 1960; Wall and Merrill, 1964) that give the proportions of carbohydrate, fat, and protein of all the common foodstuffs as determined by chemical analysis. The calorific values of the various items of food in a meal can be calculated by weighing carefully each of the main items and then looking up in the table the proportions of carbohydrate, fat, and protein in these items. By simple multiplication the total amounts of carbohydrate, fat, and protein in the diet are obtained, and the total calories are calculated by multiplying each of these totals by the appropriate "Atwater factors," given above. By this means the 24-hr intake of energy can be determined for an individual or group of individuals. However, studies (Widdowson et al., 1954) have shown that the correlation in an individual between the energy input and the energy output on a particular day is not close, but on a 7-day basis the correlation is much closer.

There are important limitations in this method of determining the 24-hr energy intake. There is first the uncertainty about the percentages of the various foodstuffs that are digested. Then the method of calculating the losses of energy from the protein fraction in the urine is not entirely satisfactory. The protein content of the diet is calculated by multiplying the nitrogen content by 6.25 (this factor is based on the assumption that most proteins contain about 16% of nitrogen). This is a crude approximation. It is too high for cereal protein (which forms the staple in the diet of most nonwhites in southern Africa, for example) and is too low for milk products (which figure prominently in the diets of the populations in the more affluent countries).

This method of determining the energy expenditure has its main use in comparing the 24-hr energy expenditures of different groups of workers such as miners, office workers, and so on. It is of no value for determining the energy expenditure of different physical efforts of shorter duration.

Measuring the Energy Expenditure During Muscular Effort

The energy expended by the body during muscular effort can be measured by direct calorimetry. This method requires that the total amount of heat given off by the body during the period of muscular effort must be measured. (Allowance must be made for the heat involved in the rise in body temperature which is associated with muscular effort.) Few laboratories in the world are equipped with the facilities necessary for direct calorimetry and, in consequence, the energy expended during muscular effort is generally measured by indirect calorimetry.

Indirect calorimetry is based upon the fact that, when glucose or fatty acids are completely oxidized in the body, the amount of oxygen consumed is directly related to the energy released as heat. This was shown to be true in the classic calorimetric experiments on men *at rest* by such experimentalists as Benedict, Atwater, and others early in this century. For example, in the oxidation of glucose the following equation applies.

$$C_6H_2O_6 + \quad 6\,O_2 \quad = \quad 6\,CO_2 \quad + \quad 6\,H_2O \quad + \quad \text{Heat}$$
$$(180\text{ g}) \quad (6 \times 22.4 \text{ liters}) \quad (6 \times 22.4 \text{ liters}) \quad (6 \times 18 \text{ g}) \quad 665 \text{ kcal}$$

From this equation it is clear that 180 g glucose oxidizes in 6×22.4 liters of oxygen to yield 665 kcal of heat. The calorific value of 1 liter of oxygen therefore is

$$\frac{665}{6 \times 22.4} = 4.95 \text{ kcal}$$

The ratio of carbon dioxide produced to oxygen absorbed is known as the respiratory quotient (RQ), and for the oxidation of glucose it is 1.0. Similar equations can be written for the oxidation of fat and protein.

Zunz, the famous Swiss physiologist, worked out a table for the energy yields of different foodstuffs in 1897, and these still form the basis for our calculation of the calorific value of oxygen at different RQs which is given in Table 17-1.

Table 17-1 Energy Yields from Oxidation of Foodstuffs

1 g of	O₂ Required, ml	CO₂ Produced, ml	RQ	Kcal Developed	Kcal Equivalent of 1 liter of O₂
Starch	828.8	828.8	1.000	4.183	5.047
Animal fat	2019.2	1427.3	0.707	9.461	4.686
Protein	966.1	781.7	0.809	4.442	4.600

From the Zunz tables, or the later modifications of them, the amount of carbohydrate, fat, and protein and the heat produced can be calculated from measurements of the amounts of oxygen consumed, the carbon dioxide produced, and the urinary nitrogen excreted. The detailed procedure involved in the calculations is set out in most physiology textbooks. The calculations are tedious and laborious. In 1949, Weir was the first to show that these calculations could be shortened by the use of a series of regression equations, and this approach was further developed by Consolazio et al. (1963) using

Magnus-Levy's factors. The amounts of carbohydrate, fat, and protein and the total energy can be calculated from four simple equations as follows:

$$\text{Carbohydrate, g} = 4.12 \, CO_{2m} - 2.91 \, O_{2m} - 2.56 \, N_u$$
$$\text{Fat, g} = 1.69 \, CO_{2m} - 1.69 \, O_{2m} - 1.94 \, N_u$$
$$\text{Protein, g} = 6.25 \, N_u$$
$$\text{Metabolic heat, kcal} = 1.16 \, CO_{2m} + 3.78 \, O_{2m} - 2.98 \, N_u$$

where O_{2m} and CO_{2m} are in liters (STPD), and N_u is in grams.

Weir (1949) also showed that the calculation of metabolic heat could be further shortened by assuming a constant percentage of total calories from protein intake. The only measurements needed are the corrected minute pulmonary ventilation and the oxygen concentration of the expired air. These are obtained from the following formula:

$$\text{Energy, kcal/min} = \frac{1.0548 - 0.0504 \, O_c}{1 + 0.082p} \times \text{liters vent./min}$$

where O_c is the percentage concentration of oxygen in expired air and p is the percentage of total dietary energy from protein.

This equation can be further simplified by assuming that 10% of energy comes from protein.

However, a very good approximation of the metabolic heat is obtained by assuming that the calorific value of oxygen is 4.85 kcal/liter. Consolazio et al. (1963) have compared the total energy expenditure of 12 subjects engaged in a wide variety of activities and found that the average total kilocalories, determined by the Weir formula and the Consolazio regression equation, were 2.52 and 2.49, respectively. Using a calorific value of 5 kcal/liters of oxygen intake gave a total metabolic heat of 2.63, and using a calorific value of 4.85 kcal/liter oxygen gave a total metabolic heat of 2.55.

It would appear that unless one is carrying out careful comparisons between energy input and energy output, it is, for all general purposes, adequate to use a factor such as 4.85 kcal/liter for the calorific value of oxygen. The rate of oxygen consumption is multiplied by this factor in calculating the rate of metabolic heat production for various physical activities.

Possibly the most serious criticism of any of these indirect calorimetric procedures for determining the heat production of tasks involving muscular effort is that no systematic studies have been conducted utilizing modern, rapid-responding calorimeters to validate the calorific values of oxygen at different RQ values during exercise. If this were done in association with C^{14} glucose studies, it would be possible to validate fully the assumptions made in the classic calculations of Zunz, Magnus-Levy, and others.

It should also be remembered that this method of calculating the metabolic heat is only valid under conditions where there is no anaerobic metabolism, that is, up to about 50% of the individual's maximum oxygen intake. As soon as anaerobic metabolism occurs and lactic acid is liberated into the arterial blood, the *RQ* no longer represents the ratio of carbohydrate to fat being metabolized. In fact, as is well known, the *RQ* may go above 1.0 in subjects at close to their maximum oxygen intakes.

The general conclusion we can draw from this section is that, for all practical purposes in exercise physiology, it is valid to express energy expenditure of muscular exercise in terms of liters per minute of oxygen consumption and *not* to convert this figure into energy units of kilocalories per minute or watts.

Variability in the Measurement of Oxygen Consumption

Surprisingly few studies have been made to examine the day-to-day variability in the oxygen consumption of an individual while exercising at a constant rate of external work. Nor has there been much research to determine the differences between individuals in oxygen consumption when they are exercising at a constant rate.

Passmore, and later Durnin, both of Edinburgh have made some of the best contributions to knowledge in this field. Passmore and his colleagues (Délbue et al., 1953) reported that the interindividual (that is, between individuals) coefficient of variation of 50 students at rest and when walking at 3.35 mph (5.4 km/hr) was of the order of 10%. In a later, more extensive study, they reported (Mahadeva et al., 1953) that the intraindividual (within individual) coefficients of variation on such physical activities as rest, stepping (15 times per minute on and off a stool 10 in. in height), and walking at 3 mph (4.8 km/hr) were between 5 and 8% and the interindividual coefficients of variation were between 16 and 18%.

Wyndham et al. (1966a) reported upon the intra- and interindividual coefficients of variation in oxygen consumption of 10 men trained for specific tasks when they engaged in a wide range of physical activities. These included stepping on and off a stool, pedalling a bicycle ergometer, shovelling sand, and pushing a mine car. Two different workloads were studied on each task, the rates of external work were carefully standardized, and the apparatus was repeatedly calibrated. They found, as did Passmore and his associates, that the day-to-day variability of the individual in oxygen consumption was smaller than the differences of oxygen consumption between individuals. The interindividual coefficients of variation were between 5 and 15%, whereas the intraindividual coefficients were only between 3 and 7%.

Interestingly enough the intraindividual coefficients of variation were closely similar in all of the tasks, even though the tasks varied greatly in the complexity of the physical movements involved. The situation was different when the differences between individuals in this measurement were examined. Here, the stepping task and the bicycle ergometer had the smaller coefficients, and shovelling sand, the more complex task, had the largest coefficient. These results suggest that *skill* and *training* play an important role in the differences between individuals in carrying out more complex tasks but, in the simpler physical activities such as stepping on and off a stool or riding a bicycle ergometer, differences in skill are not apparent.

This last suggestion is supported in a later study by Wyndham et al. (1967) in which they again studied the intra- and interindividual coefficients of variation in oxygen consumption on the three tasks of pedalling a bicycle ergometer, shovelling sand, and pushing a mine car. On this occasion they also studied walking at 2 mph (3.2 km/hr). The 16 subjects were trained on these tasks for a prolonged period before the study, and more careful attention was given to standardizing each task and ensuring that each man followed exactly the same procedure. As a result of extensive training and the careful standardization of the tasks, the intra- and interindividual coefficients of variation were of the same order of magnitude, most being between 3 and 8%. The largest coefficient of variation occurred in walking where the intraindividual value was 8.3% and the interindividual value was 10.3%. The smaller interindividual coefficients of variation in this study were not due to the men in the sample being more uniform in size. The subjects were chosen deliberately to cover a wide range of weight and stature; weight varied from 52 to 68 kg and height from 158 to 184 cm.

The general conclusion one can draw from these studies is that a day-to-day variability in oxygen consumption in most physical tasks of about 5% and differences between individuals of about 10% can validly be expected, but with very careful attention to standardization and training the latter figure may be halved.

Influence of Body Parameters on Oxygen Consumption

The reasons for the significant differences between individuals in aerobic power or oxygen consumption on standard physical tasks have been the subject of profound interest to exercise physiologists.

Mahadeva et al. (1953) examined the effects of age, sex, height, weight, surface area, race, and previous dietary history on metabolic rates utilizing three physical activities: rest, a standard stepping task, and walking at 3 mph (4.8 km/hr). They found that the metabolic rate was directly proportional to body weight. Factors such as age, sex, surface area, race, and previous dietary history did not have a significant effect on the rate of metabolism. In consequence, they were able to give the following regression equations for stepping and walking:

$$\text{Stepping:} \quad C = 0.066W \pm 3.02$$
$$\text{Walking:} \quad C = 1.024 + 0.47W \pm 3.70$$

where C is the rate of metabolism in kcal/min, W is the weight in kg, and the last term is the standard error of the estimate.

Further research in a number of laboratories has been carried out to determine the influence of certain specific body-size parameters and body composition on oxygen consumption in a variety of physical activities. The main factors which have been examined are weight, height, and percentage of body fat. The results are shown in Table 17-2.

Table 17-2 Correlations Between $\dot{V}_{O_2}$ and Body Weight, Height, and Fat-Free Mass

Authors	Number	Work	Liters/m $\dot{V}_{O_2}$	Weight $\dot{V}_{O_2}$	Height $\dot{V}_{O_2}$	Fat-Free Mass or % Fat $\dot{V}_{O_2}$
WALKING ON FLAT OR UP SLOPE						
Selzer (1940)	34	5.6 km/hr 8.6 % grade	1.96	0.77**	0.36*	—
Miller & Blyth (1955)	30	7.9 km/hr 10% grade	—	0.75**	0.32	0.67**
Brockett et al. (1956)	98	5.6 km/hr 0 grade	1.06	0.75**	0.28*	0.27*
Durnin (1959)	160	5.2 km/hr 0 grade	—	0.68**	—	—
	160	4.4 km/hr 10% grade	—	0.78**	—	—
Rasch et al. (1962)	21	4.4 km/hr 10% grade	—	0.65**	0.52**	0.54**
Wyndham et al. (1967)	16	4.0 km/hr 0 grade	0.74	0.76**	—	—
Wyndham et al. (1969)	80	7.3 km/hr 0 grade	1.92	0.70**	0.27*	0.71**
STEPPING ON AND OFF A BENCH						
Wyndham et al. (1966a)	10	30.5 cm × 12	0.95	0.95**	—	—
Wyndham et al. (1969)	45	30.5 cm × 24	1.28	0.62**	0.51**	0.57**
		37.5 cm × 24	1.61	0.66**	0.60**	0.58**
PEDALLING A BICYCLE OR BICYCLE ERGOMETER						
Adams (1967)	60	16 km/hr	1.17	0.76**	0.59**	0.71**
Wyndham et al. (1967)	16	173 kg/min	0.61	0.70**		
		346 kg/min	0.91	0.57**		
		693 kg/min	1.52	−0.30*		
		831 kg/min	1.82	−0.62**		

* Significant at 0.05 level of significance.
** Significant at 0.01 level of significance.

It must be borne in mind, of course, that the significant correlations between oxygen consumption and each of the body parameters shown in Table 17-2 may be due to the fact that the various body parameters might themselves be highly correlated. For example, Wyndham and Heyns (1969) showed that the correlation coefficients between weight and height were 0.58 in Caucasians and 0.71 in Bantus and between weight and fat-free mass were 0.97 in the former and 0.94 in the latter. Fortunately, it is possible to determine which of the factors is more important in the relationship where a number of body factors are all significantly correlated with oxygen consumption but also are themselves significantly correlated with each other. This is done by calculating partial correlation coefficients in which, first, oxygen consumption and weight are correlated, with the effect of height being eliminated (r_1); second, oxygen consumption and height are correlated, with the effect of weight being eliminated (r_2); and third, oxygen consumption and fat-free mass are correlated, with the effect of weight being eliminated (r_3). The results of these analyses are given in Table 17-3.

Table 17-3 Partial Correlation between Oxygen Consumption and Weight (r_1), Height (r_2), and Fat-Free Mass (r_3)

Task	r_1	Sig.	r_2	Sig.	r_3	Sig.	$\dot{V}_{O_2}$ (l/min)
CYCLING							
Wyndham et al. (1966)							
173 kg/min	0.75	S*	−0.50	NS	—	—	0.61
346 kg/min	0.71	S	−0.56	S	—	—	0.91
973 kg/min	−0.30	NS†	−0.61	S	—	—	1.52
831 kg/min	−0.32	NS	−0.17	NS	—	—	1.81
Adams (1967)							
15–17.5 km/hr	0.57	S	−0.08	NS	−0.06	NS	1.17
WALKING							
Miller & Blyth (1955)							
7.9 km/hr							
10% grade	0.71	S	−0.04	NS	0.46	S	—
Brockett et al. (1956)							
5.6 km/hr, flat	0.74	S	−0.22	S	−0.02	NS	1.06
Wyndham et al. (1970)							
7.3 km/hr, flat	0.69	S	−0.23	S	0.14	NS	1.92
STEPPING							
Wyndham et al. (1970)							
24 × 30.5 cm	0.43	S	−0.12	NS	−0.03	NS	1.28
24 × 37.5 cm	0.41	S	−0.25	NS	−0.13	NS	1.61

* S = significant.
† NS = not significant.

The general conclusion that can be drawn from these analyses was well summarized in Miller and Blyth's (1955) statement on this subject. They said, "The metabolic cost of work is predicted more accurately by gross body weight than by lean body mass, etc. The predictive value of factors other than body weight is largely due to the respective correlations with body weight."

Miller and Blyth's statement applied to walking at different speeds, to stepping on and off a bench at different rates of energy expenditure, and to pedalling a bicycle at relatively low rates of energy expenditure. However, it did not apply at high rates of energy expenditure, possibly because some of the men were in anaerobic metabolism at the higher work rates on the bicycle ergometer. It is clear from these results that it is perfectly valid to express oxygen consumption, or metabolism, in terms of body weight, but it is not valid to do so in terms of either height, or fat-free mass or, as Miller and Blyth and Mahadeva et al. (1953) showed, in terms of surface area.

The significant correlation between oxygen consumption and height with the effect of weight removed, shown by Wyndham and his associates and by Brockett et al. (1956) for walking, is of some interest. This is especially true for Wyndham et al's (1966) experiment, where the sample of 16 men was specifically chosen to represent as broad a range of weights and heights as was possible to obtain in the Bantu population of fit young men (the weights ranged from 52 to 68 kg and the heights from 153 to 184 cm), because the correlation was very high, being 0.68.

The interpretation of these results is that weight is the main determinant of oxygen consumption and, because the correlation is positive, the heavier the man the higher the oxygen consumption. Height also has a significant effect when men are walking. The significant negative correlation means that the taller the man the lower the oxygen consumption or, put in other words, for two men of the same weight, the taller man will have the lower oxygen consumption. This finding fits in well with Tanner's (1964) examination of the morphology of athletes who excel in different athletic events. He found that tall, lean men excelled in endurance events. This was also the experience of Leary and Wyndham (1965). They compared the heights and weights of international class Caucasians and Bantu middle-distance runners in South Africa with those of the general population. The results are shown in the table below.

	Number	Height, cm	Weight, kg
CAUCASIANS			
Athletes	4	177.9	67.5
Army recruits	35	175.9	71.8
BANTU			
Athletes	6	167.7	58.4
Mine recruits	88	165.9	60.5

Brockett and coworkers (1956) went into the relationship between oxygen consumption and height in some detail. They noted, first, that height and leg length were very highly related, having a correlation coefficient of 0.88. When they calculated partial correlation coefficients between oxygen consumption and height, with leg length eliminated, the correlation was no longer significant. However, the eff∶ct of leg length on oxygen consumption with height removed was still significant, the correlation being 0.29. They summarized the situation as follows: "Leg length seemed to have influence on the energy cost of walking. While this effect was small compared with that exhibited by body weight, it was nevertheless present."

With this significant relationship between oxygen consumption and leg length in mind, Cotes and Meade (1960) looked into the possibility of developing an equation to predict energy expenditure during horizontal walking that would include leg length. They reasoned as follows:

1. Energy expenditure of walking at the "natural step frequency" in a horizontal plane is linearly related to vertical lift work.
2. Vertical lift work is the product of lift per step, step frequency, and body weight.
3. The vertical lift per step is a geometric function of the length of the leg and the foot and of the pace. Energy expenditure during horizontal walking is also a linear function of the square of the forward velocity.

Cotes and Meade did not succeed in developing an equation to predict energy expenditure utilizing the factors concerned with vertical lift work, but they did produce an equation with forward velocity squared as follows:

$$E/W = 0.0386 + 4.25 \times 10^{-6}v^2$$

where E is the energy expenditure in kcal/min; W is body weight in kg; and v is the forward velocity in mph. They stated that the equation predicted the energy expenditure of their subjects to within 0.7 kcal in 95% of the cases.

Cotes and Meade's equation gives similar results to those obtained when using an equation developed by Ralston (1958) a few years earlier, which reads as follows:

$$E/W = 29 + 0.0053v^2$$

This equation can be rewritten for comparison with that of Coates and Meade in the following way

$$E/W = 0.029 + 5.3 \times 10^{-6}v^2$$

We should next consider what contribution to the variation in oxygen consumption while exercising is made by differences between individuals in body weight, height, and fat-free mass. It will be clear from the foregoing that, because of the intercorrelation between these various body parameters it is not possible to use the coefficients of determination (that is, $r^2 \times 100$) to estimate the percentage contribution of these various parameters to the overall variances in oxygen consumption. The correct approach is to calculate the total variances and the "irreducible minimum" variance in oxygen consumption and also to calculate the residual variances about the regression lines of oxygen consumption against the various body-size parameters. From these various variances it is possible to estimate the percentage of the variation between individuals in oxygen consumption which is due to differences between them in body weight, height, and fat-free mass. The general equation used is

$$Y = A \cdot Bx_1 \cdot Cx_2 \cdot Dx_3$$

where A, B, C, D are different parameters; $Y = \log \dot{V}_{O_2}$; $x_1 = \log$ weight in kg; $x_2 = \log$ height in cm; and $x_3 = \log$ fat-free mass in kg. This method of analysis was applied to the data obtained by Wyndham and Heyns (1969) on 80 young army recruits while walking at 7.4 km/hr (4.5 mph). The results are given in Table 17-4.

Table 17-4

	Parameters				Residual Variance	Accounted for
	A	**B**	**C**	**D**		
Total variance	—	—	—	—	0.00338	—
Regression on log weight	−1.258	0.845	—	—	0.00173	69%
Regression on log weight and log height	−0.895	0.993	−0.846	—	0.00165	73%
Regression on log weight, log height, and log fat-free mass	−1.142	0.168	−0.992	0.870	0.00161	74%
Irreducible minimum variance	—	—	—	—	0.00100	—

This table shows clearly that 69% of the variation between individuals in oxygen consumption while walking at 7.4 km/hr (4.5 mph) is due to the differences between them in body weight; a further 4% is due to differences between them in height; and only 1% of the differences is due to the difference between them in fat-free mass. This means that 74% of the variance in oxygen consumption can be accounted for by these body parameters and, of the three, body weight is clearly the most important parameter. Wyndham and Heyns (1969) also found similar results for men stepping on and off a stool. Adams (1967) used a similar approach to evaluate the effects of age, sex, height, body surface area, lean body mass, and body mass on the differences between individuals in oxygen consumption while pedalling a bicycle between 15 and 17.4 km/hr. He showed that weight was the most important parameter and that none of the other factors improved the predictive capacity of the regression equation of energy expenditure against body weight, which for this rate of pedalling the bicycle ergometer took the following form:

$$E = 2.34 + 0.467W \pm 0.608$$

where E is energy expenditure in kcal/min, W is weight in kg, and the last term is the standard error of the estimate.

It will be clear from what has been written in this section that body weight is the main determinant of the energy expenditure or oxygen consumption in physical tasks in which the body is moved against gravity. Comparison therefore of the energy expenditures or oxygen consumptions of individuals of different weight is best done in milliliters per kilogram per minute (ml/kg·min). However, when it is desired to compare the energy expenditures or oxygen consumptions of *two different populations* at the same rate of external work, then it is *not* valid to do so in these terms because the regression lines of oxygen consumption against body weight of the two groups might not pass through zero; and, it is only where this is the case that comparisons in terms of the ratio of oxygen consumptions to weight are strictly valid. This is illustrated by a comparison made by Wyndham and Heyns (1969) of the oxygen consumption of 80 Caucasians and 45 Bantu males running at 9.7 km/hr (6 mph). The regression lines with their 90% confidence limits are given in Figure 17-1. Calculation from the regression lines of oxygen consumption per kilogram for men of 50, 60, 70, and 80 kg shows that the ratios are constant with an increase in body weight as illustrated in Table 17.5.

Table 17-5 Maximum Oxygen Intakes in Milliliters per Kilogram per Minute for Two Populations, at Various Weights from Regression

	Body Weight, kg			
Population	50	60	70	80
Caucasian	44	43	43	42
Bantu	38	37	38	38

Because in this example the ratios between oxygen consumption and weight are constant, the two regression lines must pass through zero. It follows therefore that, in these particular samples, the ratios of mean oxygen intakes to mean weight of the two groups must also be similar to the values given above. For the Caucasians the ratio is 2.80/66.3 = 42.4 ml/kg·min and for the Bantu 2.23/58.9 = 37.7 ml/kg·min. It can readily be imagined that, if the regression line of one of the two populations did not pass through zero, the ratio would not be constant over the various weights and comparison of the two groups in terms of the ratio of mean oxygen intake to mean body weight would not be valid. The only valid procedure for comparing two populations in this regard is to compare the regression lines fitted to oxygen intakes against body weights of the two populations.

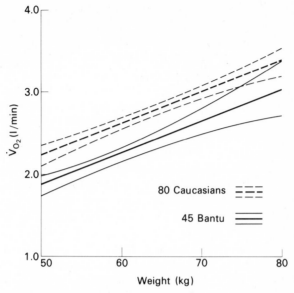

Figure 17-1. Comparison of regression lines of $\dot{V}_{O_2}$ on body weight of Bantu and Caucasians running at 9.7 km/hr (6 mph).

Predicting Oxygen Consumption from the Measurement of Heart Rate or Minute Pulmonary Ventilation

The measurement of oxygen consumption during muscular exercise presents many problems. The subject upon whom the measurement is being made has to breathe out through a system of valves and tubes into a collecting bag or into a meter (as in the Kofranyi-Michaelis or Woolf respirometers). Special apparatus and skilled staff are required for the analysis of oxygen and carbon dioxide in a sample of expired air. It is obvious that it would be of great advantage if a simpler method that was not so inaccurate that it invalidated the estimate was available for estimating the oxygen consumption. Two methods have been proposed in the physiological literature and have been examined by a number of research groups. They are the measurement of heart rate and the measurement of minute pulmonary ventilation.

Berggren and Christensen (1950) were the first to draw attention to the linear relationship between heart rate and metabolic rate. They laid down the conditions under which a measurement of heart rate can be used to predict the rate of oxygen consumption. First, because the relationship varies from individual to individual and with age, sex, and state of training, "a calibration curve has to be done for each individual." Second, the linear relationship holds for different tasks, such as running or bicycling, in which big muscle groups are used but not for tasks in which small muscle groups, such as the upper extremity, are used. Third, factors such as heat exposure and/or dehydration affect stroke volume and alter the relationship between stroke volume and heart rate and, in turn, alter the heart rate to oxygen consumption relationship. In consequence, Berggren and Christensen were led to conclude that in "using the pulse rate as an index of metabolic rate during work, one has to be careful."

The Scandinavian researchers have used heart rate as a rough indication of oxygen consumption in many industrial and sports situations, but they have been careful to calibrate the subjects on a bicycle ergometer on a number of occasions during the work or exercise period. If due regard is paid to the limitations of the method, particularly in regard to heat and dehydration, and, if careful calibration checks are carried out, then it can be regarded as a useful, but crude, method of estimating oxygen consumption. Unfortunately, however, heart rates have been used uncritically to estimate the effect of various forms of muscular activity, even under hot conditions. Sharkey et al. (1966) estimated the errors in predicting oxygen consumption from the measurement of heart rate in a variety of tasks and showed that the percentage differences between predicted and measured oxygen consumptions varied from 6 to 38% in an oxygen consumption range of 1.6 to 2.6 liters/min. The conclusion therefore is that heart rate is a valid method of predicting oxygen consumption only under very limited circumstances.

The other method of predicting oxygen consumption is by measuring the minute pulmonary ventilation. Durnin and Edwards (1955) investigated this question carefully and showed that there is a linear regression between minute ventilation and oxygen consumption over the range from 15 to 45 liters/min (BTPS). Outside of these limits the relationship is nonlinear, and therefore the prediction of oxygen consumption from minute ventilation is more difficult and less accurate. They also showed that there were large inter-individual differences in the regression lines, and thus, for reasonable accuracy, it is necessary to calibrate the individual at known work rates. Sharkey et al. (1966) came to the same conclusion. The great advantage of this method is that it is possible to collect expired air samples in either a Kofranyi-Michaelis or Woolf respirometer without interfering much with the subject's physical activity. The equipment is light and can be strapped securely to the back by means of an appropriate harness. Sharkey and his associates estimated the errors in predicting oxygen consumption from minute ventilation in a variety of tasks, with oxygen consumption ranging from 1.6 to 2.6 liters/min. The percentage differences between predicted and measured values ranged from 3 to 25%.

Two teams have compared the accuracy with which oxygen consumption can be predicted from both heart rate and minute ventilation measurements

(Sharkey et al., 1966; Datta and Ramanathan, 1969). They agree that the error of prediction is smaller when the prediction is based upon the measurements of minute ventilation than upon the measurement of heart rate. Datta et al.'s percentage differences are somewhat larger than those of Sharkey et al. quoted above, being 12–59% for heart rate and 5–21% for minute ventilation. These percentage differences are a good indication of the crudeness of these estimates of oxygen consumption and should be seen in light of the fact that the intraindividual coefficient of variation for the measurement of oxygen consumption over a wide range of tasks and levels of effort is about 5%.

Measurement of Maximum Oxygen Intake or Maximum Aerobic Power

Hill and Lupton (1923) in their studies of athletes were the first to show that oxygen consumption increases with speed of running up to a critical speed above which no further increase in oxygen consumption occurs even though the athlete is able to increase his speed of running. The rate of oxygen consumption at which this "flattening off" in oxygen consumption occurs is the maximum oxygen intake, or, expressed in other terms, the maximum aerobic power. The additional effort that the man makes at speeds above those at which the maximum oxygen intake occurs is done entirely on anaerobic metabolism. Hill and Lupton were also the first to show that in these circumstances lactic acid accumulates in the blood. Subsequently, Robinson (1938) used this approach to study the effects of age and sex on maximum oxygen intake, but the subject was only systematized and adequate criteria developed for determining maximum oxygen intake with the work of Taylor and his colleagues (1955) in the United States and Astrand (1952) in Sweden.

The direct measurement of maximum oxygen intake in the laboratory is time consuming and costly. It requires a treadmill or bicycle ergometer and the staff and equipment for the accurate measurement of the individual's oxygen consumption at a number of different workloads up to the individual's maximum physical effort. There has, in consequence, been a search for simpler and shorter methods that would give reliable estimates of the maximum oxygen intake. These have generally been based upon submaximal effort, and the two which have been most commonly used are the step test (Maritz et al., 1961) and the submaximal bicycle ergometer test (Berggren and Christensen, 1950; Andersen et al., 1965). However, even these tests require apparatus for the accurate measurement of heart rate and oxygen consumption at one or more submaximal workloads and, therefore, trained staff is needed. The need for an even simpler test which requires neither special equipment nor technical staff has led to the recent introduction by Cooper (1968) of the 12-min run or walk.

This section is concerned with the validity of the criteria for determining the maximum oxygen intake by the direct method and with the validity of the assumptions upon which the various submaximal tests are based.

Criteria for the Attainment of Maximum Oxygen Intake
by the Direct Method

A practical difficulty in determining the maximum oxygen intake by the direct method is that, although a satisfactory flattening-off of oxygen consumption with an increase in workload occurs in most fit individuals tested, this phenomenon does not occur in a certain proportion of subjects. The failure to flatten off is seen even in the intermittent procedure, where the subject rests until recovered between bouts of work; in the continuous increase of workload tests, the problem is worse. This difficulty has led to proposals of various criteria for measuring maximum oxygen intake and consideration must be given to their validity.

Taylor et al. (1955) consider that the maximum oxygen intake has been reached when (for men running at 7 mph with the grade being increased by $2\frac{1}{2}\%$ at each test) two successive determinations separated by a grade of $2\frac{1}{2}\%$ differed by less than 150 ml/min. This criterion was based upon the fact that the mean oxygen consumption increment for a $2\frac{1}{2}\%$ grade increase on 30 occasions was found to be 299.3 ml/min, with a standard deviation of 86.5 ml/min and range of 159–470 ml/min. Astrand (1952) demonstrated that in some subjects virtually no flattening-off occurred in the curve of oxygen consumption against workload, and thus he introduced the criterion of a blood lactic acid of 100 mg/100 ml blood as being indicative of the subject having reached maximum effort.

Wyndham et al. (1959) critically examined the criterion for reaching maximum oxygen intake by doing repeated measurements of oxygen consumption on 4 trained subjects at a large number of different workloads up to the individual's maximum effort. By this means they were able to satisfy themselves that oxygen consumption did in fact flatten off. They developed a mathematical equation for estimating the "true" maximum value. The equation is an exponential function of oxygen consumption against workload and requires a number of observations, especially around the flattening off point. This ideal is not attainable in most experimental situations. It is probably adequate to accept, as a valid index of the maximum oxygen intake, three oxygen consumptions at the three highest successive workloads that do not differ from each other by more than 200 ml/min; preferably, the measurements should vary in a random order about a regression line which is parallel to the horizontal axis of the graph. Although these criteria can be met in most athletic and fit subjects, many exercise physiologists will concede that it is very difficult to motivate certain categories of subjects adequately to sustain maximum or near maximum effort long enough to obtain the two or three measurements of oxygen consumption at successive increases in workload in the part of the oxygen consumption against workload curve where it has flattened off.

In the case of very unfit individuals, middle-aged, obese persons, children under ten years and primitive peoples, some relaxation of the criterion for judging maximum oxygen intake is needed. It is acceptable in these circumstances to take as the maximum oxygen intake the mean of two oxygen consumptions, obtained at two successive increases in workload which produce the maximum heart rate in the individual. In judging whether the individual has attained the maximum heart rate it should be borne in mind that age and altitude both affect maximum heart rate. Wahlund (1948) and Balke and Ware (1959), using continuous increases in workload on a bicycle ergometer, take as the maximum oxygen intake the oxygen consumption equivalent to heart rates of 170 and 180 beats/min, respectively. These procedures are certain to underestimate the maximum oxygen intake. However, on fit individuals where care is taken to use correct criteria for the attainment of maximum oxygen intake, the continuous method of determining maximum oxygen intake gives values that are closely similar to those obtained with the intermittent method (Wyndham, 1966b).

There is also some disagreement about the time after the commencement of exercise at which a valid measurement of steady state oxygen consumption can be obtained. Robinson (1938) considered that a steady state oxygen consumption is reached after 1 min 30 sec of running, whereas Taylor et al. (1955) found identical values at high levels of oxygen consumption (3.45 liters/min) for the period between 1.45–2.45 min and between 2.45–3.45 min. Wyndham et al. (1959) have contested this point. Their empirical data indicated that the rate at which steady state oxygen consumption is reached is related to the percentage of maximum oxygen intake. They found that, up to 50–60% of maximum oxygen intake, the steady state value was attained within 3 min, but above 60% of maximum oxygen intake oxygen consumption continued to rise with time. Although Astrand initially disagreed with Wyndham and his associates on this point, a figure used by Astrand and Saltin (1961a) validates Wyndham et al.'s point completely. Wasserman et al.'s (1967) careful examination of the time to steady state oxygen consumption at different workloads also validates Wyndham et al.'s contention in this regard. Clearly, some compromise on this issue has to be made in obtaining the curve of oxygen consumption against workload for determining maximum oxygen intake. If the oxygen consumption is taken too early after the commencement of exercise, a falsely low value would be obtained. In our experience expired air for the determination of oxygen consumption should be collected between the third and fourth minute at all levels of effort.

A further point which needs discussion is the nature of the exercise that should be used in order to obtain a valid measurement of maximum oxygen intake. Astrand and Saltin (1961b) and Hermansen and Saltin (1969) have looked into this question in some detail. They showed that equally high maximum oxygen intakes were obtained with cycling, running, and skiing, but cycling in the supine position and cranking a bicycle ergometer with the arms gave significantly lower values. Williams et al. (1967) have shown also that similar maximum oxygen intakes could be obtained from men pushing heavily loaded mine cars, running on a treadmill, shovelling rock, and riding a bicycle ergometer.

There has been some doubt as to whether it is possible to adapt the step test to provide maximum physical effort. Shephard et al. (1968) indicated that it is possible to do so, but other workers have not succeeded in obtaining maximum values with this technique. It is probably safe to conclude that either a bicycle ergometer or a treadmill are the most satisfactory methods of obtaining maximum physical effort. There is some contention as to whether one can obtain as high a maximum oxygen intake with the bicycle ergometer on subjects who are not accustomed to cycling or in primitive peoples who have never seen a bicycle. Wyndham et al. (1966b), Glassford et al. (1965) and, recently, Hermansen and Saltin (1969) reported significantly lower values with the bicycle ergometer than with the treadmill. Van Graan et al. (1970) could not persuade Kalahari Bushmen to exert themselves to maximum effort on a bicycle ergometer. However, in the Scandinavian countries experience with the bicycle ergometer is more favorable. Ekblom and Gjessing (1968), Swedish investigators, and Lange Andersen (1960), a Norwegian, always use bicycle ergometers and appear to be satisfied that they can obtain maximum values even with primitive peoples.

In this context a point that should be borne in mind is that athletes from different sports give higher maximum oxygen intakes on the physical activity to which they are accustomed. Thus, we found that runners gave consistently lower maximum oxygen intake values on the bicycle ergometer than on the treadmill. Most champion cyclists were clumsy runners, and they gave consistently lower values on the treadmill than on the bicycle ergometer. The mean maximum oxygen intake values of champion swimmers were lower on the treadmill and ergometer than when they swam. It appears therefore that althletes were able to bring more muscles into operation in a coordinated manner at maximum effort in the sport they were accustomed to than in an unfamiliar physical activity. This point should be borne in mind in selecting the method to use in comparing the maximum oxygen intake values of different populations and may well account for the very low values that have appeared in the physiological literature from time to time on selected population groups (Rodahl et al., 1961).

Assumptions Made in the Indirect Method of Maximum Oxygen Intake

An alternative to the direct method of measuring maximum oxygen intake was first proposed by Astrand and Rhyming (1954). In their proposal, maximum oxygen intake was estimated by means of a nomogram from the measurement of heart rate at a single level of work, stepping on and off a stool. The estimated maximum oxygen intake was based upon a number of assumptions that were implied but not explicitly stated. The first assumption was that heart rate is a linear function of oxygen consumption right up to the maximum physical effort; the second, that the straight lines for different individuals, representing the relationships between heart rate and oxygen consumption, have a common point, which is 60 beats/min at zero oxygen consumption; the third, that the deviations of individual maximum heart rates from the population mean maximum heart rate is very small; and, the fourth, that the oxygen intake of the subject at the "standard work rate deviates very little from the population mean oxygen consumption for the standard work rate." If these assumptions are valid then the following procedure, expressed in nomogram form by Astrand and Rhyming, can be used to estimate the maximum oxygen intake on an individual with precision:

> Heart rate is measured at the standard rate of stepping and the oxygen consumption is estimated from the population oxygen-consumption/work-rate graph. The measured heart rate is plotted against the predicted oxygen consumption, and this plot is joined by a straight line to the common point (60 beats/min at zero oxygen consumption) and the straight line is extrapolated to a heart rate of 128 beats/min to give an estimate of half of the individual's maximum oxygen intake (or to 196 beats/min at sea level to give the maximum oxygen intake).

Astrand and Rhyming found closely similar results between their nomogram and direct measurements on a number of different samples involving different sexes and states of fitness.

The validity of each of the points upon which the Astrand and Rhyming nomogram are based was studied in detail by Wyndham and his associates (Maritz et al., 1961). They found that two of the assumptions were fully validated. One is that maximum oxygen intake can be predicted from the mean body weight of the individual at the "standard work rate" with a variance from the population mean which is similar to the day-to-day variability in the measurement in the individual. The second is that the variation of the individual maximum heart rate from the population mean maximum heart rate is very small so that the mean population maximum heart rate (determined on a subsample of the population of, say, 20 subjects) can be employed in the test procedure without introducing significant errors in the estimate of maximum oxygen intake for the individual.

Wyndham et al. also showed that one of the premises was not strictly valid. A straight line is a good representation of the relationship between heart rate and oxygen consumption over most of the range of the measurements, but in some individuals the heart rate reaches its maximum value at lower rates of work than does the oxygen consumption. Hence, when heart rate is plotted against oxygen consumption, the curve tends toward an asymptote. Thus, the actual maximum oxygen intake by direct measurement is generally higher than that obtained by extrapolation to maximum heart rate of the straight line fitted to plots of heart rate against oxygen consumption. Wyndham et al. estimated that the order of this bias is about 0.30 liters/min. The fact that heart rate reaches its maximum at lower work rates than does oxygen consumption has since been confirmed by other workers (Davies, 1968; Rowell et al., 1964). A rather disturbing point that has been noted in recent studies on large samples of medical students, who varied very widely in their state of physical fitness, is that this tendency for heart rate to reach its maximum at lower work rates than does oxygen consumption is more marked in very unfit individuals than in fit individuals, so that the bias toward underestimating the true maximum oxygen intake is greater in the very unfit individuals.

Another premise in Astrand and Rhyming's nomogram which was not supported by Wyndham et al.'s study is that there is a common point for the heart-rate/oxygen-consumption relationship for all subjects of 60 beats/min at zero oxygen consumption. Wyndham et al. found that there was no significant difference in the oxygen consumption of 26 men at rest but that there were very significant differences in their resting heart rates and this, of course, means that the use of any common point is not valid. Wyndham et al. went on to point out that, in order to obtain a good estimate of the straight line relationship between heart rate and oxygen consumption for an individual, it is essential to make at least three measurements of heart rate and oxygen consumption at widely different work rates and that it is preferable to make four measurements. They estimated the probable error of the indirect measurement of maximum oxygen intake, using four measurements of heart rate and oxygen consumption, as a coefficient of variance of 12% compared with direct measurement. Use of the Astrand and Rhyming nomogram to estimate maximum oxygen intake on these 26 subjects gave a coefficient of variance that was approximately twice as great. Davies (1968) has also examined the validity of these criteria and gives a very similar figure for the error variance of 14%.

Comparisons of maximum oxygen intake measurements by direct and indirect methods were stimulated by the decision of the Human Adaptability Section of the International Biological Program (IBP) to make the study of physical work capacity of different populations around the world one of the main aims of the program. A number of working parties of exercise physiologists (which were attended by the writer) met to discuss methodology, and several physiology laboratories were charged with the task of comparing the various proposed methods. An initial report on these studies was made at a satellite symposium at the time of the 1968 International Congress of Physiological Sciences in Japan by Wyndham et al. (1966c). They compared estimates of maximum oxygen intake made by the indirect method with those measured directly by means of the treadmill and bicycle ergometer. They showed that the mean maximum oxygen intake of 40 fit young army recruits was 3.18 ± 0.751 liters/min on the step test, which was not significantly different from the mean of 3.21 ± 0.401 liters/min on the treadmill. However, the scatter of indirect measurements about the regression line of maximum oxygen intake per weight was about twice that for the direct measurement, and, further, there was a tendency for the indirect measurement to underestimate at low values and to overestimate at high values of maximum oxygen intakes.

Wyndham and coworkers also showed that the mean maximum oxygen intake of 40 fit young men on the bicycle ergometer was 2.89 ± 0.282 liters/min, which was significantly lower than the treadmill mean. In this case the bicycle ergometer values showed a tendency to be systematically lower than treadmill values at the higher maximum oxygen intakes. Treadmill maximum oxygen intake values measured by a method of continuous increase in speed did not differ from those measured by means of an intermittent procedure in which subjects rested between runs. Further comparisons between test methods were made by Shepard and his group in Toronto (1968), but unfortunately he introduced his own variation of the step test, which bears no relationship to the procedures of Astrand and Rhyming or Wyndham et al. His comparisons, therefore, do not help in sorting out this problem.

Some practical points that emerged from these various working parties and comparisons of tests under the IBP were

1. That the work rates for the indirect procedures should be chosen so that the heart rates do not fall below 100 beats/min nor rise above 160 beats/min. This simplifies fitting the straight lines to the plots of heart-rate/oxygen-consumption and improves the accuracy of the estimates.
2. That the bicycle ergometer can be employed for the indirect method as successfully as the step test in populations that are accustomed to cycling.
3. That the mean maximum heart rate in the population under study should be determined on a subsample of the main sample (10–20 in each ten-year age group are adequate for this purpose). In this way the effects of age and altitude can be taken into account.

Estimates of Maximum Oxygen Intake from Walking or Running Tests

The time taken to run a mile or the distance run in a set time has been used as part of a battery of tests for evaluating the "fitness" of populations of school- and college-students for some years. These tests have been of limited use because they have not always been carefully standardized, due to problems in ensuring that the subjects were well motivated, and because no attempts had been made to correlate performances in these tests with measurements of maximum oxygen intake.

Col. Cooper of the United States Air Force must be given credit for the first systematic correlation between the distance walked or run in a 12-min period and the direct measurement of maximum oxygen intake (Cooper, 1968). He studied 115 Air Force males between the ages of 17 and 52 years and between 114 and 270 lb in weight. He found a correlation of 0.84 between the distances run in 12 min and the maximum oxygen intake values on the treadmill. He gives a useful table for classifying men into different categories of cardiorespiratory fitness on the basis of the distances run or maximum oxygen intake values (Table 17-6).

Table 17-6 Levels of Cardiorespiratory Fitness Based upon 12-Min Walk or Run and Maximum Oxygen Intake (ml/kg · min)

Distance, miles	Max. $\dot{V}_{O_2}$	Fitness Level
Less than 1.0	Less than 25.0	Very poor
1.00 to 1.24	25.0 to 33.7	Poor
1.25 to 1.49	33.8 to 42.5	Fair
1.50 to 1.74	42.6 to 41.5	Good
More than 1.50	More than 51.6	Excellent

Cooper did not take account of the effects of altitude, age, or sex on these criteria, but Wyndham et al. (1971) subsequently put forward tentative adjustments. They proposed 10% be taken off the values for each decade after 40 years of age, a further 10% for females, and 10% for each 200 m above sea level. A procedure of this type could be of immeasurable importance for quick and inexpensive evaluation of the maximum oxygen intake values of different groups in the population and for comparing different populations, because all that is needed is a level 400-m track and a stop watch. However, a great deal of work is needed to validate Cooper's results and to deal with the problem of the motivation of subjects to ensure that they are making the 12-min run at their best effort.

With these points in mind and also to determine whether living at 1763 m above sea level affected the results, Wyndham et al. (1971) carried out a comparison between maximum oxygen intake measured by the direct treadmill method and by the distance run in 12-min. The sample consisted of 25 members of the laboratory staff who covered roughly the same age and weight ranges as Cooper's subjects. A correlation coefficient of 0.94 was obtained between maximum oxygen intake and the distance run in 12 min. Wyndham and his associates commented upon the need for good motivation in the subjects and upon the dangers of the 12-min run or walk to unfit men in their 50s and 60s unless they were examined medically with an exercise ECG prior to the test.

Wyndham et al. have also noted that in the 12-minute run the distances of good middle-distance runners fall above the regression line for distance run against maximum oxygen intake for the general population, which suggests either that the relationship between the two parameters is not a straight line or that different regression lines are needed for the very fit, the fit, and the very unfit. Wyndham et al. also proposed, as a check on the motivation of the subjects, that their heart rates be measured immediately after they completed the 12-min run. If the heart rate was found to be less than 160 beats/min, it would be good evidence that the subject had not exerted himself to the full extent possible, and the run should be repeated with the understanding that he try harder.

These results are encouraging for the person who wants to determine the maximum oxygen intake values of samples of school, college, or university students and lacks the equipment to make either direct or indirect measurements. This method is also useful for assessing the effect of physical conditioning programs, and so on. However, a great deal more research is needed in different age groups and sexes in order to determine the correlations between the distance run and maximum oxygen intake values before the 12-min run can be used as a valid, but crude, assessment of maximum oxygen intake.

Reproducibility of Measurements and the Effects upon Them of Physical Conditioning, Occupation, and State of Nutrition

In fit young men, maximum oxygen intake measured by the direct method is highly reproducible over prolonged periods. Wyndham and associates (Maritz et al., 1961) measured maximum oxygen intake directly at frequent intervals over a period of 4 months. They showed that the mean coefficient of variance of maximum oxygen intake of the four men was 3.5%. The coefficient of variance for the indirect method was about 12–14%. Similar observations have been made by other researchers (Davies, 1968; Rowell, 1964).

Physical conditioning also affects maximum oxygen intake. The extent of improvement is a subject of controversy because the conditioning programs studied have varied and also because the state of "fitness" and nutrition of the subjects at the commencement of the program have varied in different studies. In the usual experimental subject, the undergraduate student, the improvement in maximum oxygen intake is relatively small, averaging about 10–15% (Ekblom, 1970; Ekblom et al., 1968; Williams et al., 1967). When middle-aged sedentary subjects are subjected to a rigorous conditioning program the effect is greater and improvements of 20% have been observed (Saltin et al., 1967). Saltin et al. (1968) studied men after bed rest and, in these previously sedentary subjects, the improvement was of the order of 60% (mean of 2.43 to 3.91 liters/min). There is, however, great truth in Astrand's contention that "if you wish to be a world class athlete then you have to choose your parents carefully" or, put in other terms, world class athletes are born, not made. This does not indicate that proper physical conditioning and a specific training program cannot bring out the latent physical ability of an athlete, but a 3.0 liters/min man cannot be made into a 5.0 liters/min athlete.

Habitual physical activities have a marked effect upon maximum oxygen intake. Astrand (1956), Andersen (1966), and others have measured maximum oxygen intake in different categories of workers and have shown that men, such as lumberjacks, engaged in hard physical work have much higher maximum oxygen intakes than those engaged in more sedentary tasks. What is not clear is whether it is the men with naturally high maximum oxygen intake who gravitate to such work as lumberjacking or whether men, going into this trade in their teens, develop high maximum oxygen intakes.

The state of nutrition of the individual and the population in general affects maximum oxygen intake in one of two ways. In the underdeveloped nations there is generally a lack of first class protein during the growing period, fats are usually in short supply, and most of the calories come from cereals, which are very bulky. The people in these areas are generally of short stature and are lean with very small skinfold thickness. When these men enter industry, work hard, and are provided with a good diet, which is high in animal protein and in calories (as happens to the Bantu in the gold mines of South Africa) they gain 3.0 kg, on the average, in the first month (Wyndham et al., 1966d). Maximum oxygen intake increases from 2.3 to 2.8 liters/min but per kilogram the gain is from 42.1 to 49.0 ml/kg·min. This indicates that the men put on muscle and also improve in cardiorespiratory fitness. Probably because of nutritional factors and the harder physical work they perform, the Bantu male does not show the increase in weight nor the fall in maximum oxygen intake that the European male does after the age of 30 years. It appears that the European male pays dearly for his luxus consumption diet and sedentary habits. It seems possible that the early atherosclerosis from which the European suffers markedly reduces the ability of the ventricles of the heart to increase, or maintain, stroke volume during exercise; this, in turn, is responsible for the rapid fall in maximum oxygen intake after the age of 30 for the European. Overnutrition leads to obesity and this, in turn, to high oxygen consumption at even very low levels of effort. We then have a vicious cycle: high oxygen demands and markedly diminished maximum oxygen intake. Such a situation leads to a high incidence of coronary heart disease.

These issues have been stressed because valid comparisons of different populations can only be made in the context of knowledge of their state of physical conditioning, their habitual physical activities, and their state of nutrition. Too frequently comparisons have been made between, say, African pastoralists and European athletes without giving any of the contextual information upon which the comparison should be judged. Comparisons of maximum oxygen intake of different ethnic groups without this information are meaningless.

Relationship Between Maximum Oxygen Intake and Certain Body Parameters

The question of which body parameter is the most valid reference for maximum oxygen intake has concerned physiologists for some time. Astrand (1952) in his classic monograph reported correlation coefficients of 0.98 between maximum oxygen intake and both body weight and total hemoglobin. Since then he and Sjostrand (1953) have repeatedly claimed that total hemoglobin is the important determinant of maximum oxygen intake. This conclusion was effectively refuted by van Döbeln (1957), who showed that the high correlation between maximum oxygen intake and total hemoglobin is entirely due to the close correlation between body weight and total hemoglobin. When the partial correlation coefficient between maximum oxygen intake and total hemoglobin is calculated with the effect of body weight removed, the correlation between maximum oxygen intake and total hemoglobin is no longer significant. Van Döbeln's correlation coefficient between maximum oxygen intake and body weight was 0.75 which, as will be shown later, is much more in line with the findings of other research workers than the correlation coefficient of 0.98 found by Astrand.

Buskirk and Taylor (1957), Welch et al. (1958), and Wyndham and Heyns (1969) have examined the relationship between maximum oxygen intake and the body parameters of gross body weight, fat-free mass, and lean body mass. Wyndham et al. (1967) also looked into the relationship between oxygen intake and stature. All the studies utilized European subjects. Buskirk and Taylor's 46 subjects were highly selected; 26 were sedentary students (one had an extreme percentage fat of 34%), 15 were regular participants in sports, and 5 were cross-country runners. Welch's, et al., 28 men were test subjects at the United States Army Medical Nutrition Laboratory. Wyndham's, et al., 80 subjects were white South African army recruits who had just completed their high school courses (the studies were made in Johannesburg at an altitude of 1763 m). The physical characteristics of the various subjects

Table 17-7 Physical Characteristics of Subjects

Sample	Age, years	Height, cm	Weight, kg	Fat, %	Max. $\dot{V}_{O_2}$ Liters/m	Ml/kg·min
Buskirk and Taylor	22.1	176.3	77.5	13.9	3.58	46.2
(1957)	(2.6)	(6.1)	(15.6)	(8.9)	(0.50)	(4.8)
Welch et al.	23.1	177.0	75.3	15.1	3.73	49.5
(1958)	(1.9)	(8.0)	(9.0)	(5.8)	(0.45)	(4.3)
Wyndham et al.	19.0	174.4	66.3	13.7	3.15	47.2
(1969)	(0.84)	(5.8)	(7.3)	(8.2)	(0.40)	(6.0)

Table 17-8 Correlations between Max. $\dot{V}_{O_2}$ and Body Parameters

Sample	Max. $\dot{V}_{O_2}$ Body Weight	Max $\dot{V}_{O_2}$ Fat-Free Mass	Max. $\dot{V}_{O_2}$ Lean Body Mass	Max. $\dot{V}_{O_2}$ Height
Buskirk and Taylor (1957)	0.63	0.85	0.91	—
Welch et al. (1958)	0.54	0.64	0.65	—
Wyndham et al. (1969)	0.78	0.75	—	0.34

are given in Table 17-7, and the correlation coefficients found between maximum oxygen intake and the various body parameters are given in Table 17-8.

Buskirk and Taylor concluded, on the strength of the higher correlations between maximum oxygen intake and fat-free mass and lean body mass, that these two parameters are the important determinants of maximum oxygen intake. This conclusion is not tenable because the three parameters are highly intercorrelated, and it is necessary to calculate partial correlation coefficients with the influence of each of the parameters removed, in turn. Wyndham et al. have performed these calculations on their data, and their results are given in Table 17-9. The first two partial correlation coefficients are significant at the 5% level of significance, but the correlation between maximum oxygen intake and fat-free mass falls away. Thus, in their data Wyndham et al. find that body weight is the main determinant of maximum oxygen intake.

It is possible that the differences in the findings between Buskirk and Taylor and Wyndham et al. in this regard are due to differences in the two samples. Buskirk and Taylor specifically chose their subjects to represent as wide a range as possible of body fat percentages, whereas Wyndham's, et al., subjects were younger and were, in general, in a better state of physical conditioning. On these grounds it is probable that Buskirk and Taylor's conclusions are more generally applicable to the population at large, especially in the over 30 age level, where the range of percentage body fat is likely to be large. The general conclusion that can be drawn from these various findings is that, although it is more correct physiologically to use fat-free mass or lean body mass as the reference when expressing maximum oxygen intake, gross body weight can also be used with little loss of accuracy.

Table 17-9 Partial Correlation Coefficients between Body Parameters

Factors Correlated	Partial Correlation Coefficient
Max. Log $\dot{V}_{O_2}$/Log weight (constant height)	0.76
Max. Log $\dot{V}_{O_2}$/Log height (constant weight)	−0.22
Max. Log $\dot{V}_{O_2}$/Log fat-free mass (constant weight)	−0.06

A point of interest in Wyndham's, et al., analysis is that maximum oxygen intake has a significant negative correlation with stature when the effect of weight is removed. This indicates that, for two men of the same body weight, the taller man is likely to have the lower maximum oxygen intake. Whether the lower maximum oxygen intake of the taller man would be compensated by the lower maximum oxygen intake when walking or running, as was shown in an earlier section, is an open question.

We need next to consider how much of the variation in maximum oxygen intake between individuals is due to differences between them in these body parameters. Welch et al. calculated coefficients of determination ($r^2 \times 100$) from the correlation found by Buskirk and Taylor (1957) and Welch et al. (1958). On this basis they state that, using Buskirk and Taylor's findings, 40% of the variation between individuals in maximum oxygen intake was due to the differences between them in body weight, 72% was due to differences between them in fat-free mass, and 83% was due to differences between them in lean body mass. On their own data the differences between individuals in maximum oxygen intake due to these three body parameters was 35, 41, and 42%, respectively. However, as discussed in an earlier section, the use of the coefficient of determination in this context is invalid. The only way to determine the relative proportion of the differences between individuals in maximum oxygen intake which is due to these body parameters is to calculate multiple regression equations, the total variances, the irreducible variances, and the residual variances about the regression lines. This is done in Table 17-10.

Table 17-10 Percentage of Max. $\dot{V}_{O2}$ Accounted for by Weight, Height, and Fat-Free Mass

	Parameters				Residual Variance	Accounted for, %
	A	B	C	D		
Total variance	—	—	—	—	0.00319	—
Regression on log weight	−1.156	0.908	—	—	0.00127	70
Regression on log weight and log height	−0.861	1.029	−0.681	—	0.00122	71
Regression on log weight, log height, and log fat-free mass	−0.748	1.405	−0.610	−0.397	0.00122	71
Irreducible minimum variance	—	—	—	—	0.00046	—

Table 17-10 shows that 70% of the variation between individuals in maximum oxygen intake is due to differences between them in body weight. A further 1% of the differences between them is due to differences in height, but differences in fat-free mass do not account for any further differences in maximum oxygen intake. This means that about 30% of the variation between them in maximum oxygen intake is not accounted for by these body parameters and, presumably, is due to differences between them in state of physical conditioning, cardiorespiratory capacity, and other unspecified factors.

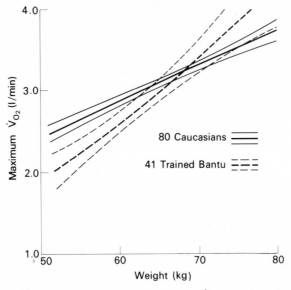

Figure 17-2.   Comparison of regression lines of max $\dot{V}_{O_2}$ on body weight of fit young and physically conditioned Bantu and Caucasians.

From the foregoing it will be clear that gross body weight is a valid reference for maximum oxygen intake when comparing individuals of different weights. However, as with oxygen intake for different rates of walking and running, it is not a valid procedure to compare the mean maximum oxygen intakes of populations by the simple ratio of mean maximum oxygen intake to mean gross body weight. It is essential to calculate regression equations for maximum oxygen intakes on body weight and confidence intervals for the two populations and base the comparisons on these regression lines. This is illustrated in Figure 17-2 for a sample of 41 fit young Bantu mine recruits, after they had been physically conditioned for hard work in the mines, and for a sample of 80 Caucasian army recruits after 3 months of physical conditioning in the recruiting center. The ratios of maximum oxygen intake to body weight of the Caucasians and Bantu were 47.2 and 45.1 ml/kg·min, respectively. Although these means were not significantly different, the regression lines with their 90% confidence limits show that the Bantu have significantly higher maximum oxygen intake values in the weight range below 60 kg. The foregoing is a perfect illustration of how invalid, in fact quite misleading, it is to compare populations by using the ratio of maximum oxygen intake to weight rather than using regression equations of maximum oxygen intake on weight if the regression lines do not go through zero.

The Measurement of Anaerobic Metabolism

The relationships between oxygen consumption, oxygen debt, and lactic and pyruvic acids, during and after muscular work at different levels of physical effort, have been a subject of investigation since the 1920s. Krog and Lindhard (1920) showed that, during recovery after vigorous exercise, the raised level of oxygen consumption fell rapidly in the initial few minutes after the exercise, stopped, and then declined more slowly to its resting level. They attributed the slow return of oxygen consumption to its resting level, which they observed during the transition from rest to work at the beginning of exercise, to the oxygen deficit. Hill and Lupton (1923) in their intensive investigation of the subject distinguished between a fast and a slow component in the recovery curve of oxygen consumption after exercise. They coined the term "oxygen debt" for the oxygen consumption in excess of the resting level during the recovery phase after exercise and attributed the entire debt to the oxidation of lactic acid. Hill and Lupton's concepts were challenged by Margaria et al. (1933). They proposed that the initial rapid fall in oxygen consumption was due to the restoration of the high-energy phosphates in muscle; they called this phase of the oxygen debt curve the alactic phase. Like Hill and Lupton, Margaria et al. attributed the slower decline of oxygen consumption to resting level to the oxidation of lactic acid.

The subject was relatively dormant until the late 1950s when Huckabee (1958) introduced the concept of "excess" lactate. He claimed that the lactic acid levels in blood were influenced by the lactic acid/pyruvic acid ratios and by the levels of pyruvic acid in the blood. From his experiments Huckabee concluded that the oxygen debt was more closely correlated with "excess" lactate than with lactic acid. His research reawakened interest in the subject and led to considerable further research, which did not substantiate his conclusions. Margaria and his colleagues were prominent in this resurgence of interest. Margaria, however, has clung tenaciously to his earlier ideas that the initial fast fall in oxygen consumption after the cessation of exercise is alactic and is due to the splitting of the high-energy phosphates ATP and CP. Margaria et al. (1964, 1966) calculated that the alactic phase of anaerobic metabolism in a 70-kg man has a capacity of about 1.5–2.0 liters of oxygen and a maximum aerobic power of 10 liters/min of oxygen consumption. They calculated, further, that the capacity of the lactic acid phase of anaerobic metabolism in a man of the same weight would be 3.2 liters of oxygen and the maximum anaerobic power would be 5 liters/min of oxygen consumption. Their values for the total oxygen debt, approximately 5 liters, are much smaller than those measured by Hill and Lupton (1923) and also by other recent workers who have recorded oxygen debts of 10 liters and more (Knuttgen, 1962; Wasserman et al., 1965; Welch et al., 1970).

Margaria's concepts have been challenged by Knuttgen (1962). He considers that the division of the recovery curve of oxygen consumption ". . . into separate lactic acid and nonlactic acid related portions (lacacid and alactic) seems oversimplistic and not in keeping with the behavior of the two dominant phases of recovery, fast and slow." He states further that ". . . a more complete understanding of the inter-related metabolic, thermal, electrolytic, and hormonal changes which the body undergoes during exercise will be necessary for its explanation." That Margaria's concepts are an oversimplification is also suggested by the recent work of Karlsson (1971) and Karlsson and Saltin (1970) on the ATP, CP, and lactate concentrations in working muscle during exhaustive exercise.

Until we have a better understanding of the physiological and biochemical changes that are associated with the different phases of the oxygen debt curve, the measurements of anaerobic capacity and maximum anaerobic power are on insecure grounds. Margaria, for example, has proposed a simple method for measuring the maximum anaerobic power and capacity (Margaria, 1967; Margaria et al., 1966). He restricts himself to measurement of the alactic phase only in his proposed method, in which the maximum speed, between the third and sixth sec from the start, of running up a staircase of 10–12 steps is measured. The lift-work in kilogram-meters per second is converted to a rate of energy expenditure on the assumption that the mechanical efficiency of all subjects running up stairs is 25%.

Margaria proposes a different method for measuring the "lactacid oxygen debt." He measures the rate of increase in lactic acid in the antecubital *venous* blood at repeated intervals during a run to exhaustion on a treadmill at different inclinations (the speeds are chosen for the different inclinations so that the subject is exhausted after between 2 and 6 min). Margaria assumes that lactic acid is evenly distributed throughout the total body water at the different times the samples are taken and, on this assumption, calculates the maximum rate of lactic acid accumulation in the body (in milligrams per liter). From the rate of accumulation of lactic acid, he determines both the maximum power and the capacity of the lactic acid phase of anaerobic metabolism.

Margaria's basic assumptions as to the clear-cut division between the two phases of anaerobic metabolism are not on secure ground, as Knuttgen has indicated. Also certain of his other assumptions are questionable. Lactic acid will not be evenly distributed throughout the total body water at the times venous blood samples are taken in his experiments. Nor is venous blood from a nonworking extremity a true measure of the lactic acid concentration. Lactic acid has been shown to be metabolized in nonworking muscle and in the splanchnic area. In addition, there are large differences between peripheral venous and arterial blood during heavy exercise.

At present, therefore, the only valid procedure for measuring anaerobic capacity and its maximum power is the laborious and tedious method of having the subject run up a slope at a rate that will exhaust him in about 5 min so that the oxygen debt may be measured directly during the recovery phase. This method has been well described by a number of authors (Knuttgen, 1962; Wasserman et al., 1965). In summary, it consists of taking samples of expired air at 1-min intervals over the first 5–10 min and at 10-min intervals thereafter until the rate of oxygen consumption has returned to its resting level. From the area under the curve, both the anaerobic capacity and the maximum anaerobic power can be calculated. This method requires the resources of a well equipped laboratory and trained technical staff.

Just as important as the measurement of anaerobic power and capacity, however, is the determination of the level of oxygen consumption, compared with the individual maximum oxygen intake, at which evidence of anaerobic metabolism is first seen. Margaria (1967), using venous blood, has stated that, "lactic acid is not produced in exercise except at very high levels of oxygen consumption, approaching the maximum aerobic power." This is certainly not the experience of other exercise physiologists using either arterial blood or arterialized blood from the finger tip warmed to 45°C.

Wyndham et al. (1962) showed that lactic acid in arterial blood increased above control levels in fit young men at between 50 and 60% of maximum oxygen intake; that in convalescent, ambulatory patients the increase occurred at about 40% of maximum oxygen intake (Wyndham et al., 1965); and that, in endurance athletes in good training, the increase is seen at between 70 and 90% of maximum oxygen intake (Strydom et al., 1967). Wyndham and his associates (Williams et al., 1967) also showed that as a result of proper training the percentage improvement in the level of oxygen consumption at which lactic acid in blood increased was greater than the percentage improvement in maximum aerobic power. These various conclusions have since been confirmed by Hermansen and Saltin (1967) and by Costill (1970).

It seems clear from the findings of these workers that it is very important to determine the percentage level of maximum oxygen intake of endurance runners at which anaerobic metabolism first occurs. The practical importance is that if one has two 1500-m runners of similar weight and maximum aerobic power, the runner with the higher percentage of maximum aerobic power at which anaerobic metabolism occurs is always at an advantage. If both men enter the final 200 m together, the runner without any lactic acid in his blood, that is, who has been running on aerobic metabolism, would be able to sprint to the tape; the other, who has been running partly on anaerobic metabolism, will be less likely to be able to increase his speed at this essential point in the race (Wyndham et al., 1969).

The measurement of lactic acid concentrations in arterial blood, or arterialized blood, is a valid method of determining the level of oxygen consumption, compared to the maximum, at which an endurance athlete begins to use anaerobic metabolism. This percentage is a good index of the state of training of the subject. The closer to the maximum aerobic power that the increase in lactic acid in the blood takes place, the better is the state of training of the athlete. It is also a useful method for evaluating the effectiveness of different endurance training programs. Unfortunately, these determinations require a well-equipped and staffed exercise physiology laboratory.

There is, however, a simpler, but cruder, method of making this measurement. Hill and Lupton (1923) were the first to draw attention to the fact that the RQ rises above 1.0 when blood lactate is raised at levels of exercise close to the individual's maximum. Issekutz and Rodahl (1961) confirmed this finding and used the increase in RQ as a criterion for judging when maximum oxygen intake was attained. Wasserman and MacIllroy (1964) showed that the RQ is relatively constant over a range of submaximal work, but it increases sharply at the same level of oxygen consumption at which lactic acid concentrations increase in the blood. The sudden increase in RQ is therefore an indication of the level of oxygen consumption at which anaerobic metabolism first occurs. Although this appears to be a valid procedure for this purpose, the method must be regarded with some reservations until a thorough and systematic examination is made of anaerobic metabolism as indicated by changes in RQ and by increases in blood lactic acid.

REFERENCES

Adams, W. C.: Influence of age, sex and body weight on energy expenditure of bicycle riding. *J. Appl. Physiol.*, **22**:539–545 (1967).

Andersen, K. L.: Work capacity of selected populations. In P. Baker and J. S. Weiner (eds.): *Biology of Human Adaptability*, Oxford, Clarendon Press, 1966.

Andersen, K. L., A. Bolsted, Y. Loyning, and L. Irving: Physical fitness of Arctic Indians. *J. Appl. Physiol.*, **15**:645–648 (1960).

Andersen, K. L., and L. Hermansen: Aerobic capacity in young Norwegian men and women. *J. Appl. Physiol.*, **20**:425–431 (1965).

Astrand, P. O.: *Experimental Studies of Work Capacity in Relation to Age and Sex.* Copenhagen, Munksgaard, 1952.

Astrand, P. O.: Human physical fitness with special reference to age and sex. *Physiol. Rev.*, **30**:307 (1956).

Astrand, P. O., and I. Rhyming: A nomogram for calculation of aerobic capacity (physical fitness) from pulse rate during submaximal work. *J. Appl. Physiol.*, **7**:218–221 (1954).

Astrand, P. O., and B. Saltin: Oxygen intake during the first few minutes of heavy exercise. *J. Appl. Physiol.*, **16**(6):971–976 (1961a).

Astrand, P. O., and B. Saltin: Maximum oxygen intake and heart rate in various types of muscular activity. *J. Appl. Physiol.*, **16**(6):977–981 (1961b).

Balke, B., and R. W. Ware: An experimental study of physical fitness in Air Force personnel. *U.S. Armed Forces Med. J.*, **10**:675–685 (1959).

Bang, O.: The lactate content of blood during and after muscular exercise in man. *Scand. Arch. Physiol.*, Suppl. 10, 1936.

Berggren, G., and E. H. Christensen: Heart rate and body temperature as indices of metabolic rate during work. *Int. Z. angew. Physiol.*, **14**:255–260 (1950).

Brockett, J. E., E. M. Brophy, F. Koniski, J. G. Mareinik, M. P. Grothear, W. A. Michalowitz, P. Kaskin, and M. I. Grossman: Influence of body size, body fat, nutrient intake and physical fitness on the energy expenditure of walking. Report No. 177. U.S. Army Nutrition Laboratory, Denver, Colorado, 1956.

Buskirk, E., and H. L. Taylor: Maximum oxygen intake and its relationship to body composition with special reference to chronic physical activity and obesity. *J. Appl. Physiol.*, **11**(1):72–78 (1957).

Consolazio, C. F., R. E. Johnson, and L. J. Pecora: *Physiological Measurements of Metabolic Functions.* New York, McGraw-Hill, 1963.

Cooper, K. H.: A means of assessing maximum oxygen intake. *J. Amer. Med. Assoc.*, **203**(3):201–204 (1968).

Costill, D. L.: Metabolic responses during distance running. *J. Appl. Physiol.*, **28**(3):251–255 (1970).

Cotes, J. E., and F. Meade: The energy expenditure and mechanical energy demand in walking. *Ergonomics*, **3**:97–119 (1960).

Datta, S. R., and N. L. Ramanathan: Energy expenditure in work predicted from heart rate and pulmonary ventilation. *J. Appl. Physiol.*, **26**(3):297–302 (1969).

Davies, C. M. T.: Limitations to the prediction of maximum oxygen intake from cardiac frequency measurements. *J. Appl. Physiol.*, **24**(5):700–706 (1968).

Delbue, C., R. Passmore, and B. Woolf: Individual variations in the metabolic cost of standardised exercises: the effects of food, age, sex and race. *J. Appl. Physiol.*, **121**:225–231 (1953).

Durnin, J. V. G. A.: The use of surface area and body weight as a standard reference in studies of human energy expenditure. *Brit. J. Nutr.*, **13**:68–71 (1959).

Durnin, J. V. G. A., and R. G. Edwards: Pulmonary ventilation as an index of energy expenditure. *Quart. J. Exp. Physiol.*, **40**:370–377 (1955).

Ekblom, B.: Effect of physical training on the circulation during prolonged exercise. *Acta. Physiol. Scand.*, **78**:145–158 (1970).

Ekblom, B., P. O. Astrand, B. Saltin, J. Stenberg, and B. Wallstrom: Effects of training on circulatory responses to exercise. *J. Appl. Physiol.*, **24**:518–528 (1968).

Ekblom, B., and E. Gjessing: Maximum oxygen intake of Easter Island populations. *J. Appl. Physiol.*, **25**(2):124–129 (1968).

Glassford, R. G., G. H. Y. Baycroft, A. W. Sedgwick, and R. B. McNab: Comparison of maximum oxygen uptake values determined by predicted and actual methods. *J. Appl. Physiol.*, **20**(3):509–513 (1965).

Hermansen, L., and B. Saltin: Blood lactate concentrations on acute exposure to altitude in R. Margaria (ed.): *Exercise at Altitude*. Amsterdam, Exerpta Medica, 1967.

Hermansen, L., and B. Saltin: Oxygen uptake during maximal treadmill and bicycle exercise. *J. Appl. Physiol.*, **26**(1):31–37 (1969).

Hill, A. V., and H. Lupton: Muscular exercise, lactic acid and the supply and utilisation of oxygen. *Quart. J. Med.*, **16**:135–171 (1923).

Huckabee, W. E.: Relationships of pyruvate and lactate during anaerobic metabolism: II Exercise and the formation of O_2 debt. *J. Clin. Invest.* **106**:255–263 (1958).

Issekutz, B., and K. Rodahl: Respiratory quotient during exercise. *J. Appl. Physiol.*, **16**:606–612 (1961).

Karlsson, J.: Lactate and phosphagen concentrations in working muscle. *Acta. Physiol. Scand.*, Suppl. 358, 1971.

Karlsson, J., and B. Saltin: Lactate, ATP and CP in working muscle during exhaustive exercise in man. *J. Appl. Physiol.*, **29**(5):598–602 (1970).

Keul, J., E. Doll, and D. Keppler: The substrate supply of the human muscle during and after work. *Experentia*, **23**:974–978 (1967).

Knuttgen, H. G.: Oxygen debt, lactate, pyruvate and excess lactate after muscular work. *J. Appl. Physiol.*, **17**:639–644 (1962).

Knuttgen, H. G.: Oxygen debt after submaximal physical exercise. *J. Appl. Physiol.*, **29**(5):650–657 (1970).

Krog, A., and J. Lindhard: The changes in respiration in the transition from rest to work. *J. Physiol.*, **53**:431–439 (1920).

Leary, W. P., and C. H. Wyndham: The capacity for physical effort of Caucasian and Bantu athletes of international class. *S. Afr. Med. J.*, **39**(7):651–655 (1965).

Mahadeva, K., R. Passmore, and B. Woolf: Individual variations in the metabolic costs of standarised exercises: the effects of food, age, sex and race. *J. Physiol.*, **121**:225–231 (1953).

Margaria, R.: Aerobic and anaerobic energy sources in muscular exercise. In R. Margaria (ed.): *Exercise at Altitude*, Amsterdam, Excerpta Medica, 1967.

Margaria, R., H. T. Edwards, and D. B. Hill: The possible mechanisms of contracting and repaying the oxygen debt and the role of lactic acid and muscular contraction. *Amer. J. Physiol.*, **106**:689–715 (1933).

Margaria, R., P. Cerretelli, and F. Mangili: Balance and kinetics of anaerobic energy release during strenuous exercise in man. *J. Appl. Physiol.*, **19**(4):623–628 (1964).

Margaria, R., P. Aghemo, and E. Rovelli: Measurement of muscular power (anaerobic) in man. *J. Appl. Physiol.*, **21**(5):1662–1664 (1966).

Maritz, J. S., J. F. Morrison, J. Peter, N. B. Strydom, and C. H. Wyndham. A practical method of estimating an individual's maximum oxygen intake. *Ergonomics*, **4**(2):97–122 (1961).

McCance, R. A., and E. M. Widdowson: The composition of foods. Spec. Rep. Ser. No. 289, Med. Res. Counc., London, 1960.

Miller, A. T., and C. S. Blyth: The relationship of body type and body fat content and the metabolic cost of work. *J. Appl. Physiol.*, **8**:139–141 (1955).

Ralston, H. T.: Energy-speed relationship and optimum speed during level walking. *Int. Z. angew. Physiol.*, **17**:277–283 (1958).

Rasch, P. J., and W. R. Pierson: The relationship of body surface area, mass and indices of energy expenditure. *Rev. Can. Biol.*, **21**:1–6 (1962).

Robinson, S.: Experimental studies of work capacity in relation to age and sex. *Int. Z. angew. Physiol.*, **10**:251–323 (1938).

Rodahl, K., P. O. Astrand, N. Birkhead, T. Hettinger, B. Issekutz, and M. Jones: Physical work capacity. *Amer. Med. Assoc. Arch Environ. Health*, **2**:499–506 (1961).

Rowell, L. B., H. L. Taylor, and Y. Wang: Limitations to prediction of maximum oxygen intake. *J. Appl. Physiol.*, **19**(5):919–927 (1964).

Rowell, L. B., K. K. Kraning, T. O. Evans, J. W. Kennedy, J. R. Blockman, and F. Kusami: Splanchnic removal of lactate and pyruvate during prolonged exercise in man. *J. Appl. Physiol.*, **21**:1773–1783 (1966).

Saltin, B., L. H. Hartley, A. Kilburn, and I. Astrand: Physical training in sedentary middle-aged and older men. *Scand. J. Clin. Lab. Invest.*, **24**: 323–334 (1967).

Saltin, B., G. Blumquist, J. H. Mitchell, R. L. Johnson, K. Wildenthal, and C. B. Chapman: Response to exercise after bed rest and training. *Circulation*, Suppl. 7, 1968.

Selzer, C. C.: Body metabolism and oxygen metabolism at rest and during exercise. *Amer. J. Physiol.*, **129**:1–13 (1940).

Sharkey, B. J., J. F. MacDonald, and L. C. Corbridge: Pulse rate and pulmonary ventilation as predictors of human energy cost. *Ergonomics*, **9**(3):233–227 (1966).

Shepard, R. J., A. Allen, A. J. S. Benade, C. M. T. Davies, R. E. di Prampero, R. Hedman, J. E. Morrison, V. Myhre, and R. Summers: Standardisation of submaximal exercise tests. *Bull. World Health Organ.*, **38**:765–775 (1968).

Sjostrand, T.: Volume and distribution of blood and their significance in regulating the circulation. *Physiol. Rev.*, **33**:202–228 (1953).

Strydom, N. B., C. H. Wyndham, and J. S. Greyson: A scientific approach to the selection and training of oarsmen. *S. Afr. Med. J.*, **41**:1100–1102 (1967).

Tanner, J. M.: *The Physique of the Olympic Athlete*. London, Allen and Unwin, 1964.

Taylor, H. L., E. Buskirk, and A. Henschel: Maximum oxygen intake as an objective measure of cardiorespiratory performance. *J. Appl. Physiol.*, **8**:73–80 (1955).

van Döbeln, W.: Maximum oxygen intake, body size and total haemoglobin in man. *Acta. Physiol. Scand.*, **38**:193–199 (1957).

van Graan, C. H., and J. S. Greyson: A comparison between bicycle ergometer and step test for determining maximum oxygen intake of Kalahari Bushmen. *Int Z. angew. Physiol.* **28**: 344–348 (1970).

Wahlund, H.: Determination of physical working capacity. *Acta. Med. Scand.*, Suppl. 215, 1948.

Wall, B. K., and A. Merrill: Composition of foods. Agriculture Handbook No. 8, U.S. Dept., Agr., Washington, 1964.

Wasserman, K., and M. B. MacIllroy: Detecting the threshold of anaerobic metabolism in cardiac patients during exercise. *Amer. J. Cardiol.*, **14**: 844–853 (1964).

Wasserman, K., G. G. Burton, and A. L. v. Kessel: Excess lactate concept and oxygen debt of exercise. *J. Appl. Physiol.*, **20**(6):1299–1306 (1965).

Wasserman, K., A. L. v. Kessel, and G. G. Burton: Interaction of physiological mechanisms during exercise. *J. Appl. Physiol.*, **22**(1):71–85 (1967).

Weir, J. B. de V.: New methods for calculating metabolic rate with special reference to protein metabolism. *J. Physiol.*, **109**:1–9 (1949).

Welch, H. E., J. A. Faulkner, J. K. Barclay, and G. A. Brooks: Ventilatory response during recovery from muscular work and its relation with O_2 debt. *Med. and Sci. in Sports*, **2**:16–19 (1970).

Welch, H. E., R. P. Reindeau, C. E. Crisp, and R. S. Isenstein: Relationship of maximum oxygen consumption to various components of body composition. *J. Appl. Physiol.*, **12**(3):395–398 (1958).

Widdowson, E. M., O. G. Edholm, and R. A. McCance: Food intake and energy expenditure of cadets in training. *Brit. J. Nutr.*, **8**:147–155 (1954).

Williams, C. G., C. H. Wyndham, R. Kok, and M. J. E. von Rahden: Effect of training on maximum oxygen intake and anerobic metabolism in man. *Int. Z. angew. Physiol.*, **24**:18–26 (1967).

Williams, C. G., C. H. Wyndham, A. J. du Raan, and R. Kok: A comparison of the physical work capacity of individuals as determined by different tasks. *Int. Z. angew. Physiol.*, **24**:102–110 (1967).

Wyndham, C. H., and A. J. A. Heyns: Determinants of oxygen consumption and maximum oxygen intake of Caucasians and Bantu males. *Int. Z. angew. Physiol.*, **27**:51–75 (1969).

Wyndham, C. H., N. B. Strydom, J. F. Morrison, J. Peter, and Z. U. Potgieter: Maximum oxygen intake and maximum heart rate during strenuous work. *J. Appl. Physiol.*, **14**:927–936 (1959).

Wyndham, C. H., C. G. Williams, and M. J. E. von Rahden: A physiological basis for the "optimum" level of energy expenditure. *Nature*, **195**:1210–1212 (1962).

Wyndham, C. H., H. S. Seftel, C. G. Williams, V. Wilson, N. B. Strydom, G. A. G. Bredell, and M. J. E. von Rahden: Circulatory mechanisms of anaerobic metabolism in working muscle. *S. Afr. Med. J.*, **39**:1008–1014 (1965).

Wyndham, C. H., J. F. Morrison, C. G. Williams, N. B. Strydom, M. J. E. von Rahden, L. D. Holdsworth, A. Joffe, and A. J. Heyns: Inter- and intraindividual differences in energy expenditure and mechanical efficiency. *Ergonomics*, **9**:17–29 (1966a).

Wyndham, C. H., N. B. Strydom, W. P. Leary, and C. G. Williams: A comparison of methods of assessing maximum oxygen intake. *Int. Z. angew. Physiol.*, **22**:285–295 (1966b).

Wyndham, C. H., N. B. Strydom, C. G. Williams, and A. J. A. Heyns: Comparison of estimates of maximum oxygen intake obtained from a treadmill ergometer and step test. In H. Yoshimur and J. S. Weiner (eds.): *Human Adaptability and its Methodology*, J.S.P.S., Tokyo, 1966c.

Wyndham, C. H., N. B. Strydom, W. P. Leary, C. G. Williams, and J. F. Morrison: The effect on maximum oxygen intake of young males of a regime of regular exercise and adequate diet. *Int. Z. angew. Physiol.*, **22**:304–310 (1966d).

Wyndham, C. H., C. G. Williams, J. F. Morrison, and A. J. A. Heyns: The influence of weight and stature on mechanical efficiency. *Int. Z. angew. Physiol.*, **23**:107–124 (1967).

Wyndham, C. H., N. B. Strydom, A. J. van Rensburg, and A. J. Benade: Physiological requirements for world class performance in endurance running. *S. Afr. Med. J.*, **43**:996–1002 (1969).

Wyndham, C. H., N. B. Strydom, C. H. van Graan, A. J. van Rensburg, G. G. Rogers, J. S. Greyson, and W. H. v.d. Walt: Estimating the maximum aerobic capacity for exercise. *S. Afr. Med. J.*, **45**:53–57 (1971).

Human Performance

Part V

SECTION EDITOR:
MAXWELL L. HOWELL
San Diego State College

Human Performance Factors

18

PAUL HUNSICKER
The University of Michigan
Ann Arbor, Michigan

Human performance could conceivably cover activities as diverse as a child learning to walk and man's flight to the moon. This chapter will be concerned with those activities generally associated with physical education programs, including the dance and the world of sports. Even with these constraints it will be obvious that the field of coverage is vast and the demands made on the human body by each activity may be quite different. Let us examine some of the possibilities.

If one looks at human performance from the standpoint of energy cost, the figures range from values as low as 3.2 kcal/min in archery to highs of 18.6 kcal/min in cross-country skiing. Variances in energy output could be attributed to differences in performance level, the intensity of competition, or the age of the participant. Aside from the human factors, the energy cost of an activity is influenced by climatic conditions such as temperature and relative humidity and by other factors such as altitude or terrain. The wide range of energy demands in sports participation makes it possible for everyone to engage in some sport, regardless of the individual's level of physical fitness.

Another criterion, the neuromuscular skill demands, could be applied to human performance, and the resulting range of demands would be equally wide. Even within the confines of a single sport the skill level of the novice is quite different from that of a world champion. If one extends the criterion to a comparison of different activities, one runs the gamut from a relatively simple motor skill such as hiking to the highly complex motor skills required in golf, basketball, or baseball. There are differences even within one sport; for example, in the case of baseball, the motor skills demanded of a pitcher are quite different from those necessary to play shortstop or to catch. Once again the fact that the participants might enjoy widely divergent neuromuscular skill patterns and still find a niche in the spectrum of sports should make sports attractive to the multitude.

A less common view of human performance is a consideration of the economic cost to the participant. Here again the range of possibilities is staggering. For a person to do some cross-country running, the cost is practically nil; but if his interests are in skiing, sailing, or horse racing, the economic drain can be prohibitive. The economics of sports have come under closer scrutiny during the past decade because of spiralling costs and more restrictive budgets. This has been particularly true in the United States where sports and physical education are so closely allied to school programs.

Although there are tremendous differences in the many facets of sports, there is a strong universality in their appeal. This is perhaps best illustrated by recognition of the fact that over 100 nations send representatives to the Olympic Games.

The foregoing paragraphs were intended to give a thumbnail sketch of the diverse nature of human performance in hopes that the reader would recognize the limitations of any subsequent attempts at generalizations. Now let us turn to an examination of the factors commonly associated with human performance. Although the topic is exceedingly complex and few traits are requisite to all manifestations of performance, selected characteristics are definitely an asset in numerous activities. The remainder of the discussion will be devoted to the identification of human factors and their relationships to physical performance. Any attempt to establish a priority order strikes the writer as an exercise in futility, consequently, a nonordered enumeration of traits will be utilized.

Human Performance Parameters

Strength

Observers of sports through the ages have been cognizant of the role of strength, and the topic has intrigued investigators in such diverse fields as physical education, psychology, medicine, child growth and development, and gerontology. Although there are still many enigmas regarding the acquisition and maintenance of strength, there is a considerable volume of literature devoted to the topic. An overview of our current knowledge in the field seems appropriate. Although no attempt will be made at a historical treatment of strength studies, it should be noted that Amar (1920) reports investigations dating back to 1699. The works of Sargent, Kellogg, Rogers, and McCloy represent landmarks in the strength literature prior to World War II. Larson (1940) differentiated between static and dynamic strength in an early factor analysis study and pointed out the low correlation between the two. This aided in understanding differences between selected physical fitness tests.

Although strength was accepted as a desirable attribute in sports prior to 1945, its importance was not really appreciated until the last 20 years. During the 1930s it was almost unthinkable for a coach to suggest weight-training techniques to increase the strength of his squad members. This was particularly true in sports such as swimming, track, and basketball. Today the practice is widespread. The studies that probably did more to direct attention to strength development and that started a fad toward isometrics were those reported by Hettinger and Müller in the early 1950s. The "instant strength" promise of isometrics was right in tune with the "instant gratification" that the public was just getting accustomed to by watching television.

In due time it became evident that isometrics alone had limited value as a training program unless you were getting a person ready to hold up a ceiling! In practically all sports performances the movements carried out are isotonic not isometric. Although the programs advocated by the proponents of isometrics had their limitations, the simple fact that a large number of people became interested in strength development regimes had a salutary effect on training programs. A plethora of periodical articles were the direct result of the renewed interest in the field of strength. Research findings supported the use of strength development programs for selected sports, and athletes in a whole host of activities began supplementing their customary training programs with strength development exercise including the use of weights and/or exercise machines. The practice even extended into competitive swimming, which would have been virtually unthinkable prior to 1940. That strength is important in selected sports is well established, and an examination of the particular activities most demanding in strength requirements is now in order.

The activity that immediately comes to mind is weight lifting. The press movements in this sport are almost exclusive feats of strength, and all the other lifts require considerable strength. Practically all the contact sports call for above-average strength output. This would include wrestling, football, boxing, hockey, combatives (such as judo), lacrosse, soccer, rugby, and others. In the category of noncontact sports that require abnormal amounts of strength one would have to list gymnastics, rowing, mountain climbing, and field events. This list of sports is in no way exclusive or an inference that other activities do not require strength; most people would agree that sports in general make strength demands. It boils down to a matter of relative requirements and the range is vast. A second category that would include strength demands above that normally exerted during the course of living would encompass sports such as baseball, basketball, swimming, skiing, handball, the racquet games (such as tennis and squash), volleyball, track, and certain phases of the dance.

Those sports calling for a lesser degree of strength would include golf, hiking, social dancing, fishing (exclusive of game fishing), croquet, and archery. Devotees of archery might well take exception to the writer's view of the strength demands of this sport by pointing out the possibility of using a bow that requires considerable strength to draw. However, this is not the type of equipment generally found in an instructional class in archery. For the bow and arrow game hunter, the strength requirements would be greater.

When one looks at selected physical education programs, one can find situations where considerable emphasis is placed on strength-producing activities. The classic examples would be the conditioning activities at the United States Marine Corps boot camps or the programs followed at an Army Ranger or Paratrooper training center. To carry out any one of these three assignments requires strength and the services do their best to see that the trainee is physically strong at the completion of his training. The conditioning programs at the Marine Corps Training Centers involve both isometric and isotonic strengthening exercises along with other activities designed to improve the other components of physical fitness.

Endurance

Even a casual reflection on sports would bring to mind the importance of endurance or cardiovascular condition. Endurance, like strength, manifests itself in a variety of ways. If one thinks of the type of endurance required to do sit-ups or pull-ups, one conjures a different concept from the endurance required for a distance swim or run. Investigators have introduced qualifying terms such as "muscular endurance" or "cardiovascular endurance" to differentiate between the two. Both types of performance call for more than a single maximum effort. Generally, if you ask the question "How many can you do," or "How long does it take to do the task," you are referring to an activity which involves a type of endurance. An examination of the sports spectrum demonstrates the importance of the endurance factor.

The endurance demands of a marathon run, wrestling, boxing, crew, distance swimming, cross-country skiing, mountain climbing, and distance running short of the marathon are all examples of sports that call for high levels of muscular endurance and/or cardiovascular endurance. Sports such as badminton, tennis, and squash racquets would also call for endurance but to a lesser degree.

Body Type

The study of body type has captured the interests of man for hundreds of years, and research workers have attempted to relate body type to predisposition to diseases, to mental, emotional, and social traits, and to sports performance. Shakespeare demonstrated a sensitivity to body type by not casting a Falstaff as Cassius in *Julius Caesar*. Most students of human nature are aware of the alleged relationships between physical type and character traits or personality traits. No cartoonist would think of depicting Santa Claus as a cadaverous looking individual or a tax collector as a jolly, rotund person. However, body type does have real relevance in terms of the kind of physical activity that can be carried out most efficiently. The difficulty arises from the simple fact that most persons are not extremes but an admixture of several types. However, it should prove fruitful to discuss some observations covering body type and sports.

In the past half century the work of Kohlrausch in connection with the 1928 Olympic athletes would represent one of the early, thorough investigations of body type and sports. The researches of Sheldon and associates (1940) did much to refine the techniques of body typing and gave subsequent workers a better research tool to work with. Cureton (1947) was one of the early and more prolific writers to use Sheldon's techniques in attempting to explain sports performance. A few obvious comments regarding body type and sports should convince even the most skeptical of the relationship between body type and sports performance.

The game of basketball is probably a prime example of where body type can be a limiting factor. A professional basketball team can be singled out in a terminal when traveling because it is one of the rare occasions when 12 to 15 young adult men whose average height is in the order of 6 ft 6 in. are seen in a single group. A professional American football team is by no means a run-of-the-mill group from a physical standpoint. It is difficult to imagine a predominant mesomorph as a marathon runner or an extreme ectomorph as a channel swimmer. It doesn't take a keen observer to note that runners have a different build from shot putters and discus throwers in track-and-field events. Even in the same sport body build differences, although less glaring, exist; the shortstop in baseball, for example, is generally a smaller man than the first baseman or the long-ball hitters in the outfield. Additional examples of the importance of body type in a sport could be cited but, like other factors in human performance, body type can be of minimal consequence.

In boxing and wrestling the body build influence is controlled to some extent by the use of weight classes in competition. In sports such as archery, handball, badminton, tennis, or golf, to name a few, men of widely diverse body builds can perform equally well. The observation would have to be qualified to exclude extremely obese individuals. In fact, the obese performer is handicapped in practically every sport with the possible exception of sumo wrestling, and this has a rather limited number of devotees.

Flexibility

Any attempt to delineate the role of flexibility in human performance is fraught with obstacles. When one considers the number of joints in the body, each with a range of movement, plus the possible number of combinations of joint movements theoretically available in human performance, the thought of attempting to define flexibility becomes a nightmare. Certainly no single criterion or test of flexibility could be applied that would adequately predict human performance. One fact that seems fairly well established is that the flexibility exhibited in human performance is highly specific in nature, and thus attempts at generalization could be misleading. With these words of caution as a preface, it is possible to cite situations in sports where a high degree of flexibility may be exhibited.

If one eliminates the gyrations of a contortionist, some forms of the dance, notably ballet and modern, call for extreme movements that definitely tax the range of movement of joints. Some of the free exercise routines in gymnastics would fall in the same category. On a limited scale the movements of the ankles of competitive swimmers, some plays that a shortstop makes in baseball, and certain shots taken by a highly skilled basketball player are all examples of above-average flexibility in isolated segments of the body. A diver or a hurdler would labor under a handicap if selected body joints were restricted in their range of movement. From a purely practical standpoint, no physical performance would be possible if the joints were completely immobile. Flexibility is the *sine qua non* of movement, and movement is the *sine qua non* of physical performance.

Coordination

The writer prefers to think of coordination in terms suggested by Fleishman (1964), namely, "it may turn out that the essence of coordination is the ability to integrate the separate abilities in a complex task." Certainly a well-coordinated movement involves perfect timing between the muscular and nervous systems. Practically without exception attempts to isolate a general motor ability or coordination factor and predict ability in sports have been discouraging. Once again the factor apparently exists in many different forms. Think of some of the kinds of coordination called for in the realm of sports.

Even when one restricts the movements performed to, say, hitting an object such as a ball, disparities occur. The task faced by the baseball hitter is not the same as that of the golfer, handball player, or tennis player. When the emphasis is shifted to another segment of the body, all relationships pale into insignificance. Think of the generally poor level of soccer ability in American youths, even those who might be highly talented in basketball, football, or baseball. The thought of predicting soccer ability from basketball ability would be ludicrous. Yet, no one would deny that talented performers in both sports are well coordinated. And one must admit both kinds of coordination are of the large muscle type.

Additional forms of coordination are present in such diverse activities as the dance, field events, bowling, badminton, gymnastics, and ice hockey. The list is far from exhaustive; it is merely an indicator of the numerous manifestations of coordination.

Speed

The term speed, like other attributes of human performance, is shrouded in confusion because of the lack of a clear-cut definition that is acceptable to all workers. Probably the simplest description restricts it to running speed as demonstrated in the dashes in track. Other more complex definitions incorporate the concepts of reaction time or the speed of the arms or hands. In any event, speed has been recognized in many forms.

One may think of speed as synonomous with the term fast. Certainly many sports observers do, and it is common to hear such descriptions as "the fast hands" of a boxer or ball player. The speed of an ice hockey puck or stick is a well-recognized phenomenon. On occasion Olympic track winners have been referred to as "the fastest human." The safety man in American football is only too aware of the speed of an opposing end or halfback who happens to catch a pass between the safety man and the goal line.

Additional manifestations of speed are seen as sudden bursts of movement in an attempt to elude a defensive player in sports. Typical examples are obvious in basketball, football, or any other game where part of the strategy involves freeing an offensive player from the covering defensive man. This kind of speed is frequently combined with a change of direction, and many observers would tab this agility.

Agility

The trait of agility usually involves speed but includes an additional dimension, namely, the ability to make a sudden change of direction or movement. Like speed, agility is important when game strategy is designed to free an offensive player. However, agility can equally be an asset in situations where no defensive player is involved. Think of when the infielder in baseball makes an outstanding fielding play by virtue of his speed and ability to change direction quickly in order to field the ball. The execution of the double-play in baseball calls for agility on the part of the shortstop or second baseman. One can cite numerous movements that involve agility in ice hockey, gymnastics, boxing, wrestling, and surf-boarding. This last sport probably demands more of the next trait to be mentioned, balance.

Balance

Any time the base of support is reduced and the subject is able to maintain control of body position, you have an expression of balance. This can be exhibited with the subject standing still, as when standing on one foot, or with the subject moving. Classic examples of activities demanding a high degree of balance would include surf-boarding, the ballet, and tight-rope walking. Other circus performers have been able to build routines which are almost exclusively balance acts.

To a lesser degree balance is important in most ball playing sports, the combatives, gymnastics, ice hockey, and skiing. The hallmark of a truly great performer often times stems from his ability to execute a movement when seemingly completely off balance. Practically every ball game of top-flight competitors will have unusual exhibitions of balance.

Intelligence

Although the world of sports is replete with performances which require a minimum of intelligence, it is nonetheless true that intelligence is needed in selected sports. The planning of strategy or the development of a game plan necessitates intellectual activity. In highly organized college or professional sports, most of the planning is left to the coaching staff, which then has the challenge of instilling these plans into the players. Even under these circumstances, however, because of the continually changing nature of events during the game, the player is frequently faced with alternatives from which he must choose the correct one. This represents a kind of intelligence and is another distinguishing characteristic amongst players. Some are looked upon as "smart" players and others are not.

Although some people have questioned the intelligence (or possibly the common sense) of anyone engaged in mountain climbing, the preparations that must precede an ascent of Mt. Everest cannot be left to a dim-wit. A similar case can be made for competitive deep-sea sailing or scuba expeditions.

An additional example of the need for intelligent choices in sports is derived from the staggering number of statistics available about past performances. The player or coach is required to be familiar with these data, and frequently decisions are based on percentages from prior games. The ability to recognize the limitations of the statistics and to make prudent choices is a sign of intelligence.

Other less common displays of intelligence occur when you have a participant or coach who is a genuine student of the sport. His analysis may call for a background in physics, physiology, or psychology. He is seriously seeking answers to the differences between good and poor performance. No one could question the need for intelligence to ferret out these answers.

Creativity

Sports are generally governed by well-defined rules and regulations, and the opportunities for creativity on the part of the player are extremely limited. In fact, many sports performances are highly repetitive and completely unimaginative. In these instances movements are practically automatic amongst high level performers. However, there are exceptions and a few activities afford the occasion to be creative, such as the routines developed in competitive figure skating and in modern dance.

Motivation

Probably one of the best practical gauges of motivation is how much time a participant is willing to devote to an activity. After all, the great bulk of adult sports participation is purely voluntary, and the player surely has other options available. The degree of motivation can vary from mild to intense, but you can be fairly certain that anyone who aspires to top-flight performance must pay the price in time and practice to achieve his goal. There is no simple answer to what motivates people and the only certain thing is that there are multiple reasons for taking part in sports.

The professional is usually playing because of the monetary returns, and these have increased handsomely over the last 20 years, thanks to television. At the other end of the scale you have the pure amateur, who takes part because of sheer love of the sport. This individual frequently invests a fair amount of his personal money without any thought of return other than the pleasure of participating. Countless sports devotees take part to improve their physical condition or because of the possible salutary health benefits derived from the sport. Large numbers engage in a sport because of the social contacts gained through the activity. To some the work-out at noon is taken as a welcomed break from the usual routine of the job. In isolated instances sports participation has been used to further business interests. Still others find the challenge of the sport sufficient reason for continuing to participate. There are probably additional motivating factors but, in any event, some type of motivation is needed for voluntary performance.

Summary

In recapitulation one can say that human performance covers a vast spectrum of activities and interests. Energy demands are quite diverse, skill requirements differ considerably, the cost of participation extends from practically zero to the high cost of owning a yacht. Sport can be a gratifying outlet for energy release to persons in all walks of life.

The enumeration and discussion of the factors required for human performance make it abundantly clear that highly talented performers in different sports could be endowed with quite dissimilar physical traits. Little mention was made of age or ability differences in sports and the human factors were viewed as operating at the better levels of performance. Obviously the demands at lower ability levels would be considerably less. Motivation to some degree is an absolute must for performance, because every movement originated first as a thought and then a decision is made to carry it out. Without motivation it would be aborted as a thought.

Table 18-1 represents an attempt to present a crude quantification of the human factors required in selected sports when performed at a fairly high level of proficiency. The factor of motivation was not included in the table because this is required for all activities, and a high degree of motivation is demanded if one aspires to top level performance. It is hoped that the coach or teacher of physical education will be aware of the vast scope of possibilities

Table 18-1 Relative Importance of Human Factors in Selected Sports*

Sport	Strength	Endurance	Body Type	Flexibility	Coordination	Speed	Agility	Balance	Intelligence	Creativity
AQUATICS										
Diving	1	1	3	3	3	1	3	3	1	1
Scuba	1	2	1	1	2	0	1	1	2	1
Swimming—distance	2	3	2	2	1	0	0	0	1	0
Swimming—sprints	3	1	2	2	1	2	0	0	0	0
Waterpolo	2	3	1	2	2	1	0	0	1	1
Water skiing	2	1	1	1	2	0	2	3	1	0
COMBATIVES										
Boxing	3	3	1	1	2	3	3	1	1	1
Judo	3	2	1	2	2	3	3	2	1	1
Wrestling	3	3	1	3	2	3	3	2	1	1
DANCING										
Ballet	1	3	3	3	3	1	3	3	2	3
Ballroom	1	1	2	2	2	1	2	2	1	2
Folk	2	2	1	1	2	1	1	1	1	1
Modern	1	3	2	3	3	1	3	3	2	3
INDIVIDUAL PHYSICAL ACTIVITY										
Bicycling	2	3	2	1	1	2	0	1	1	0
Fishing—deep sea	2	3	1	1	1	1	1	1	1	0
Fishing—lake	1	1	1	1	1	1	1	0	1	0
Hiking	1	2	1	1	1	0	0	0	0	0
Mountain climbing	2	3	1	2	2	1	2	2	2	1
Skiing—cross country	2	3	2	2	3	2	2	2	1	0
Yoga	1	2	2	3	2	1	1	3	1	1

INDIVIDUAL COMPETITION

Archery	1	0	1	1	2	0	0	1	0
Badminton	1	2	1	3	3	2	3	1	1
Bowling	1	1	0	1	1	1	0	0	0
Fencing	2	3	2	3	3	3	3	2	1
Golf	1	1	1	1	3	1	1	1	0
Gymnastics	3	2	3	2	3	1	2	3	0
Handball	2	2	1	2	3	2	2	1	0
Paddleball	2	2	1	2	3	2	2	1	0
Squash rackets	2	2	1	2	3	2	2	1	0
Table tennis	1	2	1	1	2	2	2	1	0
Tennis	2	3	1	2	3	2	2	1	0

TEAM COMPETITION

Baseball	2	1	1	2	3	2	2	1	1
Basketball	2	3	2	3	3	3	3	2	1
Cricket	2	2	1	2	3	2	2	1	0
Curling	1	1	1	1	2	1	1	1	0
Field hockey	2	2	1	2	3	2	2	1	1
Football—American	3	2	1	3	2	3	2	1	0
Lacrosse	2	3	1	2	3	2	2	1	0
Rowing	3	3	2	1	1	1	1	0	0
Rugby	3	3	1	3	2	3	2	1	0
Soccer	2	2	2	3	3	3	3	2	0

TRACK AND FIELD

Distance running	1	3	1	1	1	1	1	1	0
Field events	3	1	2	2	2	1	1	2	0
Sprints	2	3	1	1	1	3	1	1	0

* 0: little or no involvement.   1: mild involvement.   2: moderate involvement.   3: heavy involvement.

in the sports spectrum and that there is probably some activity for practically everyone regardless of his physical, psychological, or social make-up. With this as background information, the coach or teacher should be in a position to counsel students into activities more intelligently.

REFERENCES

Amar, J.: *The Human Motor*. London, George Routledge and Sons, p. 470, 1920.

Carlsten, A., and G. Grimby: *The Circulatory Response to Muscular Exercise in Man*. Springfield, Ill., Charles C Thomas, p. 129, 1966.

Cooper, K. H.: *The New Aerobics*. New York, M. Evans and Co., p. 191, 1970.

Cureton, T. K., F. W. Kasch, J. Brown, and W. G. Moss: *Physical Fitness Appraisal and Guidance*. St. Louis, C. V. Mosby, p. 566, 1947.

Damon, A., R. A. McFarland, and H. W. Stoudt: *The Human Body in Equipment Design*. Cambridge, Mass., Harvard University Press, p. 360, 1966.

Dill, D. B.: Assessment of work performance. *J. Sports Med. Phy. Fitness*, **6**:3–8 (March, 1966).

Durnin, J. V. G. A., and R. Passmore: *Energy and Leisure*. London, Heinemann Educational Books, p. 166, 1967.

Fleishman, E. A.: *The Structure and Measurement of Physical Fitness*. Englewood Cliffs, N.J., Prentice-Hall, p. 207, 1964.

Fleishman, E. A., P. Thomas, and P. Munroe: The dimensions of physical fitness —a factor analysis of speed, flexibility, balance, and coordination tests. Office of Naval Research, Contract No. 609(32) Technical Report 3, Yale University, September, 1961.

Franks, B. D. (ed.): *Exercise and Fitness—1969*. Chicago, The Athletic Institute, p. 282, 1969.

Handler, Philip (ed.): *Biology and the Future of Man*. New York, Oxford University Press, p. 936, 1970.

Hettinger, T.: *Physiology of Strength*. Springfield, Ill., Charles C Thomas, p. 84, 1961.

Hunsicker, P.: Arm strength at selected degrees of elbow flexion. Wright Air Development Center Technical Report 54–548, Aero Medical Laboratory, Wright-Patterson Air Force Base, Ohio, p. 58, 1955.

Hunsicker, P.: A study of muscle forces and fatigue. Wright Air Development Center Report 57–586, Aero Medical Laboratory, Wright-Patterson Air Force Base, p. 47, 1957.

Hunsicker, P., and R. J. Donnelly: Instruments to measure strength. *Res. Quart.*, **26**:408–420 (December, 1955).

Hunsicker, P., and G. Greey: Studies in human strength. *Res. Quart.*, **28**:109–122 (May, 1957).

Jokl, E.: *Medical Sociology and Cultural Anthropology of Sport and Physical Education*. Springfield, Ill., Charles C Thomas, p. 165, 1964.

Kato, Kitsuo (ed.): *Proc. Int. Cong. Sport Sci., 1964*. Tokyo, The Japanese Union of Sport Science, p. 624, 1966.

Karus, H., and W. Raab: *Hypokinetic Disease*. Springfield, Ill., Charles C Thomas, p. 193, 1961.

Kroemer, K. H.: Human strength: terminology, measurement, and interpretation of data. Aerospace Medical Research Laboratory, Wright-Patterson Air Force Base, Ohio, p. 26, May, 1970.

Kroemer, K. H. E., and J. M. Howard: Problems in assessing muscle strength. USAF:AMRL-TR-68-144, 1970.

Kroemer, K. H. E., and J. M. Howard: Toward standardization of muscle strength testing, *Med. Sci. Sports*, **2**:224–230 (Winter, 1970).

Larson, L. A.: A factor and validity analysis of strength variables and tests with a test combination of chinning, dipping and vertical jump, *Res. Quart.*, **11**:82–96 (December, 1940).

Larson, L. A., and R. D. Yocom: *Measurement and Evaluation in Physical Health and Recreation Education.* St. Louis, C. V. Mosby, p. 507, 1951.

McCloy, C. H.: Factor analysis methods in the measurement of physical abilities. *Res. Quart. Suppl.*, **6**:114–121 (October, 1935).

O'Shea, J. P.: *Scientific Principles and Methods of Strength Fitness.* Reading, Mass., Addison-Wesley, p. 165, 1969.

Sharkey, B. J.: Intensity and duration of training and the development of cardiorespiratory endurance. *Med. Sci. Sports*, **2**:197–202 (Winter, 1970).

Sheldon, W. H., S. S. Stevens, and W. B. Tucker: *The Varieties of Human Physique.* New York, Harper and Bros., p. 347, 1940.

Skinner, B. F.: *Beyond Freedom and Dignity.* New York, Alfred A. Knopf, p. 225, 1971.

Steinhaus, A. H.: *Toward an Understanding of Health and Physical Education.* Dubuque, Iowa, Wm. C. Brown, p. 376, 1963.

Assessment Procedures for Human Performance

19

URIEL SIMRI
Wingate Institute of Physical Education and Sports
Netanya, Israel

In recent years we have witnessed a tremendous surge in sport medicine, yet this field has, thus far, failed to meet the needs of mass testing of physical fitness, tending to enclose itself in the shrines of science. Without downgrading the important achievements of recent years, it should be pointed out that sport medicine has failed to come up with a feasible physical fitness test for the masses, feasible that is from the points of view of time, cost, facilities, equipment, and professional manpower. The area of mass testing is still primarily left to the physical educator. The scientific value of mass testing of physical fitness has been debated frequently in recent years. There is no doubt that these tests are less accurate than those performed in research laboratories, yet, as long as no other and better means of mass testing is available, physical performance tests are here to stay. At present, there seems to be no choice but to standardize valid, reliable, and objective physical performance tests and to gain maximum data on the physical fitness of the healthy individual from these. Standardized mass testing is needed to set up national norms and to serve the purpose of international comparisons; these norms would direct the individual, the teacher, and the coach in their work of enhancing physical fitness.

The following physical performance tests are recommended for ages from 6 to 32 only. Further study is needed for performance tests for other age groups. The tests have been selected as representing the more important and measurable aspects of physical capacity, for example, static, dynamic, and explosive strength; speed; agility; flexibility; and cardiovascular and muscular endurance. In the choice of items, an attempt was made to minimize the effects of specific physical skills. Yet even basic abilities are, no doubt, learned, and it should be realized that cultural differences may have their share of influence. The recommended battery of tests does not test all aspects of physical fitness. Tests for such components of physical fitness as balance, coordination, reaction time, and so on, may be added in order to achieve a more complete measurement. Nor is it implied that all the recommended tests should be considered mandatory. Each suggested test consists of an independent unit that does not depend on any other test. The administrator of the tests can therefore adjust his testing to his own specific needs.

The number of suggested tests has been restricted to eight in order to enable the administrator to complete the series in one day. It is recommended to begin with the sprint and to continue in sequence with the standing long jump, the hand-grip test, pull-ups, the shuttle-race, sit-ups, the trunk forward flexion, and to complete the tests with the distance run. If the tests are given on two separate days, it is best to devote one day primarily to the outdoor tests (sprint, standing long jump, distance run) and the other day to testing indoors.

This order of testing is not coincidental. Speed, for instance, is best tested at the beginning of a series of efforts and should be followed by the test for explosive strength. The endurance test is usually so demanding that a prolonged rest is recommended following it; therefore, it should be placed at the end of the testing session.

The subjects taking the test should be in suitable dress, for example, light shorts, vest, and rubber-soled shoes. Bare feet may be permitted. Spiked shoes must not be worn. All testers and all subjects should be adequately trained in the details of the events prior to the start of the test session. Preparation of the testers is of utmost importance if reliable results are to be obtained. Preparation of the subjects is important because the tests are demanding. For that reason, the tests should be undertaken only by healthy and well-motivated subjects. The results of the tests should be entered into a unified score sheet. However, if subjects move individually from test to test, score sheets should be prepared separately for each event.

Anthropometric differences, such as height and weight, may influence some of the test items. To attempt to adjust administrative details to take account of these differences, however, would be impractical. It would involve many arbitrary decisions and might not improve the comparability of scores. It is, therefore, considered more desirable to use balanced judgment in the evaluation and interpretation of individual or group results when comparing such results with overall norms of performance.

Another point that should be discussed is whether the scores on the various physical fitness tests should be summarized by establishing one total physical index. Such a procedure has been favored in recent years by Fleishman (1964, p. 139) and by Ruskin and Yatsiv (1969, p. 6). When creating their indices, these authors assumed that all components of physical fitness carry the same weight, an assumption which can be justified only by administrative convenience. This writer tends to agree with Ricci (1967, p. 235) that a single physical fitness score is desirable but, at present, unattainable. Keeney (1960, p. 29) goes even further, claiming that a common basis for comparison of the physical fitness of various people is a meaningless endeavor.

At the same time, it seems necessary to determine the relative ability of each person in the various components of physical fitness. For that reason norms, percentile charts, or scoring tables for various tests have been established, as in the American Association for Health, Physical Education, and Recreation (AAHPER) test (AAHPER, 1965), and these can well be summarized in a profile chart. Such a profile chart provides an immediate view of the relative capacity of the subject in each of the various components so that strong and weak points may be determined according to established norms.

Dynamic Strength and Muscular Endurance

Dynamic strength is the ability of the individual to move, lift, and support the weight of the body. When such strength is required to function repeatedly and in a strenuous and exerting manner, its overall capacity is influenced by (local) muscular endurance. When referring to dynamic strength in daily practice, that reference is usually not to one maximum effort; therefore, the factor extends into the area of muscular endurance. Very often the terms "dynamic strength" and "muscular endurance" have been used interchangeably leading Simons et al. (1969, p. 352) to suggest a new term, namely "functional strength."

Fleishman (1964, p. 65) considers dynamic strength the most general strength factor, and points out that the best measures of dynamic strength are tests in which the arms are required to move or support the weight of the body repeatedly and continuously. However, there is some evidence for the existence of a separate dynamic strength factor of the trunk muscles, and therefore batteries of physical fitness tests include more than one dynamic strength test. It should be pointed out, however, that no separate tests are needed for the flexor and extensor muscles of the arms. As Fleishman (1964, p. 72) puts it, "push-ups added to pull-ups contribute little new information regarding dynamic strength."

According to Fleishman (1964, p. 64), pull-ups up to the maximum limit of ability have the highest loading of the dynamic strength factors. However, there seems to be no consistent advantage to endurance limit tests over time limit tests (for instance, maximum number of pull-ups in 30 sec). Simons et al. (1969, p. 352), on the other hand, prefer the flexed-arm hang to the pull-ups, although most experts look upon this test only as a substitute for subjects unable to perform the pull-ups, namely children, girls, and women.

The pull-up is one of the more reliable tests, reliabilities of up to 0.96 having been reported for it (Less, 1969, p. 11). Its greatest disadvantage is that it does not suit both sexes or young children. Although Johnson and Nelson (1969, p. 273) recommend the test for boys from the age of 10 upward, the International Committee for Standardization of Physical Fitness Tests (ICSPFT) is more cautious and recommends the test only for boys from the age of 12 upward.

The pull-up test requires perhaps more standardization than any other test because it has been performed in many different ways. The main issue has been that of the grasp for the pull-up. Some prefer the overgrasp on the basis that it is the more natural method of pulling one's weight up. Others claim that the undergrasp is justified because it is easier; as all flexors participate in it, there are therefore fewer zero scores (Meshizuka, 1967, p. 20) and the distribution of the scores is better (Johnson and Nelson, 1969, p. 273). Meshizuka (1967, p. 20) reports a very high correlation between pull-ups with the overgrasp and the undergrasp, and if the overgrasp is preferred by the ICSPFT (and by many others) this is only for reasons of tradition.

Clarke (1967, p. 152) and Mathews (1968, p. 71) recommend performing pull-ups on rings. The rings are grasped in a position in which the arms are supinated, and therefore this grasp resembles the undergrasp of the bar. However, some effort is spent on keeping the rings steady, and this effort is not adequately measurable. For that reason, this recommendation is not widely accepted.

Another major difference in the administration of the pull-up is in the scoring. Some experts like Clarke (1967, p. 153), Fleishman (1964, p. 167), and Mathews (1968, p. 71) recommend scoring half points for incomplete or incorrect performances, although Mathews suggests a maximum of only four such scores. This suggestion is based on the fact that, even in incomplete and incorrect performances, some strength is shown and this effort should be scored. Those who object to this partial scoring claim that only completed and correct attempts can be measured in a reliable and objective way. Among those who score only the completed and correct attempts, in which the chin is brought above the bar, the body is not swung, no kicking motion is performed with the legs, and the body is extended fully after each pull-up, are the ICSPFT and the AAHPER. The ICSPFT also has a regulation that a subject who has failed to raise his chin above the bar on two successive attempts must stop the test.

Other administrative details are usually agreed upon. The pull-up should be performed on a 2–5-cm bar or beam set high enough to prevent the tallest subject from touching the ground in a hanging position. The subject (with chalked hands) steps from a stool to a hanging position with fully extended arms, and he must return to that position after each pull-up. Each subject is given only one trial, which continues as long as he does not pause for an appreciable time or fail to raise his chin above the bar on two successive attempts. The administrator of the test can prevent swinging and kicking motions by holding an outstretched arm across the thighs of the subject or by standing in front of him. The test can also be administered by the partner-judge system in order to facilitate faster testing.

The flexed-arm hang is the counterpart to the pull-up for children up to 12, girls, and women. This test has replaced the so-called modified pull-up in recent years (not only in the AAHPER test) because of the difficulties in administering the modified pull-up in a reliable and objective manner. The flexed-arm hang test has a reliability of 0.90 (Johnson and Nelson, 1969, p. 276) and its main weakness is that many zero scores are reported for girls aged 6–7 (Meshizuka, 1967, p. 20). For this reason the AAHPER recommends this test only for girls over 10, but at the moment no better test is available for young girls.

The flexed-arm hang differs from the pull-up in that the subject attempts to hold his chin above the bar as long as possible, and the score is measured in full seconds. The chin must be kept clear of the bar; once the chin rests on the bar or passes underneath it, the test is complete.

As mentioned earlier, there is a special test to measure the dynamic strength of the trunk muscles. This is usually done by measuring the strength of the abdominal muscles because no reliable tests for the back muscles are available. Fleishman (1964, p. 128) and Simons et al. (1969, p. 356) recommend leg lifts as the test for the trunk muscles. However, Simons et al. (1969, p. 330) report a reliability of only 0.71 for this test, and such limited reliability makes this test seem unacceptable. Fleishman (1964, p. 67) claims that the "hold half sit-up" is a better test than the traditional sit-up, but Simons et al. dismiss this test as unreliable. It seems, therefore, that the sit-up, for which a reliability of 0.94 is reported (Johnson and Nelson, 1969, p. 278), is the best test available, especially since Fleishman (1964, p. 64) himself admits that its loading with the dynamic strength factor is as high as that of the other tests. Few share the doubts of Johnson and Nelson (1969, p. 278) that the test is suitable for children from 10 years of age only.

The administration of the sit-up also requires significant standardization, the main issue being the starting position. Originally the sit-up was performed with straight legs, but at present flexed knees (at approximately right angle) are preferred in order to negate the strong iliopsoas muscle as much as possible and to test primarily the abdominal muscles. A secondary issue is the length of the test. Maximal testing has been abolished as being too time consuming and has been replaced by tests for 30, 60, or 120 sec. The first length of test is recommended here, since the correlation between the three is very high. Use of the shortest test period will save time with no loss of reliability.

The other details of the test are as follows: the subject lies on his back on a mat (or any flat, preferably soft, surface) with feet about 30 cm apart. The hands, with fingers interlocked, are placed on the back of the neck and must remain in that position throughout the test. A partner kneels between the subject's feet and presses down on the subject's instep to keep the heels in contact with the mat. The partner can serve as judge and scorer and thereby facilitate mass testing. The score is the number of sit-ups completed in 30 sec. A sit-up is completed when the elbows touch the bent knees. Upon completion, the subject must return to a position in which his back and hands touch the mat. Using an elbow to push up is not permitted; however, pausing to rest is permitted.

Explosive Strength

There is quite a divergence in the definitions of the physical fitness factor of explosive strength. There is even little agreement on the name of the factor itself, and many still prefer the old term "muscular power" to the newer term "explosive strength." Although Johnson and Nelson (1969, p. 80) define the factor as "the ability to release maximum force in the fastest possible time," Fleishman (1964, p. 130) refers to it as "the ability to expend a maximum of energy in one or a series of explosive acts." Elsewhere, however, Fleishman (1964, p. 66) refers to "one explosive act" only.

When a series of explosive acts is included in tests of explosive strength or power, these tests include speed tests, as indicated in Fleishman's (1964, p. 66) findings. However, for a test of a single explosive act, such as the standing long jump and the vertical jump, correlations with speed tests, such as sprints from 25 to 50 m, range from -0.77 (Celikovsky, 1967, Pt. II, p. 17) to $+0.69$ (Celikovsky, 1967, Pt. I, p. 53). The wide dispersion of results between those extremes indicates that no obvious correlation of great significance exists between the two.

Whatever the difference of opinion concerning the definition of explosive strength or power, there is total agreement that it makes up an independent factor of physical fitness. Fleishman (1964, p. 29) claims that separate, though highly correlated, explosive strength factors for arms and legs exist and, because of that correlation [Simons et al. (1969, p. 334ff.) report correlations up to $+0.57$], it may be sufficient to measure one of the two in a limited series of field tests. Most experts prefer the measurement of the explosive strength of the legs to the explosive strength of the arms, although Glencross (1966, pp. 358–59) doubts the validity of both of the most popular tests, namely, the standing long jump and the vertical jump.

A correlation of $+0.72$ has been reported between the standing long jump and the vertical jump (Glencross, 1966, p. 335) and a high reliability for both has also been found. For the standing long jump, reliabilities from 0.88 (Simons et al., 1969, p. 330) to 0.96 (Glencross, 1966, p. 355) have been reported; whereas for the vertical jump, the reported reliabilities range from 0.84 (Simons et al., 1966, p. 330) to 0.98 (Cooper, 1945). One reason why explosive strength tests of the legs are preferred to those of the arms may well be that those of the arms are much less reliable. [Fleishman (1964, p. 59) reports a reliability of 0.93 for the softball throw, which this writer failed to reproduce.]

In spite of the fact that Glencross (1966, p. 358) has shown by his factor analysis that the standing long jump involves more jumping ability (technique) than the vertical jump, many physical educators prefer the standing long jump as a test for explosive strength. In their opinion the standing long jump test is not only easier to perform but also much more reliable, than research may indicate, than the vertical jump. These physical educators claim that, whereas the vertical jump is of great value whenever performed for the first time, in mass testing involving a retest situation subjects cannot be prevented from not extending fully in the basic standing position in order to improve their results. As early as 1940, van Dalen (1940, p. 112) reported such inaccuracies in the common measuring techniques of the vertical jump.

The standing long jump is best performed on a flat nonslip surface. Noguchi (1967, p. 12) has found jumps into a sand pit to be of a significantly lower reliability. Each person should be permitted two attempts (the better one to count), a number found to be sufficient for reproducibility by Marmis et al. (1969, pp. 240ff.). As most subjects jump almost perpendicular to the takeoff line, perpendicular measurement from the rearmost point of contact of the heels to the takeoff line is considered accurate enough. In order, however, to minimize the influence of track-and-field rulings and to measure explosive strength primarily, any attempt in which the subject overbalances backward should be discounted and another attempt should be given. It should also be pointed out that the feet must remain in contact with the ground until the moment of takeoff, and should take off simultaneously. However, preparatory backward swings of both arms are permitted. Noguchi (1967, p. 14) reports a high correlation between jumps with and without shoes.

A few words remain to be said about the vertical jump, which enjoys a wide use as a test of explosive strength. This test was first suggested by Dr. Dudley A. Sargent (1921) and is therefore also known as the "Sargent Jump." The vertical jump is customarily scored as the distance jumped, but in recent years formulas taking into consideration the body weight, in order to calculate work/power, have been introduced. In order to minimize the effects of technique and of extraneous movements, it has also been suggested that a full squat with one hand behind the back be used as a starting position. It should be pointed out that the vertical jump has been less standardized than the standing long jump. For instance, measurement of basic height has alternately been performed with the subject standing sideways to the wall and with the subject facing the wall and lifting one or two arms. Measurement of the distance jumped without using a wall (and chalk on the tip of the fingers), as was originally planned, has almost been eliminated due to difficulties in reliable measurement or of obtaining a special piece of apparatus, such as the

Leapmeter. If the vertical jump is used as a test, it is recommended that the basic height with the subject facing the wall and lifting both arms be measured because this measurement is the most reliable.

Before continuing our considerations about testing of physical fitness, it should be mentioned that, recently, the claim has been made that biomechanical factors should be taken into account when testing strength, and that, in fact, one should measure force and not strength (Ricci, 1970, p. 28). As pointed out earlier, such an approach may turn out to be impractical.

Static Strength

Static strength is universally recognized as an independent factor of physical fitness. It is best defined by Fleishman (1964, p. 30) as "the exertion of a maximum force for a brief period of time against a fairly immovable object." The fact that static strength is an independent factor of physical fitness is best demonstrated by the fact that the most popular mass test of static strength, namely, the hand-grip test, shows no higher correlation than +0.30 with any other physical fitness test (Fleishman, 1964, p. 60), with the exception of other tests of static strength. Even though Simons et al. (1969, pp. 334ff.) found correlations of up to +0.43 with an explosive strength test (standing long jump) and of up to +0.53 with a dynamic strength test (pull-ups) in certain age groups, the correlations for larger populations are much smaller.

One question that is frequently raised is whether the static strength of various muscle groups should be measured separately. This is probably not worthwhile due to the high correlations among the scores.

The two most popular tests of static strength are the hand-grip and arm-pull dynamometers. Fleishman (1964, p. 59) and Simons et al. (1969, p. 330) agree that the hand grip is more reliable (the former reports a reliability of 0.91), yet Simons et al. (1969, p. 356) claim that the arm-pull dynamometer has a higher loading of the static strength factor. Most experts, however, prefer the hand-grip dynamometer, perhaps because the difference in loading is not great. Ishiko (1967, p. 5) has shown that the hand-grip test is reliable from age six upward, and this may be another reason for the preference of this test.

Some authorities, such as Ishiko (1967, p. 5), prefer that the hand-grip test be performed on both hands. Others, like Ruskin and Yatsiv (1969, pp. 17ff.), claim that, because the correlations between the scores of both hands are as high as +0.76 in male students and +0.72 in female students, this is unnecessary and subjects should be tested with their preferred hand only. Ishiko (1967, p. 5) has reported average differences of 1 kg in 6 year olds and of 3 kg in 11 year olds between the scores of both hands. Ruskin and Yatsiv (1969, pp. 70ff.) report average differences of 1.43 kg in male students and 2.17 kg in female students. Himaru and Meshizuka (1967, p. 9) have suggested the use of a double-hand dynamometer to make separate measurements unnecessary, but their suggestion has not been accepted widely.

The hand-grip test is best performed with an adjustable grip dynamometer, since subjects with small palms are at a disadvantage with nonadjustable dynamometers. Dynamometers should be recalibrated before testing. In the test itself, two attempts should be allowed, a number shown by Ishiko (1967, p. 5) to be sufficient for reliability. The better score is to count and should be recorded in full kilograms.

The subject should chalk his hands, take the dynamometer comfortably in the appropriate hand, hold it in line with the forearm, and let it hang down by the thigh. The second joint of the hand should fit snugly under the handle and take the weight of the instrument. It is then gripped between the fingers and the palm at the base of the thumb. The firmly held dynamometer should be raised clear of the body, and neither the hand nor the dynamometer should be permitted to contact the body or any other object during the test. During the squeezing of the dynamometer, the arm should not be allowed to swing or to perform a pumping motion. A fresh trial should be allowed if any of the aforementioned rules is broken. For motivational reasons, it is recommended that the test be performed with the dial facing the subject.

Speed

The physical fitness factor of speed has been controversial in recent years. As early as 1951 Larson and Yocom (1951, p. 161) pointed out that speed was highly correlated with muscular power. In later years, Fleishman (1964, p. 71) went as far as claiming that there was a difficulty in isolating a separate speed factor and that there seemed to be no general speed factor. This view is not accepted by one and all, and only recently Simons et al. (1969, p. 354), using the technique of factor analysis like Fleishman, have definitely recognized a distinctive factor of speed. It should be added here that, whereas those who tend to recognize a distinctive factor of speed refer to speed of movement (such as running) on a straight line, others, like Fleishman (1964, pp. 32, 83), refer to various factors of speed, including speed of change of direction, a factor considered by many to belong to the fitness factor of agility.

Tests of speed of running are not only relatively easy to perform but also tend to motivate most people favorably. However, proper distances must be chosen for the tests in order to minimize the influence of other physical fitness factors, such as muscle power or explosive strength. Havlicek and Cechvala (p. 17), using a photoelectric time registration device, have suggested 50 m as the ideal running distance for boys 11–18 and 40 m as the ideal distance for girls of the same age group. Whereas the speed of the boys improves from year to year in this age group, Havlicek and Cechvala claim that the average girl reaches her peak of speed at the early age of 13. This writer had similar findings when analyzing the results of thousands of girls who took the Israeli Sport Badge Tests; however, in this case, the peak in the 60-m race was reached at the age of 14 and was followed by a plateau in achievement which lasted 3 years. It should be pointed out that, for administrative convenience, many prefer to administer the same test, namely, 50 m, for boys and girls in spite of the abovementioned findings.

Theoretically, a test using the flying start should be preferred to one using the crouching start in order to minimize the effects of technique. However, the flying start is difficult to measure in mass testing procedures, and therefore a standing start is usually used as a compromise. Celikovsky, Hladil, and Gaislova (1967, pp. 53ff.) reported correlations of +0.85 and upward between the results of races with a flying start and races with a standing start in boys and girls aged from 6 to 18, but for inexplicable reasons these correlations are down to around +0.50 in boys and girls aged 12.

Speed of running tests can be administered to single persons or to couples. Matsuda (1967, p. 17) reported no significant differences in the results of 40 youngsters aged 6 and 45 youngsters aged 12, whom he tested in both ways. He suggests, however, that this may be the result of pairing of uneven runners, which caused the winner to slow down at the tape. If for nothing else, testing of couples in running is suggested as a time-saving device. It is further recommended to allow each subject two attempts in this event, the better one to count, as suggested by Marmis et al. (1969, p. 245), but adequate rest (at least 10 min) should be allowed between races.

The races should be held on a flat and straight surface, subdivided into lanes. Races should be held on days with no extreme temperatures, rain, or great wind velocity (above 2 m/sec). A starting pistol or a visual device should be used for starting, and one timekeeper to each runner is desirable. Times are recorded in tenths of a second.

Agility

Agility has been defined as "the ability of the individual to change positions in space" (Larson and Yocom, 1951, p. 161). Needless to say the number of possible changes of body positions in space is endless, and therefore the clear distinction of the composition of the physical fitness factor of agility is, to say the least, very difficult. However difficult agility may be to distinguish, it definitely exists as a factor in physical fitness, although it may not be a completely independent factor.

Expert opinion claims that the most important elements of agility are change of direction and change of height of movement. For that reason, the shuttle run serves as one of the better tests for agility, provided that the distance of the run is not such that the factor of speed becomes a determinant.

Expert opinion considers the distance of 10 m to meet this criteria. Furthermore, when the 10-m race is accompanied by the need to change the height of movement, the importance of the factor of speed diminishes even more. This can be assured by requiring the runner to pick up a wooden block or to put down a block at each turn. When this is the case, the runner has, in fact, just enough time to straighten up before he must begin to lower his body toward the following handling of a block.

Three changes of direction at 180 degrees are considered sufficient to test one's agility, and therefore the shuttle run includes four stretches of 10 m. At the first and third turn, a wooden block ($5 \times 5 \times 5$ cm) is picked up from a circle tangent to the line; at the second turn and at the end of the race (both at the starting line) a block is put down at a similar circle behind the opposite line. The diameter of the circles should be 50 cm, and their purpose is to prevent throwing the blocks and to provide a means for more accurate measurement.

The dependence of the shuttle run on speed can be determined by the correlation between scores in it and scores in a 50-m dash. Celikovsky, Hladil, and Gaislova (1967, pp. 53ff.) reported, for groups of boys and girls aged 6, 12, and 18, correlations ranging from -0.015 to $+0.543$, with an average of $+0.359$ for the six groups, a fact that indicates a relatively low loading of the factor of speed on this agility test. Ishiko and Kurimoto (1973, pp. 54ff.) reported more stable correlations, ranging from $+0.533$ to $+0.708$ for similar age groups, but Ruskin and Bar-Or (1973, p. 31), on the other hand, reported an unexplainable high correlation of $+0.99$ for 40 boys, aged 10 to 14.

Finally, it should be pointed out that experience has shown that, when the test is repeated after a sufficient period of rest, a significant number of people improve their scores; therefore, this procedure is recommended. Scores are measured in tenths of a second, and the better of the two times is recorded. To facilitate testing, the subjects should start from alternate sides, in order to eliminate the carrying of the blocks back each time.

Flexibility

Flexibility is the ability to move part or parts of the body in a wide range of movement. There has been some argument that flexibility is related to other factors of physical fitness. [Fleishman (1964, p. 31), for instance, relates flexibility to speed.] However, it seems not only to be an independent factor but, in addition, flexibility of a certain joint does not necessarily lead to flexibility in other joints. This writer tends to agree, therefore, with Simons et al. (1964, p. 354) who recognize flexibility as an independent factor and disagree with Fleishman (1964, p. 31), who divides flexibility into extent flexibility and dynamic flexibility. The matrix drawn by Ruskin and Yatsiv

(1969, pp. 15–16) seems to indicate similar findings to those of Simons et al.

It should also be pointed out that in normal subjects flexibility depends primarily on the structure of the joints and not on the (passive) ability of muscles to stretch; therefore, one should not speak of muscle flexibility as some writers do. Along the same line, it should be remembered that it has been shown [for instance, by Mathews (1968, p. 293)] that flexibility is not related to lower limb length, as some people mistakenly believe.

Our main interest lies in extent flexibility, and various tests have been proposed for that purpose. Fleishman (1964, pp. 77–78) suggests trunk extension backward (abdominal stretch), forward flexion of the trunk (toe touching), and twist-and-touch, in which he sees the best of the three tests followed by the trunk extension. Simons et al. (1969, p. 356) and Kasch and Boyer (1968, p. 21), on the other hand, recommend the sit-and-reach test (flexion of the trunk in a sitting position), the latter claiming that the trunk extension test is not reliable (Kasch and Boyer, 1968, p. 22).

It seems, therefore, that trunk extension is not only an unnatural movement but also one difficult to measure accurately. The scores of the twist-and-touch and of the sit-and-reach can be influenced to a large extent by motion in the knees and by the position of the legs in general. The same holds true, to a certain extent, for the forward flexion of the trunk, but in this case the control of the knees by the tester seems to be easiest and most convenient.

Therefore a test of forward flexion of the trunk is recommended with the tested person standing on a stable chair (with his toes on the edge of the chair). This enables the person to reach beyond his toes. Experience has shown that the average person scores better on his second attempt; therefore, each person should be given two attempts, the better one to count. The test administrator may assist the subject (by pressure on his knee) in keeping his knees straight and should not allow any jerking movement. Such a movement tends to cause a flexion in the knees, and therefore the Scott-French version of this test (Scott and French, 1950, p. 181) is not recommended. Measurement in centimeters is made on a ruler placed perpendicular to the chair seat and marked 0–100 cm. This ruler is placed so that the 50-cm mark is level with the top surface of the chair. Readings are made with the aid of a wooden marker, which slides down the ruler.

A warning should, however, be given that jerking movements in this test may cause, in the long run, damage to the lower spine. To avoid such movements the tested person should be required to hold the final position of his reach for at least 2 sec. It should also be pointed out that some doctors even go as far as rejecting the forward flexion of the trunk and recommend the sit-and-reach test, claiming that jerking possibilities are more limited in this test.

The ICSPFT accepts the sit-and-reach test as an alternative test to the test from the standing position. Simri and his coworkers (1971, 1973) reported correlations ranging from $+0.82$ to $+0.94$ between the two tests for different age groups, the correlation increasing with age. This test is performed with the soles leaning on a 35-cm box in order to facilitate easier measurement undisturbed by the toes. In other aspects this test resembles the previous one.

Correnti from the University of Rome suggested in 1971 the introduction of a device which would neutralize the effect of the relative length of the extremities and negate the possible factor of fear while bending forward on an elevated platform. The author, however, found that this device was less applicable for mass testing and in any case produced, at least in adults, results that correlated highly with the ICSPFT tests.

The flexion of the trunk is chosen as the test for flexibility because this movement is the one of greatest importance in human motion. It should, however, be reemphasized that good flexibility in the hip and the spine does not necessarily indicate good flexibility in any other joint. When only one test of flexibility is recommended, this is done as a result of administrative limitations. In clinical tests, for instance, the physiotherapist will definitely examine the flexibility of each joint separately, but this would be beyond the limitations of mass testing of physical fitness. In clinical practice, apparatus like the flexometer and the electrogoniometer may be used for more accurate measurement.

Cardiovascular Endurance

Cardiovascular endurance could be defined as the capacity of the individual to maintain strenuous activity of a number of muscle groups or of the whole body for a prolonged period. By "prolonged period" we mean a sufficient duration to demand a resistance to fatigue. Cardiovascular endurance could be subdivided into aerobic capacity and anaerobic capacity. Shepard (1969, p. 2), who looks upon cardiovascular endurance as a (if not the) major factor in physical fitness, is of the opinion that it is the determining factor in human efforts which last between 1 min and 1 hr. Slightly different time limits are quoted by other sources, but in any case most human efforts fall into this class.

Cardiovascular function can be measured not only in the research laboratory but also under field conditions. This is usually done by having the subject exert himself in a running event and timing his effort. Differences of opinion exist whether to measure primarily aerobic or anaerobic capacity under such conditions or whether to measure a mixture of the two. Fleishman (1964, p. 36) expressed his doubts whether endurance in long-distance races is anything more than a specific run factor, but this opinion is not shared by many.

Balke (1960, pp. 50–52), Cooper (1968, p. 35), and Shepard (1969, p. 102) obviously prefer a test of (primarily) aerobic capacity when they respectively suggest tests of 15 min running, 12 min running, and 1 or 2 miles running. It should be pointed out, however, that most test administrators prefer timing a test for a constant distance to measuring the distance for a constant-time race.

The most reliable direct measurement of cardiovascular endurance is that of maximal oxygen intake, and this measurement has a high correlation with long-distance races. It does not show such a correlation with shorter distances and for that reason, Shepard (1969, p. 102) objects to the 300-yard running test of the Canadian Association for Health, Physical Education and Recreation (CAHPER) and the 600-yard run-walk of the AAHPER.

The point is often made that long-distance races are too demanding or even dangerous for small children. Ikai (1967, p. 28), for instance, reported that the better students in the 6–7 age group show what he considered too great an oxygen debt after a 600-m race. Hanne et al. (1968, p. 16) found significant negative signs as a result of a 600-m race even in children at the age of 12 and above. Ikai (1967, p. 28) also believes that the child in this age group has pacing difficulties in a longer race and considers this race as too difficult for 6–7-year-old boys. It should be noted, however, that the pacing difficulties seem to diminish the longer the race, and the greater the role of aerobic capacity (instead of anaerobic capacity). On the other hand, Hollman and his associates (1965, pp. 265ff.) reported that they did not observe any disharmony in muscular and cardiovascular development of young children and, following their and similar recommendations, aerobic capacity tests are indeed being performed on children.

The ICSPFT recommends running tests, although walking is permitted when necessary. The importance of maintaining a steady speed should however, be stressed by the test administrator. It is felt that such a procedure would raise the reliability of the test, in comparison with the reliability of 0.80 reported by Fleishman (1964, p. 128) for the 600-yard run-walk. The distances recommended by the ICSPFT are 1000 or 2000 m for men and boys 12 years and over (the physiologists of the ICSPFT prefer the 2000-m test), 800 or 1500 m for women and girls 12 years and over, and 600 m for children under 12 years.

The different distances suggested above stem to a certain extent from cultural differences. Whereas most committee members agreed to the physiological findings, many felt that nonetheless, in their own particular culture, it would be difficult to introduce races for longer distances.

The endurance test should be performed under weather conditions ensuring normal and comparable results, which is to say that it should not be performed under extreme weather conditions. The track should be flat, in reasonable condition, and measured along a line 15 cm out from the inner-most edge of the lane. The score is the time, to the nearest half second, needed to complete the course, and the test should preferably be timed by a stop

Table 19-1 Comparison of Physical Fitness Performance Test Batteries of Recent Years

	Fleishman (1964)	AAHPER (1965)	CAHPER (1966)	Simons et al. (1969)	ICSPFT (1971)
Dynamic strength	Pull-ups	Pull-ups (male) Flexed-arm hang (female)	Flexed-arm hang	Flexed-arm hang	Pull-ups (male) Flexed-arm hang (female, children)
Trunk strength	Leg lifts	Sit-ups (maximum, straight legs)	Sit-ups (60 sec)	Leg lifts	Sit-ups (30 sec, bent knees)
Explosive strength	Softball throw	Softball throw	—	Vertical jump	Standing long jump
Static strength	Hand-grip	Standing long jump	Standing long jump	Arm-pull dynamometer	Hand-grip
Speed	100-yd shuttle run[1]	50 yd	50 yd		50 m
Agility	Cable jump	40-yd shuttle-run (blocks)	40-yd shuttle-run (blocks)	50-m shuttle run	40-m shuttle-run (blocks)
Flexibility	Turn and reach[2] Bend, twist, and touch[3]	—	—	Sit and reach	Forward flexion trunk or sit-and-reach
Endurance	600-yd run-walk	600-yd run-walk	300 yd	1-min step test	600–800–1000–1500–2000 m
Balance	One-foot balance	—	—	(Need established)	—
Limb agility	—	—	—	Plate tapping	—
Eye-limb coordination	—	—	—	Stick balance	—

[1] Fleishman considers this a test of dynamic strength.
[2] Test of extent flexibility.
[3] Test of dynamic flexibility.

watch. Judging the event can be done by assigning a timekeeper (with a stop watch) to each runner. Alternately, a partner-judge system could be used, in which each runner is assigned a partner-judge who notes the time of arrival according to the loud readings (of each second) of the timekeeper, who holds the only stop watch. This time is later reported to a recorder.

Especially for longer distances, the funnel-touch method can be used. The advantage of this method is that four judges (one timekeeper, one recorder, one "toucher," and one scorer) can judge a great number of runners. In this method the finishing runner enters a roped funnel and is given, upon crossing the finishing line inside the funnel, a numbered index card that indicates his place in the race. At the same time, the three other judges record the time of the runners according to their placing in the following manner. The time-keeper reads each second aloud, the "toucher" taps lightly on the shoulder of the recorder whenever a runner crosses the finishing line, and the recorder enters the time of each tap in a ready timing form (by a simple check mark). After the race is over the names of the runners are registered while collecting their placing cards from them.

REFERENCES

AAHPER Youth Fitness Test Manual. rev. ed., Washington, AAHPER, 1965.

Balke, B.: *Biodynamics in Medical Physics*, Chicago, Yearbook Publishers, 1960.

Celikovsky, S. et al.: *The Study of Motor Performance and the Study of the Relation between Motor Performance and Work Capacity determined by Physiological and Physique Measurements*, Prague, Charles University, 1967.

Clarke, H. H.: *Application of Measurement to Health and Physical Education*, 4th ed., Englewood Cliffs, N.J., Prentice-Hall, 1967.

Cooper, B.: *The Establishment of General Motor Capacity for High School Girls.* Microcard Doctoral Dissertation, State University of Iowa, 1945.

Cooper, K. H.: *Aerobics.* New York, Bantam Books, 1968.

Fleishman, E. A.: *The Structure and Movement of Physical Fitness*, Englewood Cliffs, N.J., Prentice-Hall, 1964.

Glasser, J. (ed.): *Biodynamics in Medical Physics.* Chicago, Yearbook Publishers, 1960.

Glencross, D. J.: The nature of the vertical jump and the standing broad jump. *Res. Quart.*, 37(3):353–359 (October, 1966).

Hanne-Paparo, N. et al.: *The Achievement of 12–15 Year Old Boys in Races for 600 and 1500 Meters and their Physiological Reactions to these Races.* Israel, Wingate Institute, 1968.

Havlicek, I., and J. Cechvala: *The Study of Adequate Running Distances for the Different Age Groups.* Prague, Charles University.

Himaru, T., and T. Meshizuka: Proposal of double-hand grip-strength dynamometer. In *Reports on Reexamination of Performance Tests by ICSPFT in 1966*, Tokyo, Japanese ICSPFT Members, 1967.

Hollmann, W. et al.: Die Entwicklung des Kardio-pulmonalen Systems bei

Kindern und Jugendlichene des 8. bis 18. Lebensjahr. *Sportarzt Sportmed.*, **16**(7):255–260 (July, 1965).

Howell, M. L., and W. R. Morford: *Fitness Training Methods*, Toronto, CAHPER.

Ikai, M.: Study on the endurance running test of elementary school pupils (age 8–11 years). In *Reports on Reexamination of Performance Tests by ICSPFT in 1966*, Tokyo, Japanese ICSPFT Members, 1967.

Ishiko, T.: Reexamination of grip-strength measurements. In *Reports on Reexamination of Performance Tests by ICSPFT in 1966*, Tokyo, Japanese ICSPFT Members, 1967.

Ishiko, T., and E. Kurimoto: Two studies on the ICSPFT test battery. In *Proceedings of the ACSPFT and the ICSPFT—1972*. Israel, Wingate Institute, 1973.

Johnson, B. L., and J. K. Nelson: *Practical Measurements for Evaluation in Physical Education*. Minneapolis, Burgess, 1969.

Kasch, F. W., and J. L. Boyer: *Adult Fitness, Principles and Practice*. Greeley, Colo., All American Productions, 1968.

Keeney, C. E.: A professor of biology proposes a new definition of physical fitness as work capacity. *J. Health Phy. Educ. Recreation*, **31**(6):29–30 (September 1960).

Larson, L. A., and R. D. Yocom: *Measurement and Evaluation in Physical Health and Recreation Education*. St. Louis, Mosby, 1951.

Less, M.: Bhina le'jecholet motorit shel studentim be'chinuch gufani. *Hachinuch-hagufani*, Israel, **25**(6):10–12 (September–October 1969).

Marmis, C. et al.: Reliability of multi-trial items of the AAHPER youth fitness test. *Res. Quart.*, **40**(1):240–245 (March 1969).

Mathews, D. K.: *Measurement in Physical Education*, 3rd ed., Philadelphia Saunders, 1968.

Matsuda, I.: Relation between standing start and flying start in 50 meter speed run. In *Reports on Reexamination of Performance Tests by ICSPFT in 1966*, Tokyo, Japanese ICSPFT Members, 1967.

Meshizuka, T.: Local muscular endurance—examination of pull-ups and flexed-arm hang. In *Reports on Reexamination of Performance Tests by ICSPFT in 1966*, Tokyo, Japanese ICSPFT Members, 1967.

Noguchi, Y.: Reexamination of measuring procedures of standing long jump. In *Reports on Reexamination of Performance Tests by ICSPFT in 1966*, Tokyo, Japanese ICSPFT Members, 1967.

Ricci, B.: For a moratorium on 'physical fitness testing.' *J. Health Phys. Educ. Recreation*, **41**(3):28–30 (March 1970).

Ricci, B.: *Physiological Basis of Human Performance*. Philadelphia, Lea and Febiger, 1967.

Ruskin, H., and O. Bar-Or: Correlations between physical performance, physiological and anthropometric variability in boys (ages 10–14). In *Proceedings of the ACSPFT and the ICSPFT—1972*. Israel, Wingate Institute, 1973.

Ruskin, H., and G. Yatziv: *A Study of the Standardization of Physical Performance Tests for Males and Females Aged 19–31*. Jerusalem, Hebrew University, 1969.

Sargent, D. A.: The physical test of a man, *Amer. Phys. Educ. Rev.*, **26**(4):188–194 (April 1921).

Scott, G. A., and E. French: *Evaluation in Physical Education*. St. Louis, Mosby, 1950.

Shepard, R. J.: *Endurance Fitness*. Toronto, University of Toronto, 1969.

Simons, J. et al.: Construction d'une batterie de tests d'aptitude motrice pour garcons de 12 a 19 ans, par la methode de l'analyse factorielle. *Kinanthropologie*, 1(4):323–362 (Octobre 1969).

Simri, U. et al.: A comparison between the flexibility tests of Correnti and of the ICSPFT. In *Proceedings of the ACSPFT and the ICSPFT—1972*. Israel, Wingate Institute (1973).

Simri, U. et al.: Hashvaah ben Mirchane Gmishut bamishor Hachitzi, Hachinuch-hagufani. *Israel*, 8(4–5):7–9 (August 1971).

Van Dalen, D. B.: New studies in the Sargent jump. *Res. Quart.*, 11(2):112ff. (May 1940).

Validity of Human Performance Assessments

20

RICHARD BRIAN ALDERMAN
The University of Alberta
Edmonton, Alberta

MAXWELL L. HOWELL
San Diego State University
San Diego, California

Validity* in any kind of measurement and evaluation is always a key issue. Its importance revolves around the basic dilemma of whether or not the test measures precisely what it purports to measure. This dilemma is especially acute in physical fitness testing because the measurements are, of necessity, indirect. This is to say (and this will be enlarged upon in a later section), that when one measures performance in "push-ups," one is obtaining valid information only on the individual's ability to do push-ups and this may, or may not, be related to his level of physical fitness. In other words, once the individual has completed his push-ups, the experimenter must make an intuitive leap from this information to the theoretical construct of physical fitness. Thus, it is necessary to obtain evidence linking various performance measures to the attribute or attributes from both a practical and a conceptual point of view.

Initially, the focus of this chapter will be on the particular relationship between motor performance testing and the theoretical construct of physical fitness and whether or not such performance measures are valid indicators of physical fitness. Of secondary interest, but emanating from and clarifying this issue, is a discussion of the generality versus specificity controversy in

---

* For an extensive discussion of validity that is particularly good for students in physical education refer to Helmstadter, G. C.: *Principles of Psychological Measurement*. New York, Appleton-Century-Crofts, 1964.

performance testing. It is hoped by the authors that this particular approach will provide some clarification to the reader.

Motor Performance Testing of Physical Fitness

Physical fitness evaluation by means of performance testing has been a popular professional pastime for many years. Some of the better known test batteries are as follows:

1. Army Physical Fitness Test (War Department, 1946)
   Outdoor test
   a. Pull-ups
   b. Squat jumps
   c. Push-ups
   d. Sit-ups
   e. 300-yard run
   Indoor test
   a. Pull-ups
   b. Squat jumps
   c. Push-ups
   d. Sit-ups
   e. Indoor shuttle run or 60-sec squat thrusts
2. United States Air Force Physical Fitness Test (Larson, 1946)
   a. Pull-ups
   b. Sit-ups
   c. 300-yard shuttle run (outdoor)
   d. 25-yard shuttle run for 250 yards (indoors)
3. Navy Standard Physical Fitness Test (Bureau Naval Personnel, 1943)
   a. Squat thrusts for 1 min
   b. Sit-ups
   c. Squat jumps
   d. Push-ups
   e. Pull-ups
4. WAC Physical Fitness Test (War Department)
   a. Knee dips or full dips
   b. Sit-ups
   c. Wing lifts
   d. Squat thrusts
5. American Association of Health, Physical Education, and Recreation (AAHPER) Youth Fitness Test (AAHPER, 1965)
   a. Pull-ups (boys) or flexed-arm hang (girls)
   b. Sit-ups
   c. Shuttle run

    d. Standing broad jump

    e. 50-yard dash

    f. Softball throw for distance

    g. 600-yard run-walk

6. Canadian Association of Health, Physical Education, and Recreation (CAHPER) Fitness-Performance Test (CAHPER, 1966)

    a. Sit-ups in 1 min

    b. Standing broad jump

    c. Shuttle run

    d. Flexed arm hang

    e. 50-yard dash

    f. 300-yard run

7. Fleishman Physical Fitness Test (Fleishman, 1964)

    a. Extent flexibility

    b. Dynamic flexibility

    c. Shuttle run

    d. Softball throw

    e. Handgrip

    f. Pull-ups

    g. Leg lifts

    h. Cable jump

    i. Balance test

    j. 600-yard run-walk

8. International Committee for Standardization of Physical Fitness Tests (ICSPFT)

    a. 1000-m run-walk (men-boys, 11 years plus) or 800-m run-walk (women-girls, 11 years plus) or 600-m run-walk (boys and girls, 11 years minus)

    b. 50-m sprint

    c. Pull-ups (men-boys, 11 years plus) or flexed-arm hang (boys-girls, 11 years minus) (women-girls, 11 years plus)

    d. Grip strength

The similarities of these test batteries are obvious. We see the same items occurring with monotonous regularity with no attempt at justification for their inclusion other than that a particular item measures a particular "factor" or "component" of physical fitness. In fact, a virtually unavoidable criticism of these instruments is that they measure performance which may or may not be highly related to physical fitness. For example, does the person who has a high level of motor performance ability (that is, high scores on the items in the test battery) automatically have a high level of physical fitness? Fleishman (1964), who makes a useful distinction between ability and skill, observes that individual performance depends not only on what developed traits a person brings to the task but also on how well he has learned the

particular task. If this is the case ～ ～ we certainly believe that it is, then, are
we not merely obtaining a measure of the individual's motor ability and/or
skill rather than a measure of his physical fitness? The natural development
from this question is thus "... what is physical fitness?" Although the
purpose of this chapter is not concerned with defining "physical fitness," the
question is a valid one with respect to justifying human motor performance
testing as a measure of physical fitness.

It is contended that the answer to this basic dilemma of definition lies in
the domain of construct validity, with the resulting claim that physical
fitness can only be considered as a construct. If this justification is legitimate,
then motor performance testing in the evaluation of physical fitness has
scientific validity. However, in order to gain validity in human measurement,
it has now become necessary to designate precisely which type of validity is
being established. The American Psychological Association Committee on
Psychological Tests, in its Technical Recommendations (1954), divides
validity studies into predictive validity, concurrent validity, content validity,
and construct validity. The first three types are familiar to test designers in
that they are concerned with criterion-oriented procedures intended to
establish the test items as a sample of a particular universe. Construct validation, on the other hand, is involved whenever a test is to be interpreted as a
measure of some attribute or quality which is not operationally defined
(Cronbach and Meehl, 1955). Of particular importance is the fact that
construct validity is not designated only by the methodological framework
of the investigation but also by the orientation of the investigator. This is of
paramount importance in the area of physical fitness where physiological,
psychological, and performance fitness measures exist in profusion.

Therefore, proceeding on the assumption that physical fitness *cannot* be
adequately defined to everyone's satisfaction, it would appear that construct
validation is the only answer. As Bechtoldt (1951) observes, "criterion-
oriented validity involves the acceptance of a set of operations as an adequate
definition of whatever is to be measured." When it is believed that no fully
valid criterion is available and one cannot avoid having to relate every
criterion to a more ultimate standard, then one *must* become interested in
construct validation. The same criticism, in the sense of a lack of unanimity,
holds for content validation. Construct validation must be the procedure
whenever no criterion or universe of content is accepted as entirely adequate
to define the quality to be measured. Such is the case with physical fitness.
Nowhere in the literature is there agreement on a definition of physical
fitness; thus, although it is not our purpose to provide one in this chapter, an
attempt is made to lay the foundations for regarding physical fitness as a
construct.

"A construct is some postulated attribute of people, assumed to be
reflected in performance." (Cronbach and Meehl, 1955.) Any person, at any

time, can be expected to possess, or n̶ ̶ ̶ ̶ssess, a qualitative attribute or structure or to possess some degree of a quantitative attribute. Each of these assumptions is consistent with the manner in which we regard physical fitness. Constructs usually carry associated meanings expressed in such statements as: "Persons who possess this attribute will in situation X, act in a manner Y (with a stated probability)." (Cronbach and Meehl, 1955.) The logic of construct validation is invoked whether the construct is highly organized or extremely loose.

Thus, when considering the construct of physical fitness in motor performance testing, the investigator must concern himself with problems of the following general nature: What constructs account for variance in test performance? (For example, is it abdominal strength or trunk flexibility which is the cause of variance in sit-up test performance?) When does a construct become a definable quality, trait, or attribute? (For example, once the separate variances of the several constructs involved in sit-up performance, that is, static strength, dynamic strength, flexibility, leg length, learning, and so on, are estimated, can we make a statement about physical fitness?) What constructs does a test actually measure? How does a person who scores high in one item and low in another item differ from a person who has these scores reversed? What are acceptable, valid criteria in the evaluation of physical fitness?

Answering these types of questions can best be approached through various construct validation procedures, among which are included group differences, correlation matrices, factor analysis, internal structure studies, and studies of changes over occasions. That is, construct validation takes place when an investigator believes that his instrument (that is, test) reflects a particular construct, to which are attached certain meanings. The proposed interpretation generates specific testable hypotheses, which are a means of confirming or refuting the claim. Physical fitness as a construct then can, it is felt, be examined from this point of view. Exactly which procedures, which combination, or which order of procedures should be used is the subject of the next section of this chapter, where specificity and generality are considered.

The Specificity-Generality Issue

Without in the least advocating either one of these theoretical positions, it is imperative that investigators in the area of motor performance testing and physical fitness be made aware of the advantages and disadvantages of both positions. One must examine the methodological thinking, the scientific rationale, the scientific legitimacy, and the explicit contributions of each of these positions when interpreting test results. Only after these requirements are met can one make inferences under the label of physical fitness.

The Specificity Position

The basic dilemma of this issue is perhaps highlighted by the work of Franklin Henry and others on specificity and by Fleishman and others on factor analysis. Henry (1960), for example, has summarized on the basis of evidence presented by Cozens (1929), Seashore, Buxton, and McCollom (1940), Rarick (1937), and Cumbee (1954, 1957) that ". . . it is no longer possible to justify the concept of unitary abilities such as strength, endurance, coordination and agility, since the evidence shows that these abilities are specific to a particular task or activity." This position of specificity implies that the performance of an individual in one type of physical activity gives only a light indication of the rank he will hold in the performance of another task. As Henry and Rogers (1960) have stated, ". . . it must be conceded that coordinations are highly specific—it is largely a matter of chance whether an individual who is highly coordinated in one type of performance will be well or poorly coordinated in another."

In recent years, such studies as those by Smith (1961a, 1961b) and Lotter (1961) have further substantiated the hypothesis that individual differences in motor coordination abilities are highly specific to the act under consideration. Individual differences may be considered demonstrated when the differences in score *between* individuals in the test or retest are large as compared with differences *within* the individual from time to time as measured by fluctuations in his test and retest scores. Hence the reliability coefficient is a measure of the magnitude of individual differences present (Henry, 1949). It is, then, only possible to say that true individual differences exist after testing a large number of individuals who score consistently high whereas others score consistently low. For example, Cozens (1929) demonstrated the point of high specificity of individual differences in physical performance when he found intercorrelations of 0.231 between accuracy in the football pass and the basketball free-throw goals and of 0.282 between the standing broad jump forward and the standing broad jump backward. In fact, over the last 30 years there are very few reported intercorrelations between even the most similar skills that exceed 0.65, with the largest percentage ranging from zero to around 0.40.

The essential conclusion, after constantly examining evidence of such low intertask correlations is that there is no such unitary function as coordination, flexibility, motor ability, agility, and so on. There is, also, no such thing as *the* coordination test or *the* test of explosive power. This view is especially emphasized when one considers the correlation coefficient as an estimate of the variance that is held in common between two variables. A particularly good demonstration is the situation that exists between pull-ups and push-ups (Morford, 1964). These two tests are most often used to measure the muscular endurance of the arms (some say body). The intercorrelation between these particular tests is usually around $r = 0$. significant but moderately low correlation. Upon squaring the coefficient can be seen that 34% of variance is held in common (namely, explained) between the two tests, whereas 66% of the variance is considered specific (namely, unexplained) to one or the other of the two tests.

The correlation relationships between either of these endurance measures and other commonly used endurance measures, that is, bent-arm hang, bent-arm push-up, rope climb, and parallel bar dips, are again all very low. Obviously the tests do not measure the same thing. That is, although one has a measurement of a subject's chinning ability, one does not necessarily have an indication of the same individual's rank within the group when performing a bent-arm hang. Yet, all these items are recognized as measures of muscular endurance. Actually, when chinning performance is listed, the only information one does have is how many pull-ups the individual can manage, and, for certainty, that is *all* one knows. Any claim to having secured a measure of muscular endurance from this performance cannot be logically supported.

Furthermore, most of these performance items are quite sensitive to contamination by numerous other independent variables. For example, the vertical "jump and reach" test shows a perfect learning curve with repeated trials (Henry, 1956b). In fact, with junior high school girls, it requires 3 days of practice of several trials per day to bring an individual to plateau (Pacheco, 1942). Yet, typically, we use this test, the best of three trials usually, to assess an individual's explosive strength regardless of the contamination of performance by learning. Vertical jump performance is also contaminated by short periods of warm-up exercise and also by prior muscle stretching and massage. So, not only are these performance scores unrelated to each other, but one testing may not even be a good indicator of the individual's ability or capacity.

In essence, then, the specificity position is that one cannot make inferences from various performance measures to loosely defined constructs when the amount of relationship between the measures is low and when the reliability of individual differences in these measures is either unreported or ignored. To ascribe a performance to a construct requires much more intensive investigation than the mere labeling of underlying factors.

The Generality Position

The generality position, based primarily on the results of factor analytic procedures, is concerned with the identification of components underlying physical proficiency and the recommendation of appropriate test procedures to measure these components. This is a clear attempt to link performance measures with theoretical constructs described as basic factors. This is exactly what must be done in the area of human motor performance testing when the final objective is the identification and definition of a construct, like physical fitness. However, it is important to remember at this point that the construct of physical fitness is in turn made up of a framework of theoretical constructs, namely, strength, endurance, agility, flexibility, and so on. This is the *crux* of the issue: how *valid* are the factors identified by the factor analysts when one is interpreting motor performances in terms of broad, categorical capacities? For example, should a trait such as strength first be identified as a factor of physical fitness or should it first be examined, identified, and defined in and of itself? The former approach takes one only so far, whereas the latter requires much more intensive investigation. With respect to how much import the identification of factors has in the investigation of abilities, Bechtoldt (1951) had this to say:

> ". . . factor analysis is a technique of interdependency analysis where all variables are coordinate and treated alike, and factor analysis is inappropriate where variables are distinguished as independent and dependent as Fleishman does, and, in fact, as all experimental psychologists do. In other words, factor analysis is descriptive, not predictive. It is not hard, therefore, to see why differential psychology and its primary tool of factor analysis [has] fail[ed] to excite experimental psychologists who are dedicated to the old fashioned scientific goal of predictive laws. Differential psychology simply has failed to come up with fruitful techniques that experimental psychologists can use for the individual differences in the laws they seek. The failure, however, is not only in technique but in analytical thinking about the interrelationships of learning variables and individual differences, and here both differential and experimental psychology are derelict."

This view is reinforced by Thurstone's (1947) comment that ". . . factor analysis is only a halfway house between uncharted psychological domains and hypotheses for the experimental laboratory. . . . After all, investigators . . . have somehow managed to develop fruitful hypotheses and laws for complex phenomena without factor analysis."

In the light of these searching comments, one would consider Fleishman's (1964) recent publication on the components of physical fitness as having real benefit in descriptive terms as it applies to motor performance testing. That is, as a contribution to clarifying the status of performance levels in various motor task items, the study is extremely valuable. However, can one logically go further and infer scientifically that the basic factors that account for these performances have been identified?

Factor analysis begins with a complete set of intercorrelations between all the test items believed to be measures of, or related to, the factors under consideration. A successful analysis results in the "isolation" of a number of factors or components, which are said to account for the major part of the content of the tests analyzed. As described by Fleishman (1964), factors represent clusters or groupings of tests based on high intercorrelations among those tests. From this grouping of tests, a factor score, that is, an average score taken from only those tests that correlate highly with each other, is obtained. This represents the correlation of each test with a factor. Finally, those tests that fail on the same factor (that is, those with high factor loadings on one factor and little or zero in other factors) are examined *subjectively* to see what they have in common. From this judgement the factor is then "named" in terms of the common requirements assumed.

To this point, except for reservations about the naming of factors and the size of the correlation coefficient that they consider high, there is little disagreement between specificists and factor analysts. However, at the next step contention begins because it is here that the factor analyst proceeds to compute an index of how much of the performance on each test is accounted for by the common factors. This is called the test's communality (h^2) and turns out to be the sum of the squares of the test's factor loadings. Mathematically, then, one can reproduce all the original correlations from the factor loading on each factor. Fleishman notes that all tests will have some specificity, that is, some portion of performance will not be accounted for in terms of common factors, but implicitly states that the specificity of these test items is less than their communality. This is a contentious issue.

Whenever correlational analysis is dealt with, two aspects are of immediate concern: (1) the size of the correlation coefficient and its implications for the *amount* of relationship that exists between the two variables, and (2) the statistical significance of the correlation coefficient from zero. Aspect (2) is highly dependent on a large number of subjects tested, and significance can be gained with low order correlations. Although these coefficients tell us that the relationship is significantly different from no relationship, they tell us very little of the specific make-up of the proportions of the relationship. In order to gain this information we must look at the amount of common variance that is shared by the two variables being correlated, that is, aspect (1), the amount of relationship that exists. This is done simply by squaring the coefficient and multiplying by 100. For example, a correlation of 0.40 indicates that only 16%, $100 \times (0.40)^2$, of the variance is held in common and 84% is specific to one or the other of the two variables.

Significance from zero becomes less informative in this context. If large portions of the common variance are unexplained, the fact that the minute portion of explained variance is significant from zero tells little of the make-up of the relationship. Of additional importance in this connection is that the size of the relationship is severely limited by the reliability of individual differences in each variable. If reliabilities are low, then the correlation coefficient between the two variables is inflated; that is, it seems much higher than it actually is. On the other hand, if the reliabilities are quite high, then a low correlation can *only* be attributed to the lack of variance held commonly. These points *must always be considered* when one is handling correlations.

This caution is especially necessary when considering the size of factor loadings. There seem to be no set criteria for evaluation of the size of these factor loadings except that they are probably accepted on the basis of statistical significance, which, as already has been pointed out, depends on large numbers of subjects (N). This is of prime importance because it is through factor loadings that the factors are determined. Furthermore the communality is inflated by squaring and adding in of nonsignificant factor loadings. For example, say the level of significance at the 0.05 level requires 3.6 for $N = 50$, and the factor loadings on a particular item are 0.75, 0.25, 0.15, 0.05, and 0.35. Then h^2 (communality) $= (0.75)^2 + (0.25)^2 + (0.05)^2 + (0.35)^2 = 0.77$, which is a moderately high accounting of performance. However, all these factor loadings are nonsignificant except the 0.75, so that in effect one is summing nonsignificant factor loadings and inflating the total variance accounted for. Therefore, the specificity ($b + r^2 - h^2$) is grossly underestimated. This point should be seriously considered until an exact definition of a significant factor loading is determined.

Thus, when one deals only with the amount of relationship, one is *not* theorizing but only speaking relatively about generality. There is no doubt in our minds that common factors do exist but, without going into further multivariate analysis and construct validity, it is unjustifiable to talk about generality existing when it is swamped by specificity. It is also impossible to know the exact common variance accounted for without knowing the reliability of individual differences in each variable. Without this rarely reported information, it is impossible to calculate how much of the observed variance is made up of error. The amount of generality and its converse, specificity, is directly dependent upon the reliability of the individual differences. When it is high, we can say with some assurance that the variance unaccounted for (that is, the residual) is specific. When one has a list of factor loadings that single out an item or series of items to describe the factor, and the loadings on the factor account for less than 50% of the common variance in the item or items, then how can one say the factor has been identified.

It is at this point that we rest our case. Factor analysis is an important step on the way to determining the make-up of human motor performance, but it is only important in that we consider it a part of the determining process.

REFERENCES

Adams, J. A.: Motor skills. *Ann. Rev. Psychol.*, **15**:181–202 (1964).
American Association of Health, Physical Education, and Recreation: *AAHPER Fitness Test Manual* (rev. ed.). Washington, D.C., 1965.

Bass, R. I.: An analysis of components of tests of semicircular canal function and of static and dynamic balance. *Res. Quart.*, **10**:33–52 (May, 1939).

Bechtoldt, H. P.: Selection. In S. S. Stevens (ed.): *Handbook of Experimental Psychology*, New York, Wiley, pp. 1237–1267, 1951.

Bechtoldt, H. P.: Factor analysis and the investigation of hypotheses. *Percept. Mot. Skills*, **14**:319–342 (1962).

Bureau of Naval Personnel, Training Division, Physical Fitness Section. *Physical Fitness Manual for the U.S. Navy*, 1943.

Canadian Association for Health, Physical Education and Recreation: *The CAHPER Fitness-Performance Test Manual*, Ottawa, 1966.

Cronbach, L. J., and P. E. Meehl: Construct validity in psychological tests. *Psychol. Bull.*, **52**:281–302 (July, 1955).

Cozens, F. W.: *The Measurement of General Athletic Ability in College Men*. Eugene, Ore., University of Oregon Publication, Physical Education Series, 1929.

Cumbee, F.: Factorial analysis of motor coordination. *Res. Quart.*, **25**:412–428 (December, 1954).

Cumbee, F.: Factorial analysis of motor coordination variables for third and fourth grade girls. *Res. Quart.*, **28**:100–108 (May 1957).

Cureton, T. K.: Flexibility as an aspect of physical fitness. *Res. Quart.*, Suppl., **12**:381–390 (May, 1941).

Fleishman, E. A. *The Structure and Measurement of Physical Fitness*, Englewood Cliffs, N.J. Prentice-Hall, Inc., 1964.

Henry, F. M.: Condition ratings and endurance measures. *Res. Quart.*, **20**:126–133 (1949).

Henry, F. M.: Future basic research in motor learning and coordination. *Coll. Phys. Educ. Assoc., 59th Ann. Proc.*, pp. 68–75, 1956a.

Henry, F. M.: Evaluation of motor learning when performance levels are heterogeneous. *Res. Quart.*, **27**:176 (1956b).

Henry, F. M.: Specificity versus generality in learning motor skills. *Coll. Phys. Educ. Assoc. 61st Ann. Proc.*, pp. 126–128, 1958.

Henry, F. M.: Influence of motor and sensory sets on reaction latency and speed of discrete movements. *Res. Quart.*, **31**:459–469 (1960).

Henry, F. M., and D. E. Rogers: Increased response latency for complicated movement and a "memory drum" theory of neuromotor reaction. *Res. Quart.*, **31**:448–458 (1960).

Howell, M. L., and R. B. Alderman: The measurement of physical fitness by human performance. Paper presented at the American College of Sports Medicine, Las Vegas, March 1967.

Hull, C. L.: The place of innate individual and species differences in a natural science theory of behavior. *Psychol. Rev.*, **52**:55–61 (1945).

Jones, M. B.: Practice as a process of simplification. *Psychol. Rev.*, **69**:274–294 (1962).

Larson, L. A.: Some findings resulting from the Army Air Forces physical training program. *Res. Quart.*, **17**:114–164 (May, 1946).

Larson, L. A., and R. D. Yocom: *Measurement and Evaluation in Physical, Health, and Recreation Education*. St. Louis, C. V. Mosby Co., 1951.

Lotter, W. S.: Specificity or generality of speed of systematically related movements. *Res. Quart.*, **32**:55–62 (March, 1961).

Morford, W. R.: Motor ability—physical fitness and specificity of human motor performance. *Alberta Teachers' Assoc. Bull.*, **4**:32–52 (1964).

Pacheco, B. A.: Effectiveness of warm-up exercise in junior high school girls. *Res. Quart.*, **13**:259 (1942).

Rarick, L.: An analysis of the speed factor in simple athletic activities. *Res. Quart.*, **8**:89–92 (December, 1937).

Seashore, H. G.: The development of a beam-walking test and its use in measuring development of balance in children. *Res. Quart.*, **18**:246–250 (December, 1941).

Seashore, H. G.: Some relations of fine and gross motor abilities. *Res. Quart.*, **13**:259–274 (October, 1942).

Seashore, R. H., C. E. Buxton, and I. N. McCollom: Multiple factorial analysis of fine motor skills. *Amer. J. Psychol.*, **53**:251–259 (1940).

Smith, L. E.: Reaction time and movement time in four large muscle movements. *Res. Quart.*, **32**:88–94 (March, 1961a).

Smith, L. E.: Individual differences in strength, reaction latency, mass and length of limbs and their relation to maximal speed of movement. *Res. Quart.*, **32**:203–220 (May, 1961b).

Technical recommendations of psychological tests and diagnostic technique. *Psychol. Bull. Suppl.*, **51** (2, Pt. 2):1–38 (1954).

Thurstone, L. L.: *Multiple-Factor Analysis.* Chicago, Ill., University of Chicago Press, 1947.

War Department: Physical training. W.D.F.M. 21–30, January, 1946.

War Department: *WAC Physical Fitness Test.* Washington, D.C.

The Development of Work Capacity and Physical Fitness

Part VI

SECTION EDITOR
E. ASMUSSEN
The University of Copenhagen

Individual Differences

21

LARS HERMANSEN
Institute of Work Physiology
Oslo, Norway

Man's capacity to perform muscular work is determined by several independent factors, the following being considered of great importance: energy
output (that is, aerobic and anaerobic processes), neuromuscular function
(that is, muscle strength and technique), and psychological factors (that is,
motivation, fighting spirit). All these factors are involved in almost all types
of labor or physical exercise. However, the relative importance of the
different factors varies to a large extent from one activity to another. The
relative importance is, for instance, dependent upon the type of work and the
duration and intensity of the work. In some occupations, for instance, light
industry work or office work, the energy-liberating processes are taxed to a
minor extent, while motivation or working technique may play a more
important role. In other types of activities (jobs), such as farming, forestry,
or construction work, large muscle groups are engaged in prolonged exercise
at a relatively high work intensity. Consequently, the energy-liberating
processes are taxed to a large extent.

It is also well known that physical performance capacity is higher in
men than in women and lower in children than in adults. Furthermore, after
20–30 years of age there is a fairly steady decrease in physical performance
with increasing age. Thus, it can be concluded that the individual's capacity
to perform physical work varies to a large extent from one subject to another.
Furthermore, the requirements of the different factors underlying physical
work capacity vary greatly with different work tasks. Therefore, objective
measurements of the individual's physical performance capacity have been
shown to be of great importance in different fields in modern society. For
instance, one of the major goals in rehabilitation therapy is to bring the
patient back to his job in the best possible condition. Evaluation of the
patient's physical performance capacity during convalescence in order to
achieve this goal more rapidly must be determined by objective criteria. The

395

same need for objective measurements of the individual's physical performance capacity is present in many other fields, for example, in different
sports events, in industry, and in the military.

This chapter will focus on the variability in physical performance capacity
in large groups of subjects with special reference to sex, age, and level of
physical activity.

Determination of Physical Performance Capacity

Whenever the physical performance capacity of different individuals or
groups of subjects is to be evaluated, the methods employed for estimation
are of primary importance. The great majority of tests for estimation of
physical performance capacity can be grouped broadly into (1) physical
fitness tests and (2) physiological tests. These two main approaches have
certain advantages and disadvantages, and both have been used in the present
study.

Physical Fitness Tests

Competitive sport events represent the classical test of physical performance capacity. The physical performance of the subjects may be determined objectively in meters (centimeters) or minutes (seconds). For the
present study the track-and-field events discussed below were used.

Sprint Running (60-m). The running was performed in the following way:
Three subjects were involved in each heat. The start was taken from a standing
position. The time was measured with conventional stop-watches and expressed in seconds and tenths of a second. Each subject was allowed only one
trial.

Endurance Running (1500 m). The endurance run was performed on a
400-m track. Fifteen subjects participated in each heat. The time was taken
for each subject and expressed in minutes and seconds. Each subject was
given only one trial.

Long Jump. Each subject was allowed to choose his own length of
approach, and the take-off was made from a take-off board, 1 m × 1 m. The
length of the jump was measured in centimeters. Each subject was given three
trials, and the best result was recorded.

High Jump. The high jump was performed in a large gymnastic hall, the
length of the approach ranging from 10 to 20 m. The take-off and the jump
were made at right angles to the bar. The height of the bar was increased in
steps of 5 cm, and each subject was allowed to have three trials at each
height.

Throwing a Small Ball. The test was performed on a grass field. The
diameter of the ball was approximately 6 cm and the weight 50 g. The throw
was measured in meters. Each subject performed three times, and the best
result was recorded.

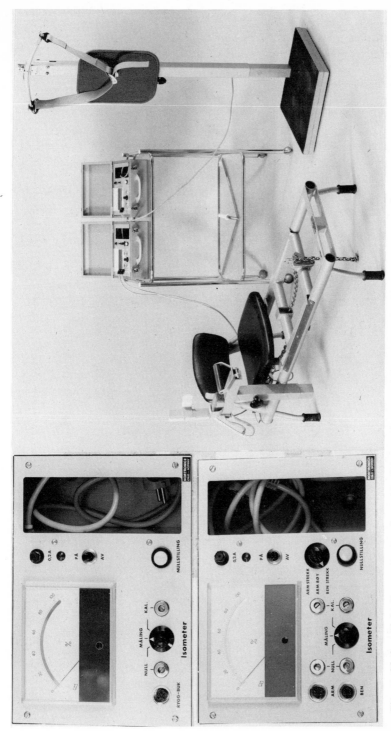

Figure 21-1. *Right.* Dynamometers for measuring muscle strength in arm flexors, arm extensors, abdominal, and back muscles, and knee extensors. *Left.* Enlargement of the instrument panel.

Throwing a Large Ball. The large ball was thrown on a grass field. The diameter of the ball was approximately 22 cm and the weight 425 g. The throw was measured in meters. Each subject was allowed three trials, with the best result being recorded.

Physiological Tests

Determination of Maximal Oxygen Uptake. Maximal oxygen uptake constitutes the most commonly used index of physical work capacity. In the present investigation two different methods were used to measure the maximal oxygen uptake, that is, the direct and the indirect methods.

Oxygen uptake was measured directly (that is, the direct method) during maximal uphill running of the treadmill, using the Douglas bag method. A

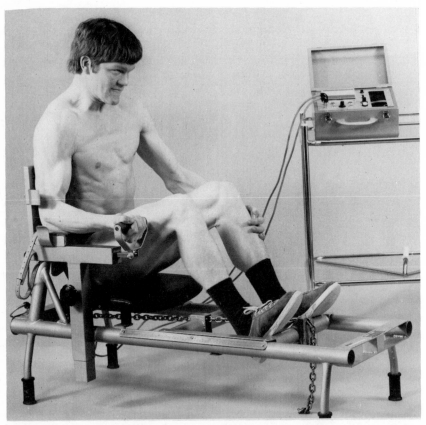

Figure 21-2. Standard position for measuring the muscle strength in the arm flexors. When the muscle strength of the arm extensors is measured, the hand of the subject is turned 180°.

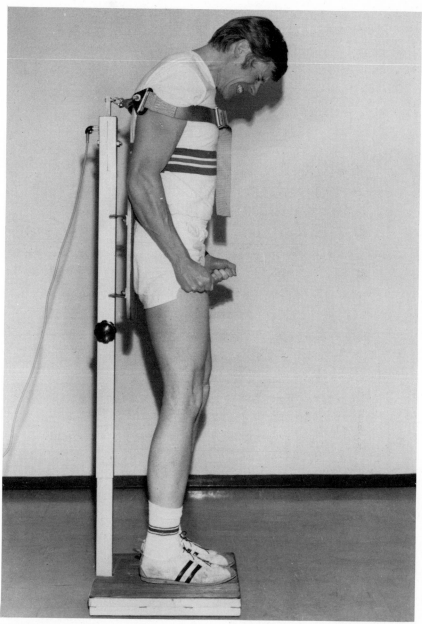

Figure 21-3. Standard position for measuring the strength in the abdominal muscles.

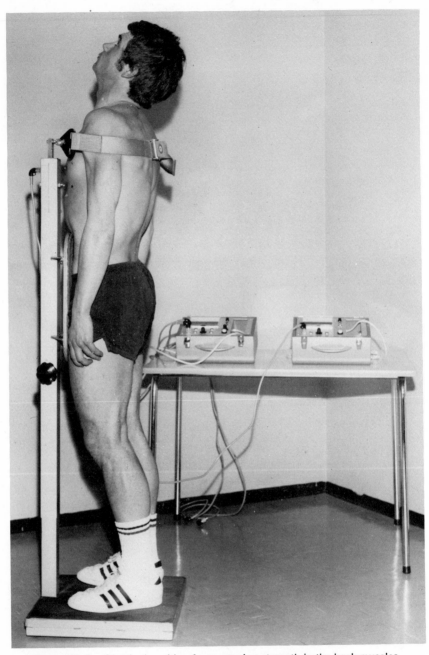

Figure 21-4. Standard position for measuring strength in the back muscles.

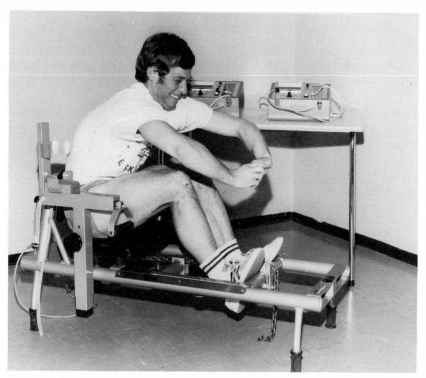

Figure 21-5. Standard position for measuring the muscle strength in the knee extensors.

further description of this method and procedure are given by Hermansen and Saltin (1969). In a large group of subjects ($N = 801$) the maximal oxygen uptake was calculated from measurements of heart rate and workload during submaximal bicycle exercise, according to the method of Åstrand and Rhyming (1954).

Determination of Muscular Strength. Objective evaluation of muscle strength can be undertaken in several ways. In general, the methods usually are divided according to the conditions under which the muscles are activated during the actual test (Asmussen, 1967). If the muscles are maximally stimulated and contracted against an outer resistance that is impossible to move, the maximal force produced is a measure of the muscle strength. This maximal muscle force is defined as the maximal isometric muscle strength.

In the present investigation maximal isometric muscle strength is measured in the following muscle groups: arms, flexors, arm extensors, abdominal muscles, back muscles, and knee extensors. The dynamometers and the standard positions used for the measurements are shown in Figures 21-1 through 21-5.

Variability in Physical Performance Capacity of Young Healthy Subjects

Among healthy men and women there exists a wide variation in all bodily functions underlying physical performance capacity. This wide variation exists in both sexes and at all age groups and may partly be explained by differences in body dimensions. However, considerable differences remain even when the subjects are compared on the basis of body weight or body height.

In order to make a reliable description of the total variation in a population, large numbers of carefully selected subjects need to be investigated. However, since most accurate and reliable tests are very time consuming, both for the investigators and the subjects, population studies on a large scale basis are difficult to carry out. Partly owing to these difficulties, more simple test procedures have been developed. However, the accuracy of most of these simpler methods is not very good. Consequently the results must be evaluated with these limitations in mind.

Maximal Oxygen Uptake of Young Norwegian Men

In Norway a large number of young men every year are assigned to military services with widely varying physical demands. Obviously, from a

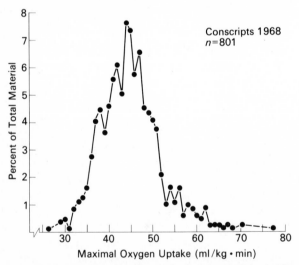

Figure 21-6. Distribution of the values for maximal oxygen uptake (ml/kg·min) in 801 young Norwegian men. (Mean age 18.9 years.) The mean value was 45.0 ml/kg·min. Maximal oxygen uptake is calculated from measurement of heart rate and workload according to the method of Åstrand and Rhyming (1954).

Table 21-1 Mean Values (±Standard Error and Standard Deviation) for Age, Height, Weight, Heart Rate During Submaximal Bicycle Exercise (i.e., 900 kgm/min)* and Calculated Maximal Oxygen Uptake in Three Groups of Subjects

Groups	Number of Subjects	Age, years	Weight, kg	Height, cm	Heart rate, 900 kgm/min	Max. Oxygen Uptake l/min	ml/kg·min
Oslo	724	18.92 ± 0.02 0.60	68.93 ± 0.18 8.57	178.89 ± 0.13 6.11	160.40 ± 0.56 15.17	2.90 ± 0.02 0.51	44.96 ± 0.26 6.99
Höytorp	18	18.83 ± 0.06 0.25	70.17 ± 3.25 13.42	179.17 ± 1.65 6.81	156.20 ± 3.37 13.91	3.01 ± 0.11 0.47	46.28 ± 1.79 7.37
Ulsteinvik	59	18.75 ± 0.05 0.37	69.61 ± 0.95 7.26	179.00 ± 0.78 5.91	159.51 ± 1.92 14.63	2.92 ± 0.06 0.44	44.41 ± 0.74 5.60
Total	801	18.92 ± 0.02 0.58	68.95 ± 0.30 8.58	178.91 ± 0.21 6.11	160.35 ± 0.53 15.10	2.90 ± 0.02 0.50	44.95 ± 0.24 6.90

* kgm/min = kilogram meters per minute.

military point of view it is important to match the individual's physical capabilities with the actual demands of the tasks.

In 1968 maximal oxygen uptake was estimated in 801 young men using the indirect method (that is, maximal oxygen uptake was predicted from measurements of heart rate and workload on the bicycle ergometer). Of these subjects 724 lived in the area of Oslo, 59 were studied on the west coast of Norway, and 18 were studied in the southeast part of Norway. The results are given in Table 21-1 and in Figure 21-6.

This study offers an ideal opportunity to investigate the variability in physical performance capacity (that is, maximal oxygen uptake) in a large and relatively homogeneous group of subjects. As will be seen from Table 21-1, the mean values for maximal oxygen uptake were approximately the same in all three groups, although the number of subjects in the three groups varied between 18 and 724. The range of variability in the total material for maximal oxygen uptake is illustrated in Figure 21-6. It will be seen that the maximal oxygen uptake, expressed as milliliters per kilogram of body weight per minute (ml/kg·min) varied between 26 and 77, the mean value being 45.0 ml/kg·min. It should be emphasized that, although this material was gathered from a relatively large number of subjects, it is impossible to indicate definite limits for the normal values. So far, there is no agreement on definitions of normality in this field.

Maximal Isometric Muscle Strength of Young Norwegian Men

As indicated earlier the individual's physical performance capacity depends on several factors. Maximal oxygen uptake is supposed to be the best

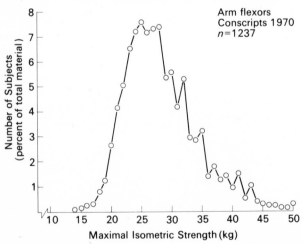

Figure 21-7. Distribution of the values for maximal isometric muscle strength of the arm flexors in 1237 young men. Mean values for age, height, and weight are given in the text.

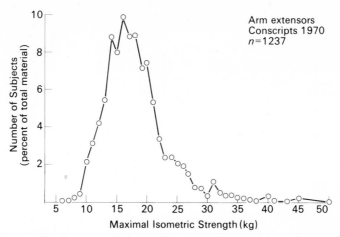

Figure 21-8. Distribution of the values for maximal isometric muscle strength of the arm extensors in 1237 young Norwegian men. Mean values for age, height, and weight are given in the text.

single determinant of the individual's physical work capacity. However, muscle strength is another important parameter. In 1970, maximal isometric muscle strength was determined in 1237 young men, using the dynamometers described earlier (Figures 21-1 through 21-5). The average values for age, height, and weight in these subjects were 19 years and 1 month, 179 cm, and 69.2 kg. The results are given in Figures 21-7 through 21-11. As seen from

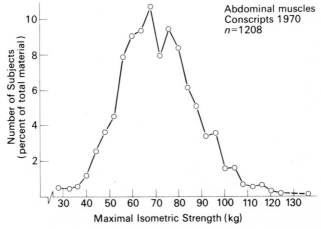

Figure 21-9. Distribution of the values for maximal isometric muscle strength of the abdominal muscles in 1208 Norwegian men. Mean values for age, height, and weight are given in the text.

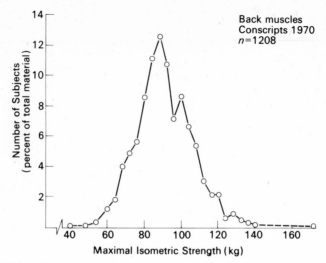

Figure 21-10.   Distribution of the values for maximal isometric muscle strength of the back muscles in 1208 young Norwegian men. Mean values for age, height, and weight are given in the text.

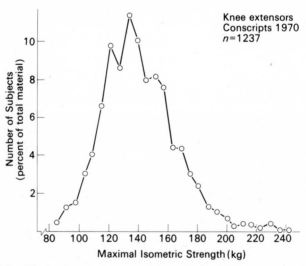

Figure 21-11.   Distribution of the values for maximal isometric muscle strength of the knee extensors in 1237 young Norwegian men. Mean values for age, height, and weight are given in the text.

these figures, the values for maximal isometric muscle strength vary considerably from one individual to another and for all the muscle groups tested. It should, however, be emphasized that these results are not corrected for differences in body size. Consequently, the large variation may be at least partly explained by variation in body size. On the other hand, it may be pointed out that, even when muscle strength is expressed as force per unit surface area, there is a considerable variation from one subject to another (Ikai and Fukunaga, 1968). The basis for this variability is not yet known.

Figure 21-12 shows the results obtained from measurements of maximal isometric strength in athletes. So far, only a few athletes from a limited number of sport events have been investigated. However, the result of this investigation clearly showed that the degree of training is another important factor, which also may explain part of the large variations observed in the young men.

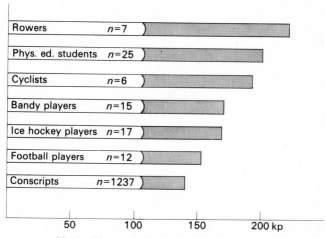

Maximal Isometric Strength, Knee Extensors

Figure 21-12. Mean values for maximal isometric muscle strength of the knee extensors in different groups of trained and untrained subjects. (*n* denotes the number of subjects in each group.)

Variability in Physical Performance Capacity in Relation to Sex and Age

Maximal Oxygen Uptake in Relation to Sex and Age

Studies from several laboratories have demonstrated that maximal oxygen uptake and related physiological parameters (that is, pulmonary ventilation, cardiac output, and so on) show considerable variations with sex and age (Hermansen and Andersen, 1965; Robinson, 1938; Åstrand, 1960; Åstrand, 1952).

Figure 21-13 gives the mean values from direct measurements of maximal oxygen uptake in different groups of schoolchildren and adults of various ages and occupations. Altogether 243 individuals participated in these studies. The general health condition of the subjects was good. None of the subjects was an athlete, but most of them participated regularly in outdoor activities. The schoolchildren also participated in the regular physical education program of the schools (that is, two times 45 min a week). The general age effect characteristics are in agreement with observations in earlier studies (Robinson, 1938; Åstrand, 1952).

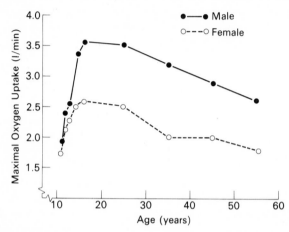

Figure 21-13.   Mean values for maximal oxygen uptake in different groups of untrained schoolchildren and adults.

It can be seen (Figure 21-13) that the maximal oxygen uptake increases with increasing age both in boys and girls during childhood. It should be noted that the mean values for maximal oxygen uptake in boys are higher than in girls at all age groups. The difference was not statistically significant; however, this observed trend is in agreement with several other studies and also with the better endurance capacity of the boys in running 1500 m (see Figure 21-17) in the present study. The maximal oxygen uptake (liter/min) was found to increase in the female subjects up to the age of 15 years. Between 15 and 25 years of age, the maximal oxygen uptake was approximately constant, but from then on a gradual decrease with increasing age was observed. The mean values for the male subjects showed almost the same pattern of development. The peak value was found at the age of 17 years, and during the next 10 years almost no change could be demonstrated. However, after the age of approximately 30 years, an almost linear decrease in the mean values was observed.

In adult life, the values for maximal oxygen uptake are approximately

30% lower in women than in men. This difference is at least partly explained by the fact that women are smaller than men. If the values for maximal oxygen uptake are corrected for differences in body size (that is, expressed as milliliters per kilogram per minute), the difference is reduced from approximately 30% to 15%.

It is also known (von Döbeln, 1957) that women have approximately 10% larger fat deposits than men. Thus, if the values for maximal oxygen uptake are expressed as milliliters of oxygen per kilogram of fat-free body weight, the difference between men and women is reduced to about 5%.

It should also be emphasized that the intragroup variability is very large, not only in young male subjects (see Figure 21-6) but also in schoolchildren and older age groups. There is also a considerable overlap between male and female subjects at all age levels.

Athletic Performance Capacity in Relation to Sex and Age

The athletic performance capacity of man has been a subject of considerable interest for centuries. In fact, athletic competition in different sport events represents the classical test for measurement of man's physical performance capacity. However, the results obtained in these tests are markedly influenced by previous practice and training. Consequently, it is difficult to carry out a reliable analysis of the physiological functions that determine the subject's physical performance capacity on the basis of these tests. On the other hand, testing of athletic performance capacity may be of considerable interest as a pedagogic tool for increasing motivation, for instance, in schoolchildren.

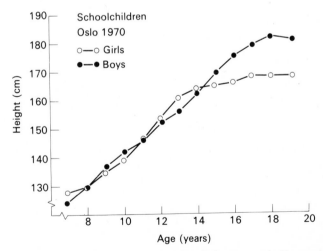

Figure 21-14. Mean values for body height in relation to age in Norwegian school-children.

In 1970, athletic performance capacity was studied in 1014 school-children, between 7 and 19 years of age, from nine different schools in the area of Oslo. The methods and procedure for the tests were described earlier in this chapter (pages 396–401). The sampling of the subjects was performed by taking one whole class from four different schools at each age level. The mean values for body height and body weight in relation to age are given in Figures 21-14 and 21-15.

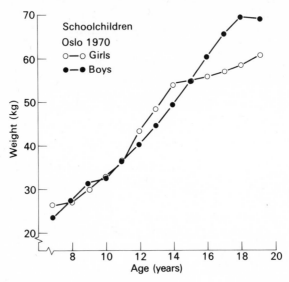

Figure 21-15. Mean values for body weight in relation to age in Norwegian school-children.

The mean values for body height varied from 125 to 181 cm in the boys and from 128 to 168 cm in the girls between the seventh and nineteenth year of age. As seen from Figure 21-14, body height increased at approximately the same rate in both girls and boys up to the age of 13 years. From then on, the body height of the girls started to level off, whereas in boys it continued to increase almost linearly up to the age of 18 years. The mean values for both girls and boys at the age of 19 years were almost identical to the mean values for adult Norwegian men and women.

The changes in body weight (Figure 21-15) of boys and girls showed almost the same general pattern of development as that for body height. However, there was a tendency toward a higher rate of increase between 11 and 14 years of age and a lower rate of increase between 14 and 19 years of age in body weight in the girls than in the boys.

The results of the athletic performance tests are given in Figures 21-16 through 21-21. Spring test results are shown in Figure 21-16. The mean value

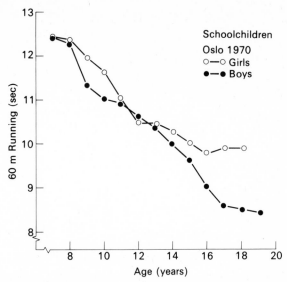

Figure 21-16. Mean values for physical performance (that is, time for running 60 m) in relation to age in Norwegian schoolchildren.

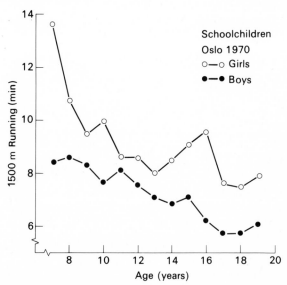

Figure 21-17. Mean values for endurance capacity (that is, time for running 1500 m) in relation to age in Norwegian schoolchildren.

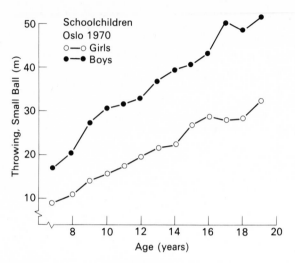

Figure 21-18. Mean values for physical performance (that is, throwing a small ball) in relation to age in Norwegian schoolchildren.

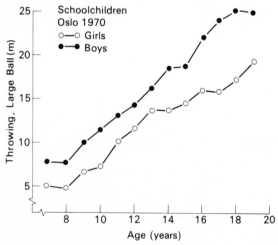

Figure 21-19. Mean values for physical performance (that is, throwing a large ball) in relation to age in Norwegian schoolchildren.

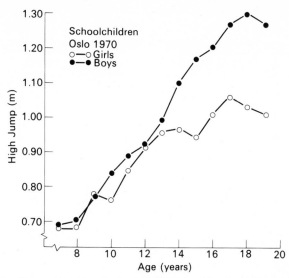

Figure 21-20. Mean values for physical performance (that is, high jump) in relation to age in Norwegian schoolchildren.

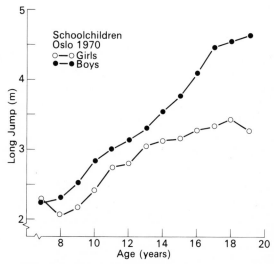

Figure 21-21. Mean values for physical performance (that is, long jump) in relation to age in Norwegian schoolchildren.

(that is, time) for running 60 m was 12.4 sec for both boys and girls at the age of 7 years. The corresponding values at the age of 18 years were 8.5 and 9.9 sec for boys and girls, respectively. It will be seen that the mean values were approximately the same in both sexes up to the age of 12 years. From then on, the mean value for the girls started to level off, whereas in the boys the mean value continued to decrease (that is, the physical performance capacity was increasing).

The results of the endurance test are given in Figure 21-17. As seen from the figure, the mean values for running time at 1500 m were lower in the boys than in the girls at all age levels. It should also be emphasized that, in contrast to what was found in the sprint test, the changes in endurance capacity in relation to age seem to show almost the same pattern in both sexes.

In the ball-throwing tests (Figures 21-18 and 21-19), the physical performance capacity increased almost linearly from the seventh to the nineteenth year of age both in boys and girls. In the jumping tests (Figures 21-20 and 21-21), however, the physical performance capacity increased almost linearly in both sexes up to the age of 12–13 years (that is, puberty). From then on the results of the girls started to level off, whereas the results of the boys continued to increase almost at the same rate as before puberty.

Thus, there seem to be differences in the pattern of development of physical performance capacity in relation to age in the different sport events. These differences are shown very clearly when comparing the pattern of development in Figure 21-19 and Figure 21-20 (that is, throwing the small ball and high jumping). At present, no obvious explanation can be given for the observed differences.

Ethnic Group Differences in Physical Performance Capacity

Man's capacity for prolonged severe muscular exercise is an important determinant of survival and successful living in a stressful climate. To make a living off the land in an arctic area certainly involves hard physical work in the process of gathering and hunting for food, making adequate housing, and so on. On the other hand, the inhabitants of a tropical or subtropical area do not need to perform hard work in order to construct strong or solid houses or to collect the necessary amount of food for living. Therefore, it is possible that exposure to a cold and stressful climate has produced strong and physically fit individuals, and that physically weaker individuals are able to survive to a larger extent in a warm and pleasant climate.

If this hypothesis is correct, one would expect that the physical performance capacity of people living in an arctic area should be higher than that of the people living in a tropical climate. The level of physical performance capacity in terms of maximal oxygen uptake has recently been established in a sample of nomadic Lapps in the northern part of Norway (Finnmark).

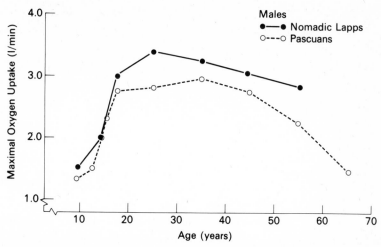

Figure 21-22. Mean values for maximal oxygen uptake (liter/min) in male Pascuans and nomadic Lapps.

Similar studies have also been performed on the inhabitants of Easter Island in the South Pacific (that is, the Pascuans). These studies make it now possible to compare two ethnic populations living in very contrasting climates.

The maximal oxygen uptake for these two populations are given in relation to sex and age (Figures 21-22 through 21-25). Since the body size of the subjects in both populations differs, the maximal oxygen uptake was expressed both as liters per minute (Figures 21-22 and 21-23) and in milliliters per kilogram per minute (Figures 21-24 and 21-25). The typical age effect characteristic, which is shown in many other studies (Robinson, 1938; Åstrand,

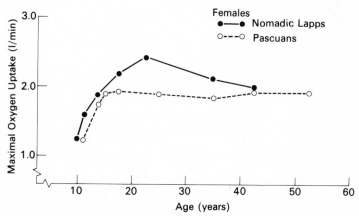

Figure 21-23. Mean values for maximal oxygen uptake (liter/min) in female Pascuans and nomadic Lapps.

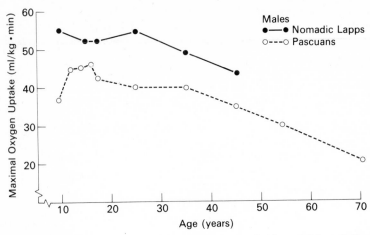

Figure 21-24. Mean values for maximal oxygen uptake (ml/kg · min) in male Pascuans and nomadic Lapps.

1960; Åstrand, 1952), was observed also in these two populations. However, a small difference in the age curve between the two populations was found.

The maximal oxygen uptake (in liters per minute) increased with increasing age during childhood in both populations (Figures 21-22 and 21-23). The Lapp males reached a peak in the maximal oxygen uptake values in the middle twenties (Figure 21-22). From then on, a gradual decrease in these values was observed. The Pascuan males (Figure 21-22) reached their peak of physical performance capacity at an earlier age, that is, 18 years, and this level was almost unchanged until the age of 40 years. After this age, a pro-

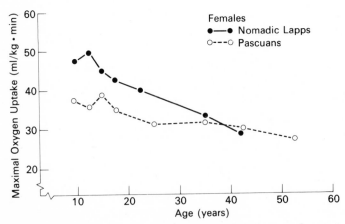

Figure 21-25. Mean values for maximal oxygen uptake (ml/kg · min) in female Pascuans and nomadic Lapps.

nounced decrease was observed, and the rate of decrease was somewhat higher than that observed in the Lapps. The Lapp women (Figure 21-23) reached a peak in the maximal oxygen uptake values early in the twenties, followed by a gradual decrease with increasing age. The corresponding values (in liters per minute) for the Pascuan women (Figure 21-23) increased to about 15 years of age. From then on, almost no change in maximal oxygen uptake in relation to increasing age could be demonstrated.

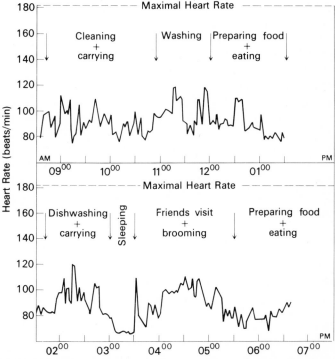

Figure 21-26. The heart rate curve of a Pascuan woman during a day. Age, 29 years; height, 167 cm; weight, 60 kg; maximal oxygen uptake, 35.8 ml/kg·min.

Compared on the basis of body weight (Figures 21-24 and 21-25), that is, maximal oxygen uptake expressed as milliliters per kilogram per minute, it appears that the nomadic Lapps possess a higher capacity to perform muscular exercise. This observation was consistent for all age groups of the male subjects and also in the women up to the age of 30 years.

This rather large difference in maximal oxygen uptake supports the hypothesis that climate and living habits may influence the individual's capacity to perform prolonged severe exercise. The habitual physical activity associated with life in the two contrasting environments is certainly different.

The nomadic Lapps, particularly adult men and young unmarried women, are physically active during a large part of the day, working with their reindeer. On the other hand, most people in the Easter Island community had a rather sedentary life. The daily pattern of activity was studied in a few Pascuan subjects by using a radiotelemetric system for measurements of the heart rate throughout a whole working day. The results obtained in a 29-year-old woman are presented in Figure 21-26 as an example. The results may be classified as a typical curve for a person living a sedentary life. Unfortunately, similar data on the nomadic Lapps are not available. However, it is well known that the Lapps are walking or running (or both) for a fairly long period of time almost every day.

It is not possible at present to give a definite explanation for the observed differences in maximal oxygen uptake between the nomadic Lapps and the Pascuans. It is, however, well known from several studies (Saltin and Åstrand, 1967; Saltin et al., 1968) that increased physical activity (training) increases the maximal oxygen uptake. On the other hand, it is also known that inactivity causes the maximal oxygen uptake to decrease (Saltin et al., 1968). Thus, the difference in the daily physical activity level between these two populations is probably the most important factor contributing to the observed difference in physical performance capacity. However, other factors, such as nutrition or the incidence of acute or chronic diseases, may also be of importance.

REFERENCES

Asmussen, E.: Measurement of muscular strength. *Försvarsmed.*, 3:152 (1967).

Åstrand, I.: Aerobic work capacity in men and women with special reference to age. *Acta Physiol. Scand.*, Suppl., 49:169 (1960).

Åstrand, P-O.: Experimental studies of physical working capacity in relation to sex and age. Copenhagen, E. Munksgaard, 1952.

Åstrand, P-O., and I. Rhyming: A nomogram for calculation of aerobic capacity (physical fitness) from pulse rate during submaximal work. *J. Appl. Physiol.*, 7:218 (1954/55).

Hermansen, L., and K. L. Andersen: Aerobic work capacity in young Norwegian men and women. *J. Appl. Physiol.*, 20:425 (1965).

Hermansen, L., and B. Saltin: Oxygen uptake during maximal treadmill and bicycle exercise. *J. Appl. Physiol.*, 26:31 (1969).

Ikai, M., and T. Fukunaga: Calculation of muscle strength per unit cross-sectional area of human muscle by means of ultrasonic measurement. *Int. Z. angew. Physiol.* (einschl. Arbeitsphysiol.), 26:26 (1968).

Robinson, S.: Experimental studies of physical fitness in relation to age. *Arbeitphysiol.*, 10:251 (1938).

Saltin, B., and P-O. Åstrand: Maximal oxygen uptake in athletes. *J. Appl. Physiol.*, 23:353 (1967).

Saltin, B., G. Blomqvist, J. H. Mitchell, R. L. Johnson, K. Wildenthal, and C. B. Chapman: Response to exercise after bed rest and after training. *Circulation*, **37/38**: Suppl. VII, 1968.

von Döbeln, W.: Maximal oxygen uptake, body size and total hemoglobin in normal man. *Acta Physiol. Scand.*, **38**:193 (1957).

Potentials for Development

22

HOWARD G. KNUTTGEN
Boston University
Boston, Massachusetts

The general purpose of this chapter will be to examine the existing evidence concerning the possibilities for bringing about improvement in the factors related to physical performance. Because the status of a particular function prior to a training or conditioning program has an important bearing on potential for change, the discussion will include values obtained from the so-called "normal average healthy" population whenever available.

It should be emphasized that the author does not believe in a single entity of physical fitness nor in any wholesale evangelistic endorsement of the development of large functional capacities principally as an end rather than as a means. Every sport and every work situation demands a different combination of functional capacities and, therefore, the fitness of an individual must be specific to the particular task (Knuttgen, 1969). The decision as to whether an individual cares to develop certain capacities in order to perform better or more fully enjoy sport and work should be a personal one.

At the same time, the author does believe that functional capacities could very well be considered as factors in the assessment of a person's quality of health. In this way, a person with greater strength and endurance would be described as healthier because of his greater capacity for physical performance and the lessened physiological response to submaximal physical challenges. The presence of disease, injury, or infirmity would still play an important role in this assessment, but mere absence of them would not constitute a terminal point in such an evaluation. With the exception of instances where a government, school system, or other group decides that this form of health (large functional capacities) should be mandatory or something to strive for, the choice should remain with the individual.

The physiological capacities for physical performance affect the way in which an individual can exhibit force, power, and endurance and can conduct certain coordinated movements with precision. The force (or strength) that a person can maximally exert in any one of the myriad movements of the skeleton is actually the torque created by the skeletal muscles expressed through the bony levers. When this force is expressed through a distance, it can be expressed as work or work equivalents. When this force is repeatedly expressed through a distance, work is performed at a certain rate and additional physiological factors come into play. The expression is one of power. Endurance is the term used for the ability to maintain a certain exertion or work intensity (power) for a period of time and, again, additional factors play roles of importance.

The expression of strength is principally dependent upon the muscle mass involved or, more specifically, the physiological cross section of the muscles creating the force. Other factors, such as initial length of the muscles, mechanical advantage, and type of contraction (shortening, isometric, or lengthening) are also important. Muscle contraction is under the direct control of the central nervous system and, therefore, subject to the various facilitory and inhibitory events that can affect the eventual level of stimulation. The latter aspect will be considered psychological in nature and not considered in this discussion.

The expression of power is a matter of the rate at which energy can be released in the muscle cells. The energy-release processes are often categorized according to whether or not the presence of oxygen is directly involved and termed aerobic or anaerobic, respectively. Because the processes requiring constant delivery of oxygen (aerobic) can account for a quantity of energy release per unit of time (that is, rate of release) different from that of the so-called anaerobic processes, the capacity of an individual for energy release (and power) can be discussed as two interrelated capacities, aerobic and anaerobic.

The energy for contraction is held to come directly from the cleavage of adenosine triphosphate (ATP). Therefore, the quantity of ATP that exists in a muscle cell, although very small, constitutes a potential for maintaining contraction. The other compounds found in skeletal muscle cells, which are employed in the processes that resynthesize ATP during contraction (creatine phosphate, glycogen, glucose, and free-fatty acids), constitute tremendously larger sources of energy. The availability of these compounds at the beginning of exercise (stored in the muscle cells) and the rates of uptake of glucose and free-fatty acids delivered by the blood will determine the length of time that activity can be maintained. The circumstances of muscular activity as regards length of each contraction, number of contractions per unit of time, and relative work load will impose various sets of demands on the active muscle cells and, therefore, affect endurance in various ways. The availability of oxygen, the buildup of metabolic waste products, and the alteration of the interior milieu (for example, pH) are also possible sources of fatigue for the muscle cell.

Provided a person has the muscular strength to perform a particular movement, the precision with which the movement is performed will be principally the function of the nervous system. Again, this will be considered psychological in nature, and precision will not be included in the present discussion.

Strength

Because of the effects of a variety of conditions upon the expression of muscular force or strength in the human, the determination of maximal values is extremely difficult. First of all, the type of contraction (shortening, isometric, or lengthening) will be of importance. It has been shown in both isolated animal muscle and in intact human beings that eccentric (lengthening) contractions generate the greatest forces, concentric (shortening) contractions the lowest maximal values, with maximal values for isometric contractions falling in between (see Asmussen, 1968; Asmussen et al., 1965).

Secondly, it should be pointed out that all contractions express their forces through the movement of skeletal levers, and the effectiveness is measured as moment of force (or torque) rather than force *per se*. Therefore, the position of the lever becomes important as it affects both the relative strength of the muscle and its mechanical advantage by means of the angle of attachment.

A third complicating factor in strength measurement is the fact that muscle responds to stimulation from the nervous system and, therefore, maximum volitional strength is greatly affected by psychological factors (Ikai and Steinhaus, 1961). Most strength training studies have neglected this consideration. It is, therefore, impossible to determine to what extent strength gains observed during the course of the training programs are due to physiological change in the skeletal muscle cells and to what extent due to altered psychological factors.

It is generally held that human skeletal muscle can exert a force of somewhere between 4 and 6 kg/cm^2. The torque is then dependent on the factors discussed above. There is an apparent sex difference when similar movements and, therefore, muscle groups are compared for men and women. The difference is most probably due to differences in body proportions and not in the quality of muscle tissue itself.

It is difficult to compare values reported in the literature because of the differences in subjects, test methods, and methods of recording (for example, force versus torque). The fact that the human skeleton is capable of hundreds of separate movements also complicates the attempt to discuss standards. That so many separate movements exist is an extremely important consideration in light of the finding that the correlations among strengths of various movements in groups of individuals are extremely poor (Tornvall, 1963). In other words, individuals cannot and should not be assessed for "strength" on the basis of the measurement of a few movements. Standards must be developed for each movement.

The type of exercise program necessary to develop strength is still another consideration. The type of contractions (concentric, isometric, or eccentric), the duration of each contraction, the resistance, the number of repetitions, and the number of exercise bouts per week are not well-studied in this respect and create the possibility for thousands of different programs. The one factor that seems to stand out is that the force developed by the muscle during its contraction must be relatively high (close to its maximal) during the exercise program in order to bring about maximal change.

The controversy over the value of isometric compared to dynamic contraction lingers, although the greatest part of the confusion appears to have been clarified. The possible advantage of isometric contraction over concentric contraction in strength training was first pointed out by Asmussen (1949). The results of Hettinger and Müller (1953) with one isometric contraction per day held for 6 sec at two thirds maximal tension appeared sensational at the time of publication but have not been confirmed. The first of a number of studies to challenge their observations and conclusions was that of Peterson (1960). Apparently, higher relative tensions and a greater number of contractions are needed in each exercise session.

Reports have appeared where strength gains of as high as 41% of original values have been reported within 5 weeks, but most studies report a rate of gain of 3–6% per week. One factor contributing to the differences is the variety of programs involved. Once again, the question can be raised as to the relative contributions of physiological as opposed to psychological factors. Two related considerations that must be considered when discussing potential for rate of gain and eventual maximal increase are the ages and initial levels of strength of the individuals involved. As a general rule, one would expect a lower potential for improvement with either older persons and/ or higher initial levels of strength as compared to norms for the age group.

Power

If activity is begun at an extremely high intensity, such as to bring about exhaustion within a few minutes, the muscle cells cannot obtain and/or the metabolic events cannot proceed rapidly enough to utilize oxygen. Therefore the events of the tricarboxylic acid cycle (Krebs cycle) and respiratory chain cannot support the demands of ATP resynthesis. Other metabolic events (glycolysis) can, however, proceed with ATP resynthesis without oxygen, the rate at which this can take place constituting a sort of anaerobic capacity for power. Added to this, the high-energy phosphate compounds, themselves, constitute a small reservoir of energy that does not demand the immediate presence of oxygen for utilization. If aerobic energy release is defined as energy involving delivery of oxygen from the lungs, the oxygen bound to myoglobin and dissolved in the tissue fluids could, while supporting oxidative processes, also be considered as part of the "anaerobic" picture.

If values of 4.8 mmole/kg and 18.0 mmole/kg wet muscle are employed for ATP and creatine phosphate concentration, respectively, in resting skeletal muscle, a person utilizing 15 kg of muscle (as in a man running) has an anaerobic potential of less than 4 kcal from this source (assuming 11 kcal/mole high-energy phosphate). By other methods, Margaria et al. (1964) have estimated the total energy available through anaerobic sources as 95 and 220 cal/kg (total body weight) for processes not involved in lactate formation and resulting in lactate formation, respectively. They also predicted the maximal power for these same mechanisms as 45.0 and 21.5 kcal/hr·kg (total body weight).

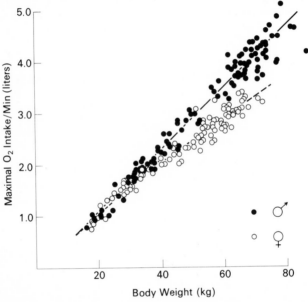

Figure 22-1. The relationship of maximal oxygen consumption to body weight: open circles, female subjects; closed circles, male subjects. [From P.-O. Åstrand: *Experimental Studies of Physical Working Capacity in Relation to Sex and Age*. Copenhagen, Munksgaard, 1952.]

Presumably, the various factors that participate in "anaerobic" power can be altered and, therefore, an increase in this capacity can be brought about. Two studies have observed such increased capacity as a result of high-intensity training (Cunningham and Faulkner, 1969; Margaria et al., 1964) but, as the subjects also increased the time they could perform the "anaerobically" supported power, the contribution of psychological factors (for example, tolerance of discomfort) is uncertain. There are no data available at the present time to permit discussion of the physiological mechanisms of improvement.

Considerable research has been devoted to aerobic energy release and the capacity for aerobic power. A very strong positive relationship exists between body size and maximal oxygen consumption and, therefore, between age and maximal oxygen consumption prior to attainment of physiologic maturity. The latter shows variation among different populations and occurs, on the average, a few years earlier for females than for males but in both cases takes place in the late teens.

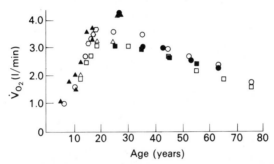

Figure 22-2. The relationship of maximal oxygen consumption to chronological age for male subjects from various nationality groups.

Data from the following sources:

Open triangles: K. König, H. Reindell, J. Keul, and H. Roskam: Untersuchungen Über das Verhalten von Atmung und Kreislauf im Alter von 10–19 Jahren. *Int. Z. angew. Physiol.,* **18**:393–434 (1961).

Closed triangles: P.-O. Åstrand: *Experimental Studies of Physical Working Capacity in Relation to Sex and Age,* Copenhagen, Munksgaard, 1952.

Open circles: S. Robinson: Experimental studies of physical fitness in relation to age. *Arbeitsphysiol.,* **10**:251–323 (1938).

Closed circles: I. Åstrand: Aerobic work capacity in men and women with special reference to age. *Acta Physiol. Scand.,* Suppl., **49**:169 (1960).

Open squares: H. von Valentin, H. Venrath, H. von Malinckrodt, and M. Gürakar: Die Maximal Sauerstoffaufnahme in den verschiedenen Altersklassen. *Z. Alternforsch.,* **9**:291–308 (1955).

Closed squares: R. A. Binkhorst, J. Pool, P. van Leeuwen, and A. Bouhuyd: Maximum oxygen uptake in healthy nonathletic males. *Int. Z. angew. Physiol.,* **22**:10–18 (1966).

Open hexagons: H. G. Knuttgen: Aerobic capacity of adolescents. *J. Appl. Physiol.,* **22**:655–658 (1967).

Therefore, if maximal oxygen consumption is plotted against body size, a strong positive relationship is found (Figure 22-1). If, on the other hand, capacity for aerobic power is plotted using age (Figure 22-2), it is seen that an increase occurs until attainment of physiological maturity and, after the age of approximately 25 years, a slow decrease occurs through the later years of life (data are from four nationality groups with no special state of physical conditioning). Data are more limited on women but show generally a lower capacity in this regard, after puberty, which is principally attributed to lower hemoglobin concentration and less physical activity in daily life among women.

The capacity for aerobic energy release is one consideration but, if this power is to be put to use in any form of locomotion, the capacity should be expressed in terms of some unit of body size. Such expression would also present the capacity in qualitative form and conform to the concept of capacity as a partial index of degree of health. The physical parameter most often employed is body weight and, therefore, the qualitative determination of power is expressed as oxygen consumption (in milliliters per kilogram of body weight per min).

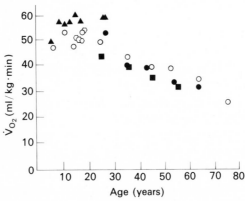

Figure 22-3. The relationship of maximal oxygen consumption equated for body weight to chronological age in male subjects. Sources and symbols as in Figure 22-2.

The data cited above appear quite different when expressed in this manner (see Figure 22-3). It can be seen that there is very little qualitative change in the aerobic capacity per kilogram in the general population through the first 25–30 years of life. Thereafter, a slow decrement occurs.

We can then consider aerobic capacity as an index of working (power) capacity and consider aerobic capacity per unit body weight as an index of fitness. Since studies have shown that human beings have become larger (height, weight, and so on) through the centuries, the average person has therefore had an increase in aerobic power and work capacity purely on the basis of size increment alone. From a health standpoint, aerobic capacity is not a meaningful item of data until it is expressed per unit of body size. The fact that individuals from different populations presently have a maximal oxygen consumption averaging approximately 3.5 liters/min and that certain

champion athletes have been measured at 6.0 liters/min gives us little information. If humans double in body size in the next 1000 years, an aerobic
capacity of 7.0 liters/min would quite possibly be commonplace in the
general population.

It is of greater interest to note that, from the youngest age groups studied
(lower elementary school grades) through groups in their late twenties, the
average values for aerobic capacity per unit body weight hover around
50–55 ml/kg·min. The observation that champion athletes in endurance
sports (for example, cross-country skiing, distance running) exceed 80 ml,
in spite of some variations in body size, indicate a possible upper limit for
humans. This extremely high standard must be considered as a combination
of tremendously high intensity training programs and of genetics (inheritance).

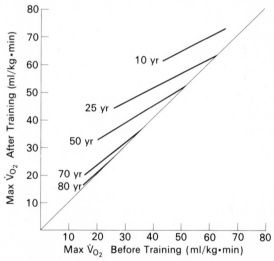

Figure 22-4. Changes in maximal oxygen consumption which can be expected after
10 or more weeks of intensive, endurance-type conditioning. It can be observed that
persons of higher age begin at lower quantitative values and can expect smaller quantitative increases. [From G. Grimby and B. Saltin: Fysisk träning: fysiologiska effecter.
Läkartidningen, **67**:4530–4539 (1970).]

In a discussion of the potential of an individual to improve his aerobic
capacity, two extremely important factors must be considered: the person's
age and the person's starting level of fitness for large-muscle endurance
activity. In general, the lower the age and the lower the initial level the greater
the potential for improvement as measured quantitatively (increase in
ml/kg·min) or qualitatively (percent of initial value). This is vividly shown in
a figure presented by Grimby and Saltin (1970) from a composite of data
from a number of studies (see Figure 22-4). This does not say, of course, that

a person with low fitness in this respect has a greater chance to attain higher terminal values but relates purely to the potential for percentage increase. Therefore, a discussion of potential for improvement is meaningless unless one qualifies the conditions, principally age group and initial capacity. The figures of 10–20% are often cited as the average range of improvement following conditioning programs.

Of special interest are the observations that especially marked increases result from physical training during the immediate prepubescent and pubescent years. The factors include the ability to continue submaximal work for longer periods of time (Ikai, 1969) and increases in heart volume and aerobic capacity that exceed those which could be expected from body size increments alone (Ekblom, 1969). It would appear that, during these periods of growth, the greatest change or improvement in functional capacities for physical work can be brought about and that these changes will not regress as quickly and to as great an extent as in other age groups when training programs are suspended.

Saltin et al. (1968) found in three young healthy, but untrained, subjects (20–21 years) increases in aerobic capacity of 100% between the end of a 3-week period of bedrest and the end of a vigorous conditioning program. They were relatively inactive subjects even before the enforced bedrest so that the situation represents an extreme in the consideration of the problem of potential for improvement.

Certain physiologic factors that are known to increase and contribute to the increase in aerobic capacity are the blood volume, total hemoglobin, stroke volume, and cardiac minute volume (cardiac output). No significant changes are believed to take place in maximal oxygen extraction ($a - v\,O_2$ difference), muscle blood flow (expressed as volume of blood per minute per muscle mass), pulmonary parameters (for example, vital capacity, maximal ventilation), or the membrane component of pulmonary diffusing capacity. It might be mentioned that, in swimming, increases in vital capacity are probably important to success in competition and can result from training because of the difference in breathing pattern and resistance to lung ventilation. Less is known about the metabolic changes in skeletal muscle cells (that is, ability of cells to increase the rate of energy release and utilization of oxygen) in response to training.

A consensus of various training studies (see discussions in Ekblom, 1969; Hartley et al., 1969; Saltin, 1969; Saltin et al., 1968; Saltin et al., 1969; Siegel et al., 1970) would seem to indicate that aerobic capacity is best increased by a program of exercise at least once every 3 days. Each exercise period should consist of repeated bouts of high-intensity work lasting approximately 2–4 min (or possibly as wide a range as 1–6 min) interspersed with recovery periods (approximately 5 min duration). The number of times these bouts should be repeated is another unknown factor, but it seems safe to say that the total exercise period should last somewhere between 30 and 60 min. Within 1–2 months, a healthy inactive person should expect an increase in aerobic capacity of somewhere between 10 and 30%. If the person is older or in a state of good condition prior to beginning such a program, the increase will be proportionately smaller. For a healthy 25-year-old with an aerobic capacity of 45 ml to strive for 55 ml/kg·min would seem both attainable and reasonable; for a 45-year-old with an aerobic capacity of 35 ml to strive for 40 ml/kg·min is equally realistic. For a competitive distance runner with a capacity of 70–80 ml, an increase of 3 ml (or 4%) as a result of hard training would constitute a fantastic change.

Endurance

Although endurance may be defined in more than one way, the present discussion will employ the term as referring to the ability to maintain physical activity. The ability of skeletal muscle to maintain activity (contractions) will depend upon the length of each contraction (time), the intensity of each contraction (force), and the number of contractions per unit of time. If length of time of contraction is the criterion and resistance is the independent variable, a type of "isometric endurance" or holding time can be tested. Although the metabolic factors involved in this type of endurance have not been well researched, fatigue would apparently be due to a depletion of high-energy phosphate, with the involvement of a possible inhibition of oxidative

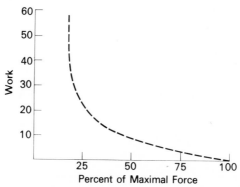

Figure 22-5. Relationship of total work that can be performed at a predetermined rate (contractions per minute) when the resistance is varied so as to elicit different forces of contraction or torque. Units of measurement are arbitrary. [Data from M. Samson: *Contribution à l'étudé ergometrique de la fatigue neuromusculaire normale et pathologique.* Paris, Foulon, 1953, and J. Sherrer, M. Samson, and A. Paléologue: Étude du travail musculaire et de la fatigue. *J. Physiol. (Paris),* **46**:887–916 (1954).]

phosphorylation because of impaired blood flow. If the resistance to contraction is low enough, the contraction should be able to be maintained indefinitely.

Rhythmic work presents a similar picture. If the number of contractions per minute is held constant and the intensity (or resistance) is varied, a curvilinear relationship is obtained when percent of maximal force is plotted against work performed (or tension × time). This curve was first described by Samson (1953) and Scherrer (1954). An example of the curve is presented in Figure 22-5. The comparable relationship of isometric endurance to relative resistance is presented in Figure 22-6 (from Scherrer and Monod, 1960), as originally presented by Monod (1956) and later confirmed by Rohmert (1960).

At the resistance where the muscle or muscle group is capable of only one contraction (1 repetition maximum or 1 *RM*) in rhythmic work, the reasons for fatigue are most likely related to local events either within the sarcomeres, at the myoneural junction, or at the muscle cell membrane. If the repetition

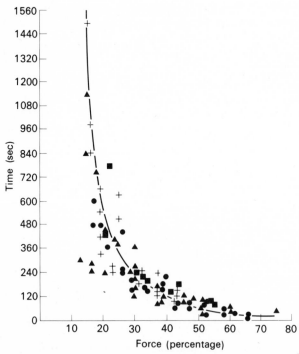

Figure 22-6. Relationship of endurance time of contraction to resistance, expressed as percentage of isometric contraction force. [From J. Scherrer and H. Monod: Le travail musculaire local et la fatigue chez l'homme. *J. Physiol.* (*Paris*), **52**:419–501 (1960).]

rate was such that the recovery time before a second contraction was attempted became insufficient to allow restitution of the necessary conditions, repetition would become impossible. At less high resistances where small numbers of repetitions are possible, a vital limiting factor is probably the rate of ATP breakdown versus the rate of ATP resynthesis. At high resistances, where only limited endurance is possible, the inadequate resynthesis processes that do take place are predominantly anaerobic. As the resistances become smaller and ability to endure increases, the resynthesis processes are predominantly aerobic.

The causes for fatigue in this range of high work intensities have not been elucidated. Depletion of high-energy phosphate and extreme alteration in hydrogen ion concentration (high concentrations of metabolic acids) in the cells are two possible factors.

At resistances and, therefore, intensities of power that can be carried on for longer periods, oxidative phosphorylation is sufficient to balance the utilization rate of high-energy phosphate. The person is working within his aerobic capacity. Endurance will then be determined by the availability of the metabolites necessary for oxidative phosphorylation, glycogen (and glucose) and free-fatty acids. The relative contributions of carbohydrate and fat are still not completely resolved. At high intensity submaximal work, the evidence seems overwhelming in favor of carbohydrate as the important energy source—in particular, the glycogen store already present in muscle at the beginning of activity. The uptake of glucose from the blood is apparently too slow to replenish the rapid breakdown of glycogen and, when the glycogen is exhausted, the limit to endurance is reached.

It has been observed that, in both trained and untrained subjects, exhaustion after exertion lasting in excess of 1 hr occurred simultaneously with depletion of the glycogen stores of the working muscles (Bergström and Hultman, 1967; Hermansen, 1967). It has also been observed that a high carbohydrate diet can cause an increase in muscle glycogen stores (Bergström et al., 1967; Hermansen et al., 1967), especially if preceded by exercise-induced glycogen depletion (Saltin and Hermansen, 1967). The high initial glycogen content then corresponds to a longer work time at high submaximal intensities (Bergström et al., 1967) or better performance (faster total pace) in distance running (Karlsson and Saltin, 1971, and Figure 22-7). The high-carbohydrate diet, especially in combination with special training procedures, can greatly affect endurance capacity for high-intensity work. The data obtained from the above references would indicate that, for a person with an average resting muscle glycogen concentration of 70 mmole/kg (wet muscle), such a regimen could easily double the glycogen concentration and double the endurance capacity for high-intensity work.

Therefore, the capacity for submaximal work can be enhanced in two ways. By increasing the capacity for delivery and employment of oxygen, a person can increase his power capacity thereby making all submaximal work intensities less stressful on a relative basis. By increasing the muscle glycogen concentration, a person can increase his capacity for continuing exercise of high intensity. In both cases, the absolute limits are dependent upon age and the relative increases dependent upon the initial level (that is, prior to training).

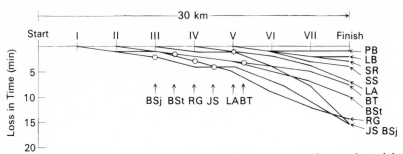

Figure 22-7. Loss in time in minutes between a 30-km race run after regular training and a mixed diet as opposed to the better time recorded in the same race run after a regimen of glycogen depletion and carbohydrate-rich diet. Time loss was recorded at 7 checkpoints and the finish. Arrows indicate estimated point of muscle glycogen depletion to 3 g/kg or less. [Courtesy of J. Karlsson and B. Saltin: Diet, muscle glycogen, and endurance performance. *J. Appl. Physiol.*, **31**:203–206 (1971).]

Another physiological cause for fatigue in submaximal work can be the result of hypoglycemia. Christensen and Hansen (1939) observed the onset of fatigue as blood sugar levels became lower during extended periods of submaximal work (probably 70% of aerobic capacity or lower). Oral administration of glucose brought about rapid return of blood sugar to normal values or above, disappearance of symptoms of fatigue, and renewed ability to continue exertion. The detrimental effect of hypoglycemia is on the functioning of the nervous system, with little or no direct relationship to local metabolic events in the muscle cell.

REFERENCES

Asmussen, E.: Training of muscular strength by static and dynamic muscle activity. 2:a Lingiaden 1949 Kongressen. Lund.: Berlingska boktryckeriet, 1949.

Asmussen, E.: The neuromuscular system and exercise. In H. B. Falls (ed.): *Exercise Physiology*, New York, Academic Press, 1968.

Asmussen, E., O. Hansen, and O. Lammert: The relation between isometric and dynamic muscle strength in man. Comm. Dan. Nat. Assoc. Infant. Paralysis, No. 20, 1965.

Astrand, I.: Aerobic work capacity in men and women with special reference to age. *Acta Physiol. Scand.*, Suppl. **49**:169 (1960).

Astrand, P.-O.: *Experimental Studies of Physical Working Capacity in Relation to Sex and Age.* Copenhagen, Munksgaard, 1952.

Bergström, J., L. Hermansen, E. Hultman, and B. Saltin: Diet, muscle glycogen, and physical performance. *Acta. Physiol. Scand.,* 71:140–150 (1967).

Bergström, J., and E. Hultman: A study of the glycogen metabolism during exercise in man. *Scand. J. Clin. Lab. Invest.,* 19:218–228 (1967).

Binkhorst, R. A., J. Pool, P. van Leeuwen, and A. Bouhuys: Maximum oxygen uptake in healthy nonathletic males. *Int. Z. angew. Physiol.,* 22:10–18 (1966).

Christensen, E. H., and O. Hansen: Arbeitsfähigkeit und Ernährung. *Skand. Arch. Physiol.,* 81:160–171 (1939).

Cunningham, D. A., and J. A. Faulkner: The effect of training on aerobic and anaerobic metabolism during a short exhaustive run. *Med. Sci. Sports,* 1:65–69 (1969).

Ekblom, B.: Effect of physical training on oxygen transport system in man. *Acta Physiol. Scand.,* Suppl. 328 (1969).

Grimby, G., and B. Saltin: Fysisk träning: fysiologiska effecter. *Läkartidningen,* 67:4530–4539 (1970).

Hartley, L. H., G. Grimby, A. Kilbom, N. J. Nilsson, I. Astrand, J. Ekblom, and B. Saltin: Physical training in sedentary middle-aged and older men, III. Cardiac output and gas exchange at sub-maximal and maximal exercise. *Scand. J. Clin. Lab. Invest.,* 24:335–344 (1969).

Hermansen, L., E. Hultman, and B. Saltin: Muscle glycogen during prolonged severe exercise. *Acta Physiol. Scand.,* 71:129–139 (1967).

Hettinger, T., and E. A. Müller: Muskelleistung und Muskeltraining. *Arbeitsphysiol.,* 15:111–126 (1953).

Ikai, M.: Training of muscular endurance related to age. *Fed. Internat. d'Educ. Phys. Bull.* 3–4:19–27 (1969).

Ikai, M., and A. H. Steinhaus: Some factors modifying human strength. *J. Appl. Physiol.,* 16:157–163 (1961).

Karlsson, J., and B. Saltin: Diet, muscle glycogen, and endurance performance. *J. Appl. Physiol.,* 31:203–206 (1971).

Knuttgen, H. G.: Aerobic capacity of adolescents. *J. Appl. Physiol.,* 22:655–658 (1967).

Knuttgen, H. G.: Physical working capacity and physical performance. *Med. Sci. Sports,* 1:1–8 (1969).

König, K., H. Reindell, J. Keul, and H. Roskam: Untersuchungen über das Verhalten von Atmung und Kreislauf im Alter von 10–19 Jahren. *Int. Z. angew. Physiol.,* 18:393–434 (1961).

Margaria, R., P. Cerretelli, and F. Mangili: Balance and kinetics of aerobic energy release during strenuous exercise in man. *J. Appl. Physiol.,* 19:623–628 (1964).

Monod, H.: *Contribution à l'étude du travail statique.* Thèse Méd. Paris, Foulon Ed., 1956.

Petersen, F. Bonde: Muscle training by static, concentric, and eccentric contractions. *Acta Physiol. Scand.,* 48:406–416 (1960).

Robinson, S.: Experimental studies of physical fitness in relation to age. *Arbeitsphysiol.,* 10:251–323 (1938).

Robinson, S., and P. M. Harmon: Effects of training and gelatin upon certain factors which limit muscular work. *Amer. J. Physiol.*, **133**:161–169 (1941).

Rohmert, W.: Ermittlung von Erholungspausen für statische Arbeit des Menschen. *Int. Z. angew. Physiol.*, **18**:123–164 (1960).

Saltin, B.: Physiologic effects of physical conditioning. *Med. Sci. Sports*, **1**:50–56 (1969).

Saltin, B., G. Blomqvist, J. H. Mitchell, R. L. Johnson Jr., K. Wildenthal, C. B. Chapman: Response to exercise after bedrest and after training, Monograph No. 23. New York, American Heart Association, 1968.

Saltin, B., L. H. Hartley, A. Kilbom, and I. Astrand: Physical training in sedentary and middle-aged and older men, II. Oxygen uptake, heart rate, and blood lactate concentration at submaximal and maximal exercise. *Scand. J. Clin. Lab. Invest.*, **24**:323–334 (1969).

Saltin, B., and L. Hermansen: Glycogen stores and prolonged severe exercise. In G. Blix (ed.): *Nutrition and Physical Activity*, Uppsala, Almqvist and Wiksell, 1967.

Samson, M.: *Contribution à l'étudé ergometrique de la fatigue neuromusculaire normale et pathologique.* Paris, Foulon, 1953.

Scherrer, J., and H. Monod: Le travail musculaire local et la fatigue chez l'homme. *J. Physiol. (Paris)*, **52**:419–501 (1960).

Scherrer, J., M. Samson, and A. Paléologue: Étude du travail musculaire et de la fatigue. *J. Physiol. (Paris)*, **46**:887–916 (1954).

Siegel, W., G. Blomqvist, and J. H. Mitchell: Effects of a quantitated physical training program on middle-aged sedentary men. *Circulation*, **41**:19–29 (1970).

Tornvall, G.: Assessment of physical capabilities. *Acta. Physiol. Scand.* Suppl. **58**:201 (1963).

Valentin, H. von, H. Venrath, H. von Mailinckrodt, and M. Gürakar: Die maximal Sauerstoffaufnahme in den verschiedenen Altersklassen. *Z. Altern-forsch.*, **9**:291–308 (1955).

Development Patterns in Physical Performance Capacity

23

ERLING ASMUSSEN
The University of Copenhagen
Copenhagen, Denmark

Work capacity and physical fitness—both expressions taken in their broadest context—are primarily expressions of motor ability, that is, the ability of the body to act as a motor, with force, power, endurance, and precision. The muscles and their lever arms, the bones, the respiratory and circulatory systems, and the nervous system are the direct anatomical-physiological prerequisites for these abilities. The development of each of these systems will integrate into the complex development pattern of a person's physical performance capacity.

Influence of Body Size on Physical Performance

Time is the most appropriate parameter for development. Time in relation to an individual may be expressed as his chronological age; thus, age becomes the most important denominator of the stage of development for any individual. In adolescence increasing age is synonymous with growth and maturation. Later, increasing age may mean increasing experience and better adaptations to environmental stresses—these latter often voluntarily endured as in training for sports—but it also may mean stagnation or the beginning of deterioration. At old age, the latter will dominate and "development" becomes negative with respect to work capacity and physical fitness.

This pattern is roughly the same for all humans. Individually it may vary in the details, being dependent on genetic and environmental modalities. Primary among the first is sex; the development patterns of boys and girls, men and women, differ in several aspects. Ethnic background is probably of importance, although often inseparably mingled with cultural factors. Acquired variations may be caused by living habits, job, food, climate, availability, and motivation for using sport facilities, and several other hard-to-define factors.

In this chapter we shall consider the general pattern of development and concentrate principally on the period in which becoming older also means growing bigger, that is, the period of adolescence. We shall omit the earliest period, which may be termed infancy, and define adolescence as the period from age 7–8 years up to 18–20 years. In order to grasp fully what is happening during this period, with respect to work capacity and physical fitness, it will be appropriate first to consider the situation as it would be if the only changes that took place were due to the fact that the individuals became anatomically bigger.

We shall therefore presuppose that growth does not cause changes in the body proportions, that, for instance, leg length will remain the same percentage of total body height throughout the period and that, correspondingly,

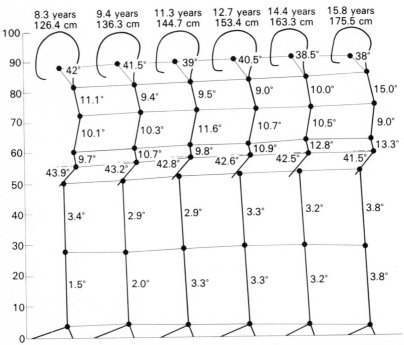

Figure 23-1.   Relative body dimensions in percentage of height of about 300 Danish boys, divided into height groups for every 10 cm of total body height. Free standing posture. Average age and height for each group are shown at the top. Numbers on the figures are angles between the vertical and the lines connecting the following measuring points (from below): Malleolus lat.; epicondylus ext.; trochanter maj.; spina iliaca post. sup.; deepest point in lordosis lumb.; top of kyphosis thor.; proc. spin. vert. cervic. VII; outer ear opening. [From K. Heebøll-Nielsen: *Tidsskrift for Legemsøvelser*, 1958, p. 41.]

all other linear measures in the body will remain the same percentage of any other linear dimensions at the end of the period as they were at the beginning. In other words, we shall assume that the smaller individuals at age 7–8 years are geometrically similar to the bigger ones of age 18–20 years. Obviously, this is not true. An 8-year-old boy "magnified" to the same height as an 18-year-old boy could easily be distinguished from the older one; for girls the difference would be even more obvious. However, for a first approach the assumption is useful. Figure 23-1 demonstrates how justifiable the assumption is but also shows that there are discrepancies in the relative measures of some of the body segments.

We shall further assume that the "material" of which the body is constructed remains the same throughout the period, that is, that bones, muscles, body fluids, and so on, remain qualitatively the same. This would mean, for instance, that the specific gravity of the organs do not change, the contractile power of the muscles per square unit is unaltered, and the composition of blood, and so on, is constant. This also is obviously not true. However, by making these assumptions it will be easier to distinguish that part of the development pattern which is due solely to dimensional changes from that which is caused by qualitative changes.

With these assumptions it is possible to make certain predictions concerning the development of strength, working capacity, and so on, on a purely theoretical basis. These predictions can be compared to actual findings and

	A	B
Heights	1	1.5
Areas	$1^2 = 1$	$1.5^2 = 2.25$
Volumes	$1^3 = 1$	$1.5^3 = 3.375$

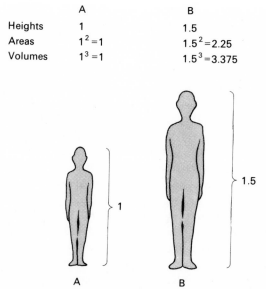

Figure 23-2. For explanation, see text.

may thus also serve to analyze some of the other factors in the pattern of development.

To facilitate comparison, let us assume that we have two individuals, A and B (Figure 23-2). A, the younger, is 120 cm tall: B, the older, is 180 cm tall. They are geometrically similar, and we assume them to be qualitatively equal. It is obvious that the height (h) of B is 1.5 times that of A. Because of their being geometrically similar, all other *linear dimensions* in B will also be 1.5 times larger than in A. This also applies to lengths of arms and legs, lever arms of the muscles in the body, length of individual muscles, their path of shortening. and so on.

All *areas* in B will have the dimensions of $1.5 \times 1.5 = 2.25$, as compared to those in A. This holds true both for outer surfaces (for example, total body surface and its components), but also for inner surfaces (for example, intestines and lungs, and for "hidden" areas such as the transectional areas of trachea, blood vessels, and muscles). *Volumes* in B will further have the dimension $1.5 \times 1.5 \times 1.5 = 3.375$ as compared to those in A and, since we assumed the same specific gravity for younger and older, this ratio will also hold true for all *weights*. Lung volumes, blood volumes, as well as body weight, muscle weights, and so on, will be 3.375 times greater in B than in A.

Certain deductions concerning some physiological functions can now be made from these facts. The maximal force a muscle can produce in contraction is, everything else being equal, proportional to its transectional area. The larger person, B, consequently should be able to develop 2.25 times more force in a muscle contraction than a smaller person, A. If he uses his greater strength in lifting weights, he will be clearly superior to A. This is diagrammed in Figure 23-3A, in which f is muscle force, b is weight of burden, a and A their respective lever arms. In equilibrium we have: $a \times f = b \times A$. Hence $b = a \times f/A$. Introducing dimensions we find that a and A, being linear dimensions will cancel out and leave $b \approx f$, and, because f is proportional to an area (h^2) we find that B can hold a weight 2.25 times as heavy as can A.

If, on the other hand, B must use his greater strength in handling his own body, w, for example, as in chinning (Figure 23-3B), he will be at a disadvantage as compared to A because his body weight will be 3.375 times greater than A's, whereas his muscle strength is only 2.25 times greater. From these or similar simple calculations, it follows that by simply growing taller—with everything else remaining equal—increasing capacity for handling *external weights* develops, whereas the capacity for handling one's *own body*, as in chinning, push-ups, and other gymnastic exercises, diminishes.

In numerous cases our muscles are used not simply for developing force but rather for producing work. Physically, work is the product of a force multiplied by the distance over which it acts. This distance is limited in the body by the length of the muscles and the bones and by the possible movements in the joints. The work must, therefore, be proportional to the linear dimensions of the body, for example, to height (h). The maximum work a muscle or a muscle group can perform is consequently proportional to the linear dimensions in the third power (h^3). In the example of Figure 23-3, maximum work would be 3.375 times greater for B than for A.

Let us consider a standing high jump (Sargent jump). The maximum work the leg and hip extensors can perform in the jump will be proportional to the height of the jumper raised to the third power (h^3). This work applied to the body mass of the jumper will determine the height of the jump. But, because body mass also is proportional to h^3, it follows that the height of the jump will be independent of the size of the jumper. "Height of jump" here means the elevation of the body's center of gravity. A jump over a bar naturally is performed more easily by a tall person whose center of gravity initially lies higher above ground level.

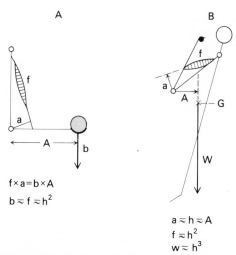

Figure 23-3. **A.** f is muscle force; b is weight of burden; a and A are lever arms; h is body height. **B.** f is muscle force; W is weight of body; G is center of gravity; a and A are lever arms; h is body height.

When *rate* of work (power) is considered rather than just work, *time* becomes a factor. Taken as the time for an event in the body (for example, the time it takes to extend the legs from a crouching position to a toe-standing position, or the time of a stride, a breath, or a heart beat) time must also be dependent on body dimensions. This can be deduced from Newton's second law, *force equals mass multiplied by acceleration ($f = m \times a$)*. Consider a stride in walking. The length (l) of a stride obviously will be proportional to the height (h) of the subject. The mean velocity of the foot will be l/t, t being the time it takes for one stride, and the acceleration a of the foot will be proportional to l/t^2. Substituting this in the formula one gets: $f \simeq m \times l/t^2$. Because in muscle force $f \simeq h^2$, in body mass $m \simeq h^3$, and in length of stride $l \simeq h$, the proportionality takes on the form $h^2 \simeq h^3 \times h/t^2$. It follows that $t^2 \simeq h^2$ and $t \simeq h$. That is, the taller an individual is the longer time it will take for any movement to be performed.

As was pointed out above, the maximum work (w) that a muscle group can perform in a single movement is proportional to h^3. Now it can be seen, that the maximum work per time unit, or the maximum power (w/t), must be proportional to $h^3/h = h^2$.

Frequency of an event is the reciprocal of the time it takes to perform the event ($fr = t^{-1}$). Consequently, $fr \simeq h^{-1}$. As the maximum speed in running is the product of stride length and stride frequency ($l \times fr$), it follows that maximum running speed will be proportional to $h \times h^{-1} = 1$, that is, it is independent of size. This has been discussed earlier, for example, by Hill (1956), who compared greyhounds and race horses, in which the necessity of being geometrically similar is nearly fulfilled. Even though smaller and larger individuals may reach the same maximal running speed, it must be remembered that, because acceleration is f/m and hence in the body proportional to h^2/h^3 or h^{-1}, it follows that large individuals will accelerate slower (for example, at the start of a race). Likewise, they will be handicapped in running uphill where potential energy $\simeq$ weight (w) is produced. Because $w \simeq h^3$ and both their maximum rate of work and their muscle force $\simeq h^2$, they will be handicapped proportional to h^{-1}.

Other events may be treated in the same way. Maximum pulmonary ventilation is, theoretically, the product of maximal tidal volume and maximal respiratory frequency. Tidal volume is proportional to h^3, frequency to h^{-1}, and maximum ventilation consequently to h^2. Maximum heart rate ought to be proportional to h^{-1}, stroke volume to h^3, and cardiac output (stroke volume $\times$ heart rate) to $h^3 \times h^{-1} = h^2$.

In summarizing what has been said above, we come to the conclusion that, even if growing older in adolescence only meant growing bigger (with no qualitative changes occurring), growth would induce considerable change in an individual's fitness for work and sport. Some of the expected changes may be summarized as in Table 23-1.

Influence of Sexual Maturation on Physical Performance

The increase in size that takes place with becoming older in adolescence is not a simple function of time. This is most clearly demonstrated by the annual increase in body height throughout the growth period (Figure 23-4). The annual increase is large during early infancy, but at age 7–8 years it has levelled off to about 5 cm/year (in a European population). But then, rather suddenly, at age 11–12 years in girls and 13–14 in boys, it increases consider-

Table 23-1 Theoretically Predicted Changes in Some Physiological Functions with Increasing Height, h

Muscle strength, used in lifting and carrying burdens	$\simeq h^2$
Ability in handling own body	$\simeq h^{-1}$
Maximum muscular work, absolute	$\simeq h^3$
Maximum muscle work per time unit (power)	$\simeq h^2$
Frequencies	$\simeq h^{-1}$
Jumping height	$\simeq h^0$
Running speed	$\simeq h^0$
Acceleration	$\simeq h^{-1}$
Vital capacity	$\simeq h^3$
Maximum ventilation, liters per minute	$\simeq h^2$
Maximum oxygen uptake per minute	$\simeq h^2$
Maximum heart rate	$\simeq h^{-1}$
Maximum stroke volume	$\simeq h^3$

ably, reaching values of 8–9 cm/year for a year or two. After this, the rate again declines steeply and reaches 0 at ages 17–19 years, the age when final adult height has been reached (Figure 23-4). The "growth spurt" at age 12–14 years is coincident with puberty and is most probably caused by a sudden increase in the production of growth-accelerating hormones from the adrenals and, in boys, from the gonads.

The time course of the height/age curve is—as it appears from the above—different for boys and girls. The final body height is also different for the two sexes; consequently, it must be expected that, for this reason alone, the

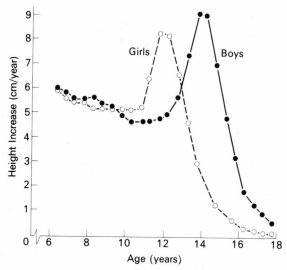

Figure 23-4. Annual increase in body height in relation to age. [Redrawn after J. M. Tanner: *Growth at Adolescence*, 2nd ed. Oxford, Blackwell, 1962.]

height-dependent functions discussed on the preceding pages would differ in later adolescence and in the adult man and woman. It must be further emphasized that ethnic and cultural groups may differ both with respect to the time course of the height/age relation and with respect to the final adult height. Differences in work capacity and fitness among such groups must vary for the simple reason of different size, following the rules summarized in Table 23-1.

Finally it may be worth while to point out that an apparently global secular change in both the time course and in the final body height has been going on for the last several decades (see Tanner, 1962). It has been observed that the "growth spurt" appears earlier and that the final height is greater now than 20–30 years ago. The reason for this development is unknown. Without doubt at least some of the improvements in athletic performances noticed at the more recent Olympic games and world competitions may be ascribed to this general increase in the size of the competitors.

With the increasing height in adolescence follows an increase in weight. Theoretically, as pointed out before, weight should increase in proportion to height elevated to the third power (h^3). This is, however, not quite so. Actual measurements show that in adolescence weight rather increases proportionally to $h^{2.7-2.9}$ (that is, a little less than expected). The reasons for this discrepancy may be several, but the fact remains that the weight increase on a percentage scale is much larger than the height increase. The implications of this have been discussed before. Here it suffices to point out that, as there are height differences between the two sexes and between different populations, there will be, percentagewise, even larger differences in weights. The consequences for several sport events are obvious and should be considered (for example, when tests are applied internationally).

Specifically, when the development of the weight/height relation is considered in relation to sex, it has been found that, while weight is proportional to $h^{2.7}$ in boys, it is close to being proportional to $h^{2.9}$ in girls. Apparently some factors related to sex influence the relationship, and it is highly probable that it has to do with the specific effect of the female sex hormone on the deposition of fat. This is clearly a deviation from the assumption made before, that is, that no qualitative changes take place with growth. For the physical fitness of girls, as compared with boys, it will have an obvious effect. In all events in which body weight plays a role (for example, in jumping, running, chinning, and so on), girls will be handicapped, even if this were the only qualitative difference. Only in one type of sports event will the increased amount of body fat be an asset, namely, in water sports. Due to the low specific gravity of fats, a girl's weight in water will be less than that of a boy of equal height. She will use less energy in keeping afloat, with more spared for propulsion.

Although the final adult body height is a fairly accurate and constant measure, which only high age may reduce, a final adult body weight is rather difficult to define. Insurance companies may have "ideal" body weights for the different heights and ages, but they have no scientific meaning. From a sportsman's point of view it is obvious that, for some sports, a relatively low body weight is an advantage (for example, high jump), whereas in others a relatively high body weight may be of advantage (for example, shot-putting).

The foregoing showed some examples of deviations from the simple dimensional rules that were laid down in the first part of this chapter—for example, the deviations in the weight/height relation due to sex. It became clear that the assumption that neither qualitative changes nor changes in proportion take place in the body during adolescence is not true once the period of sexual maturation begins. In both sexes we find at this period an increased production of sex hormones, but the composition and amounts of these hormones are different in the two sexes. Whereas the female sex hormones, besides their primary function in sexual maturation, mainly influence body weight by causing a deposition of fat, the male sex hormones have no such effect. They apparently influence physical capacity by a specific effect (not the least) on the muscles.

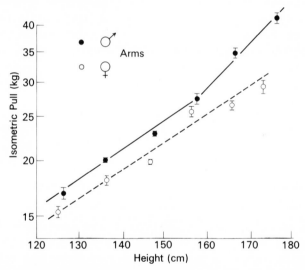

Figure 23-5. Maximal isometric horizontal pulls performed with the arm-shoulder muscles, in relation to body height. Logarithmic coordinates.

This effect is demonstrated by the failure of maximum muscle force simply to increase with h^2, as it should if only size changed with growing older. This assumption can be written: $f \simeq a \times h^2$. Using logarithms on both sides, one gets: $\log f \simeq \log a + 2 \log h$. In other words, a straight line should result if $\log f$ is plotted against $\log h$. Choosing a simple test of muscle strength (for example, an isometric pull on a handle with horizontal, 90° flexed arm) applied to one group of girls and one of boys in the age range 8–16 years and plotting the mean values for each 10 cm height increase in double logarithmic scales, the result may come out as shown in Figure 23-5. It is obvious that, whereas the results from the girls can be represented by one straight line, the results from the boys apparently best fit a line with a sudden break upward at height 150–160 cm. This height corresponds to the age of about 13 years (Danish boys), which is the age when puberty sets in. A new factor apparently becomes active in the boys at this age, and it seems justifiable to assume it is the male sex hormone. (It must be stated here, that the "break" on the log-log line of force versus height is not apparent in all muscle groups; it is especially pronounced in the upper extremities, somewhat less in the legs and trunk.)

In the pattern of development we thus have a factor besides the increase in body dimensions, namely, sexual maturity. It causes qualitative changes, so that the simple quantitative changes due to dimensions cannot alone explain the development of physical performance capacity. This factor has a detrimental effect on some physical capacities of girls because it causes the weight to increase relatively more than corresponding to the increase in height and muscle force but, in boys, it has an enhancing effect by increasing muscle force more than the corresponding increase in height and weight. Sexual maturity also influences, for example, the hemoglobin concentration in boys so that it increases from about 8 g/kg bodyweight to about 10 g/kg. This increase does not occur in girls. It is obvious that the relative physical capacities of girls and boys must change considerably from the time of puberty. The usually small sex differences in prepubescent children (see Figure 23-5) now attain considerable dimensions, partly due to the quantitative differences caused by the smaller size of females and partly due to real qualitative differences.

Influence of Maturation of Central Nervous System

Besides size and sexual maturity, still another maturational factor influences the development of working capacity and physical capacity, presumably that of the central nervous system. This results in a performance capacity increased beyond that which is due to the two other factors. This maturation factor is naturally most significant in tests that demand a high degree of neuromuscular coordination (for example, running, jumping, throwing) but can also be demonstrated in simple tests of muscular strength. A group of children of the same sex and within the same height brackets may be of rather diverse chronological age. If they are divided into two groups, an older and a younger, their mean ages may differ as much as 1.5 year. Even though they are of the same height and their muscle strength should vary

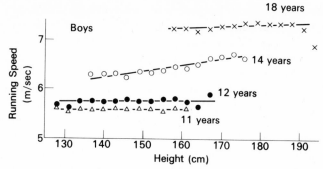

Figure 23-6. Maximum running speeds in boys of different ages as related to body height. [Computed from data of F. Bach: *Ergebnisse von Massenuntersuchungen* Frankfurt a/M, Limpert-Verlag, 1955.]

around the same mean, it will be found that the older subgroup is 5–10% stronger per year age difference.

This separate effect of age per se is probably one of the reasons for the fact that several tests of physical fitness, such as jumping, running, maximum oxygen uptakes and others, do not precisely follow the rules worked out by a dimensional analysis. However, if the number of test subjects is great enough, the various factors, such as sex, size, age, and sexual maturity, can be clearly distinguished. This is nicely illustrated in an analysis performed on the school records (Bach, 1955) of nearly 100,000 Bavarian schoolchildren. The compilation contained age, height, weight, and test results of boys and girls partaking in school competitions. By dividing them into both age groups and height groups and then plotting their running speeds against body height in double logarithmic scales, the data could be presented as in Figures 23-6 and 23-7.

Figure 23-6 shows the results from some of the boys. The two bottom lines are the results from the 11-year-old and the 12-year-old boys. Two things can be seen: (1) With age constant, the height may vary from 130 to

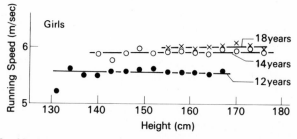

Figure 23-7. Maximum running speeds in girls of different ages as related to body height. [Computed from data of F. Bach: *Ergebnisse von Massenuntersuchungen*. Frankfurt a/M, Limpert-Verlag, 1955.]

165 cm without any change in maximum running speed. This is as predicted from the dimensional analysis on page 440. (2) Within the same height limits, boys that are 12 years old run faster than those 11 years old. This is probably the effect of the maturation with age, but the possibility that systematic training may have increased skill cannot be eliminated.

The middle curves are from boys 14 years old. As might be expected they run faster than the 12-year-old boys (although some of the difference is due to the longer distance run). But here, apparently the rule that running speed is independent of height does not hold. The taller the boys the faster they run. The most likely explanation for this deviation from the prediction is that the 14-year-old boys are in the midst of puberty. Puberty may influence running speed via its effect on muscular strength, as mentioned earlier. At the same time, it causes the "growth spurt" so that those 14-year-olds that are furthest into puberty also will be the tallest. This explanation is supported by the fact that the 18-year old boys (top curve), who have all presumably passed puberty, again show running speeds practically independent of height. It is further supported by the fact that girls (Figure 23-7) do not show a corresponding transitory deviation from the dimensional rules. The effect of age per se is again clearly seen in the girls. The surprisingly small increase from the 14-year-old to the 18-year-old girls may be due to the increase in body fat in the older girls.

A comparison of the 12-year-old boys with the 12-year-old girls shows that boys run faster than girls even before puberty. This may be a question of training, but it may also be a true sex difference.

Summary

In summarizing, it may be noted that the development of physical performance capacity during adolescence for all humans will be patterned by (1) the increase in size, (2) a maturation process by age per se, and (3) the state of sexual maturation. The third factor is different for boys and girls. For boys it means an extra increase in physical performance capacity, above that caused by the first and second factors. For girls, if anything, it means stagnation or deterioration. As for the psychological attitude toward sports, and so on, this difference may play a very important part by increasing the motivation of boys for continued training whereas girls may become frustrated because their efforts, compared to those of the boys, apparently have very little effect.

In adulthood the development of physical performance capacity is patterned by the interplay between the processes that tend to maintain, or eventually further increase capacity and those forces that slowly but unavoidably decrease one's working capacity and physical fitness. It is noteworthy that muscle strength seems to increase up to about age 30 years, even though no specific training of strength is undertaken. From that age, strength

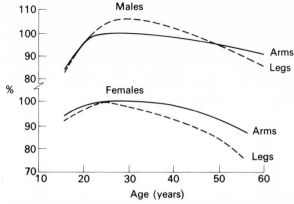

Figure 23-8. Average isometric strength in some arm- and leg-muscle groups in about 600 males and females, in relation to age. [From E. Asmussen, and K. Heebøll-Nielsen: Comm. Dan. Natl. Assoc. Infant. Paralysis, 1966.]

usually begins to decline, faster in the muscles of the trunk and legs than in the upper extremities (Figure 23-8). This pattern may be culture-dependent, that is, dependent on the type of daily work that, in an industrial population, puts smaller demands on the larger muscle groups of legs and trunk than on those of hands and arms. In a farming population the decline in muscle strength may follow quite another pattern. It is also a well-known fact that systematic training of muscle strength is able to change this general pattern completely.

Maximum work power, for example, as expressed by maximum oxygen uptake, will also decrease with age. Some of this decrease seems to be due to a gradual decrease in the maximum heart rate—from about 195 beats/min at age 20 to about 165 beats/min at age 60 years (Figure 23-9). As body weight quite often increases due to fat accumulation, the capacity for running, jumping, and so forth will decrease with age. A systematic training will delay and postpone the deterioration, and, for this and other reasons (for example, nutritional, cultural, genetic), a common pattern of this negative

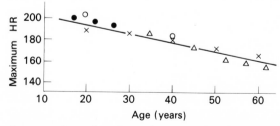

Figure 23-9. Average values of maximum heart rates in men and women, compiled from data in the literature. [From E. Asmussen and S. Molbech: Comm. Dan. Natl. Assoc. Infant. Paralysis, 1959.]

phase of development is hard to describe. With senescence the deterioration accelerates, but the age at which this happens is again individually very different.

As in so many other aspects of human life, the general pattern of development for physical performance capacity is a rather rapid increase to a maximum early in adult life and then a slow, creeping decline, ending in a final, steeper fall at the end of life.

REFERENCES

Asmussen, E., and S. Molbech: *Methods and Standards for Evaluation of the Physiological Working Capacity of Patients.* Comm. Dan. Natl. Assoc. Infant. Paralysis, 1959.

Asmussen, E., and K. Heebøll-Nielsen: *Isometric Muscle Strength of Adult Men and Women.* Comm. Dan. Natl. Assoc. Infant. Paralysis, 1966.

Bach, F.: *Ergebnisse von Massenuntersuchungen* etc. Frankfurt a/M, Limpert-Verlag, 1955.

Heebøll-Nielsen, K.: *Tidsskrift for Legemsøvelser.* Copenhagen, Dansk gymnastiklarerforening, p. 41, 1958.

Hill, A. V.: The design of muscles. *Brit. Med. Bull.,* **12**:165–166 (1956).

Tanner, J. M.: *Growth at Adolescence,* 2nd ed. Oxford, Blackwell, 1962.

Physical Fitness Measurements

Part VII

SECTION EDITOR:

J. ATHA
Department of Ergonomics and Cybernetics
Loughborough University of Technology

Agreed upon by the International Committee on the Standardization of Physical Fitness Tests convened at the International Congress of Sport Sciences, Tokyo, 1964.

Meetings

Jyväskylä, Finland	August, 1973
Cologne, Germany	August, 1972
Magglingen, Switzerland	August, 1971
Oxford, England	September, 1970
Tel Aviv, Israel	August, 1969
Mexico City, Mexico	September, 1968
Magglingen, Switzerland	August, 1967
Sandefjord, Norway	June, 1966
Tokyo, Japan	September, 1965
Tokyo, Japan	October, 1964

Contents

Introduction

Except for a few selected populations, the physical fitness and exercise tolerance of the human races of the world is unknown. Fitness for work is a changeable characteristic, probably subject through all phases of human living to improvement or reduction. The state of fitness is different in various ethnic and cultural groups. It can be expected to be influenced by such factors as age and sex, the state of nutrition, acute and chronic disease, the cultural and social patterns of living, work and physical activity, the physical environment, and heredity.

A study of the fitness and tolerance for work of human populations is an important undertaking that requires cooperation between different scientific groups. Studies performed by using standard techniques and precisely identified experimental methods will render possible descriptions of variations within any given population. By comparing culturally primitive and technically advanced societies, sedentary subjects and well-trained athletes, arctic communities and people living in temperate and tropical zones, new light will be thrown upon some of the problems outlined above.

If levels of fitness are assessed with acceptable scientific techniques, the results thus obtained may form a basis to which measurements undertaken in the future can be ubiquitously referred. Long term longitudinal survey studies will give important information about changes that might take place in respect to important aspects of the body's functioning and may be a way of demonstrating how man adapts himself to changes in his various habitats. This is an important undertaking at a time when advances in technology and economy greatly alter the traditional conditions of living of most human societies of the world.

Provided that the nutritional status is optimal, habitual physical activity seems to be the most powerful factor influencing the work capacity of a healthy subject. However, it is not known to what extent modifications of the kind under reference can be achieved by training. Young subjects are possibly able to increase their functional status more than elderly people. Results of recent research investigations certainly suggest this.

The industrialization and urbanization that is taking place at an ever-increasing rate in many countries have reduced demands for the vigorous muscular exercise previously necessitated by the process of earning a living.

451

Because of modern technology, it is now possible for an individual to spend virtually his entire life at a level of energy expenditure close to that of his resting state. The effect upon the work capacity of the body of this reduction in the daily load of life's activities is deleterious. It remains to be seen what such a decreased functional capacity means for man's health, in terms of his resistance to acute and chronic diseases, longevity, adaptability, as well as for his well-being.

Although the *International Committee for the Standardization of Physical Fitness Tests** is concerned primarily with methods of measurement, it remains well aware that fitness is an attribute of the human personality at its best. Insofar as culture emphasizes the need for an ever-increasing pursuit of excellence, fitness finds itself to be an inherent part of the culture of mankind. The work of the Committee thus relates to the humanities as well as to the exact natural sciences.

Five major areas are covered by the agreements recorded here, namely, personal background and athletic history, medical history and health status, physique and body composition, physiological responses to exercise, and general physical performance. A simple data coding system has been incorporated in the text for the convenience of those intending to program their analyses of results on the computer. It can be readily ignored by those without such plans.

Methods are described for testing the more significant elements of fitness within each area, and alternative procedures are given in cases where problems could arise because of variations among individuals or because of the restricted availability of apparatus. Although the scope of the assessment procedures outlined is wide, it is by no means exhaustive, and many good evaluation techniques are not included. Furthermore, although carefully chosen, the tests described are not to be considered essential for all test programs. As always, the researcher is advised to select carefully in order to find those items that meet his needs best.

* The International Committee for the Standardization of Physical Fitness Tests was convened at the 1964 Tokyo meeting of the International Congress of Sports Sciences.

Section 1

Personal Data and Athletic History

Section 1 is a guide to the personal information necessary if the physical fitness measurements described in the later sections are to be meaningfully interpreted. Where the results of fitness test programs are intended for local use only, much of this information may seem irrelevant. However, if the results obtained are to be compared with those of other groups, to be interpreted in the light of norms established on selected populations, or to be used in the development of data banks prior to some subsequent full scale analysis, then it is essential that the basis for these comparisons or tabulations be meticulously established.

The characteristics identified include sex, age, marital status, nature of employment, activity background, major sports interests, and levels of performance achieved. Section 1 is set out as a brief questionnaire that may either be filled in by the subject or used as the basis of a structured interview by the test administrator. In common with the other sections the answers are coded for the convenience of those wishing to record their data on computer cards ready for later analysis.

A. PERSONAL DATA

Family name: ─────────────────────────────

First name, other initials: ─────────────────────

Card serial number: ─────────────── 1 (1–2)

Study number, Subject identity number:─────── (3–6)

Examining body ─────────────────── (7–9)

──────────────────────────────

Please tick in the appropriate box, or fill in as indicated.
Ignore the number coding which is for office use.

1.0 Permanent address:───────────────
                   No.   Street   (11–14)

   ─────────────────────────
       City   County/State   (16–19)

   ─────────────────────────
          Country   (20–25)

1.1 Country of birth: ───────────────

1.2 Date of birth:*────/─────────/19──── (27–31)
             Day   Month   Year

1.3 Date of examination*:────/───────/19──── (33–36)
                Day   Month   Year

1.4 Age:────/───────── (38)
      Years   Months

1.5 Sex: Male □ = 1; Female □ = 2 (40)

1.6 Marital status: Single □ = 1; Married □ = 2;
    Widowed, etc. □ = 3

1.7 Children (number):──── (42–43)

2.0 Occupation at present: ─────────── (45–47)

2.1 For how many years?────years (49–50)

2.2 Type of work?†
     sedentary   □ = 1
     light   □ = 2
     medium-light □ = 3
     medium-heavy □ = 4
     heavy   □ = 5   (52)

2.3 Time spent working?
     hours per day ────hours
     days per week ────days
     weeks per year────weeks   (54–57)
     total hours per year (approx.) = ────hours

* See Appendix A.
† See Appendix B.

2.4 Responsibilities of your work?

    nil   □ = 1
    low   □ = 2
    moderate   □ = 3
    high   □ = 4
    don't know □ = 0

(59)
(61–63)
(65–66)

3.0 Main occupation previously:_____

3.1 For how many years?_____years

3.2 Type of work?†

    sedentary   □ = 1
    light   □ = 2
    medium-light   □ = 3
    medium-heavy □ = 4
    heavy   □ = 5

(68)

3.3 Time spent in this work on average?

    hours per day _____hours
    days per week _____days
    weeks per year_____weeks
    total hours per year (approx.) = _____hours

(70–73)

3.4 Responsibilities in this work:

    nil   □ = 1
    low   □ = 2
    moderate   □ = 3
    high   □ = 4
    don't know □ = 0

(75)

B. ATHLETIC HISTORY

DATA CARD 2

Card serial number: _____

Study number, Subject identity number:_____

Examining body:_____

2 (1–2)
(3–6)
(7–9)

4.0 Do you take part in recreational physical activity* or sport?

    yes, daily   □ = 1
    yes, weekly   □ = 2
    yes, monthly   □ = 3
    yes, occasionally □ = 4
    no   □ = 5

(11)

4.1 If no, is this because of:

    lack of interest   □ = 1
    ill health   □ = 2
    injury   □ = 3
    lack of facilities □ = 4
    lack of leaders   □ = 5
    other, specify   □ = 6

(13)

† See Appendix B.
* Gardening and similar activities involving physical activity would qualify for inclusion here.

4.2 If yes, do you take part primarily?
      for pleasure   ☐ = 1
      to improve your health   ☐ = 2
      to improve your physical condition ☐ = 3   ☐ (15)
      to gain competitive success   ☐ = 4
      other, specify   ☐ = 5

4.3 Time spent in physical activity, on average?
      hours per day ———hours
      days per week ———days
      weeks per year———weeks   ☐☐☐☐ (17–20)
      total hours per year, approx. =———hours

4.4 How many whole days each year do you spend on sport?   ☐☐ (22–23)
      ———days

5.0   Are you a professional or an amateur competitive sportsman?
      full time professional   ☐ = 1
      part time professional ☐ = 2
      full time amateur   ☐ = 3   ☐ (25)
      part time amateur   ☐ = 4
      none of these   ☐ = 5   ☐☐☐ (27–29)

5.1 What is your best, i.e. main, sport?

5.2 What level of achievement have you attained in this sport?*
      international record holder   ☐ = 1
      national record holder   ☐ = 2
      member of a national team   ☐ = 3
      member of state or major district team   ☐ = 4
      member of a town or city team, etc.   ☐ = 5
      member of a school, club, or college team, etc. ☐ = 6   ☐ (31)
      other   ☐ = 7
      Give details:—————————————

5.3 At what age did you first:

      play the sport?———years   ☐☐ (33–34)

      compete in the sport?———years   ☐☐ (36–37)

      achieved your best performance?———years   ☐☐ (39–40)

5.4 What is your second best sport? ————————   ☐☐ (42–44)

5.5 What level of attainment have you attained in this sport?*
      international record holder   ☐ = 1
      national record holder   ☐ = 2
      member of a national team   ☐ = 3
      member of a state or major district team ☐ = 4
      member of a town or city team   ☐ = 5
      member of a school, club or college team ☐ = 6
      other, specify   ☐ = 7   ☐ (46)
      Give details:—————————————

* Only record the higher or highest achievement level. If these categories do not fit
exactly, try to indicate the most appropriate equivalent.

5.6 At what age did you first:

      play the sport?_____years   (48–49)

      compete in the sport?_____years   (51–52)

      achieve your best performance?_____years   (54–55)

5.7 How many times this year will you compete in any sport in organized competitions?_____   (57–59)

Section 2

THE MEDICAL EXAMINATION

Contents

Form **A.** Medical History   Form **C.** Laboratory Tests
Form **B.** Physical Examination

The Medical Examination Committee

J. Král (Chairman), Czechoslovakia   T. Ishiko, Japan
K. L. Andersen, Norway   E. Jokl, United States
T. Azuma, Japan   Y. Kuroda, Japan
B. Corrigan, Australia   L. Samek, Czechoslovakia
V. Ganeshan, Malaysia   H. Toyne, Australia
V. Hung, Vietnam   I. Zurita, Mexico
M. Ikai (late), Japan

The aims of this medical examination are

1. To determine the level of health of the individual insofar as this is measured by freedom from injury, ailment, abnormality, or disease.
2. To establish the somatological status that indicates the limits of permitted functional testing, in particular in the young.
3. To measure the basic physical and functional state of the individual prior to his participation in stressful physiological and general performance tests.

   The medical examination should be a prerequisite to the physiological and performance tests described in Sections 4 and 5. For persons over 40 years of age a complete examination is vital and a full ECG during activity should be considered of particular importance. When the examination has been completed, the physician should express his opinion unequivocally about whether the individual should or should not undertake strenuous physiological and other performance tests.

   If, after a long lay-off period, these physiological and other tests are to be repeated, the subject's medical history during the lay-off period should be examined. Any intervening illness should be considered as grounds for repeating the entire medical examination.

   The medical examination consists of three parts: Forms A and B, with the exception of item 43.0, should be considered mandatory. Form C, with the exception of item 44.0, which is vital, should be considered optional.

458

(To be filled in by subject)

Family name: ————————————————————————

First name, other initials: ———————————————————

For office use
DATA CARD 3

		3	(1–2)
			(3–6)
			(7–9)

Card serial number: ———————————————————

Study number, Subject identity number:————————————

Examining body:————————————————————

Please tick in the appropriate box, or fill in as indicated. Ignore the number coding which is for office use.

6.0 Do you feel healthy?   Yes = 1   No = 0   Not sure = 2   ☐ ☐ ☐   (11)
    If not, specify: ———————————————————

7.0 Sleep?———hours per day
    (———hours per week): not sure ☐ = 99   (12–13)

8.0 Smoke?   Yes = 1   No = 0   Occasionally = 2   ☐ ☐ ☐   (14)

    If yes:
8.1 At which age did you start?———years; stop?———years   (15–16)
    duration = ———years
8.2 Do you usually inhale?   Yes = 1   No = 2   ☐ ☐   (17)

8.3 Number per day?   cigarettes:———
              cigars: ———
              tobacco: ———g
              chewing: ———g
    Daily total in grams* =———g   (18–20)

9.0 Alcohol, etc.?   Yes = 1   No = 0   Occasionally = 2   ☐ ☐ ☐   (21)
    If yes:

9.1 Beer?   no, rarely   ☐ = 0
       up to 1 liter/day   ☐ = 1
       more than 1 liter/day   ☐ = 2
       not sure   ☐ = 3   (22)

9.2 Wine?   no, rarely   ☐ = 0
       up to ½ liter/day   ☐ = 1
       more than ½ liter/day   ☐ = 2
       not sure   ☐ = 3   (23)

* Assume 1 cigarette = 1 g tobacco, or 25 cigarettes = 28 g = 1 oz. of tobacco.

9.3	Spirits?	no, rarely	☐ = 0	
		up to 200 ml/day	☐ = 1	
		more than 200 ml/day	☐ = 2	☐ (24)
		not sure	☐ = 3	

9.4	Coffee plus tea?	none, negligible	☐ = 0	
		up to 3 cups/day	☐ = 1	
		over 3 cups/day	☐ = 2	☐ (25)
		not sure	☐ = 3	

Yes = 1   No = 0

10.0 Frequent medicaments or drugs? ☐   ☐   ☐ (26)
If yes, specify: _____

11.0 Pains?

	Yes = 1	No = 0	
joints, muscles, tendons	☐	☐	(27)
frequent headaches needing treatment	☐	☐	(28)
abdominal pains	☐	☐	(29)
lower back pains	☐	☐	(30)
difficulties in heart region	☐	☐	(31)
difficulties in breathing (asthma?)	☐	☐	(32)
other difficulties	☐	☐	(33)

If yes, specify: _____

12.0 Eyesight:

	Yes = 1	No = 0	
abnormal	☐	☐	(34)
wears glasses	☐	☐	(35)
wears contact lenses	☐	☐	(36)
color-blind	☐	☐	(37)
nightblindness	☐	☐	(38)

Yes = 1   No = 0

13.0 Hearing: abnormal ☐   ☐   (39)

14.0 Handedness: right handed = 1 ☐
left handed = 2 ☐   (40)
ambidextrous = 3 ☐

15.0 Diseases: past and present.

	Past			Present	
	Yes = 1	No = 0	Query = 2	Yes = 3	
Chickenpox	☐	☐	☐	☐	(41)
Measles	☐	☐	☐	☐	(42)
Diphtheria	☐	☐	☐	☐	(43)
Scarlet fever	☐	☐	☐	☐	(44)
Smallpox	☐	☐	☐	☐	(45)

460

| | Past ||| Present | |
	Yes = 1	No = 0	Query = 2	Yes = 3	
Whooping cough	☐	☐	☐	☐	(46)
Rachitis (rickets)	☐	☐	☐	☐	(47)
Typhoid fever	☐	☐	☐	☐	(48)
Meningitis/or encephalitis	☐	☐	☐	☐	(49)
Poliomyelitis	☐	☐	☐	☐	(50)
Pneumonia	☐	☐	☐	☐	(51)
Pleuritis	☐	☐	☐	☐	(52)
Hepatitis (jaundice)	☐	☐	☐	☐	(53)
Frequent common cold	☐	☐	☐	☐	(54)
Frequent sore throat	☐	☐	☐	☐	(55)
Frequent influenza	☐	☐	☐	☐	(56)
Frequent tonsillitis	☐	☐	☐	☐	(57)
Herpes simplex	☐	☐	☐	☐	(58)
Otitis	☐	☐	☐	☐	(59)
Tuberculosis	☐	☐	☐	☐	(60)
Bronchial asthma	☐	☐	☐	☐	(61)
Rheumatic fever	☐	☐	☐	☐	(62)
Rheumatoid arthritis	☐	☐	☐	☐	(63)
Heart disease	☐	☐	☐	☐	(64)
Hypertension	☐	☐	☐	☐	(65)
Nephritis or pyelitis	☐	☐	☐	☐	(66)
Infectious intestinal disease	☐	☐	☐	☐	(67)
Chronic intestinal disease	☐	☐	☐	☐	(68)
Diabetes	☐	☐	☐	☐	(69)
Allergic diseases	☐	☐	☐	☐	(70)

If yes, specify: ————————————————

Malaria	☐	☐	☐	☐	(71)
Helminthosis	☐	☐	☐	☐	(72)
Other parasitic or tropical diseases?	☐	☐	☐	☐	(73)

If yes, specify: ————————————————

	Past			Present
	Yes = 1	No = 0	Query = 2	Yes = 3
Syphilis	☐	☐	☐	☐	(74)
Gonorrhea	☐	☐	☐	☐	(75)
Heavy furunculosis	☐	☐	☐	☐	(76)
Other infectious communicable diseases?	☐	☐	☐	☐	(77)

If yes, specify: _____

Card serial number: _____

Study number, Subject identity number: _____

| 4 | (1–2) |

(3–6)

16.0 Major surgery? Yes = 1 ☐ No = 0 ☐   (11)
If yes, specify: _____

17.0 Major injuries? Yes = 1 ☐ No = 0 ☐   (12)

17.1 Type: _____ Date: _____ /_____
                                    month   year

Type: _____ Date: _____ /_____
                                    month   year

17.2 Were you left with permanent handicap? Yes = 1 ☐ No = 0 ☐   (13)
Specify: _____

18.0 Have you ever been unconscious for any reason?
Yes = 1 ☐ No = 0 ☐ Not sure = 2 ☐   (14)

19.0 Family history
Have any members of your family suffered from:

	Yes = 1	No = 0	Not sure = 2	
Hypertension	☐	☐	☐	(15)
Diabetes	☐	☐	☐	(16)
Coronary diseases (infectious, angina)	☐	☐	☐	(17)
Obesity	☐	☐	☐	(18)
Serious infectious diseases	☐	☐	☐	(19)

Give details: _____

Females Only

20.0   Menstruation started?   Yes = 1   No = 0   ☐   ☐

  20.1   Age at onset?_____years

  20.2   Duration?_____days

  20.3   Regular?   Yes = 1   No = 0   ☐   ☐

  20.4   Age at cessation?_____years   Not yet = 1   ☐

21.0   Pregnancies?

      If yes, number_____,   None = 0   ☐

  21.1   Deliveries?

      If yes, number_____,   None = 0   ☐

      Date of last delivery?_____/_____/19_____
                          day   month   year

  21.2   Miscarriages?

      If yes, number_____,   None = 0   ☐

22.0   Gynecological diseases and disorders?

      Past: Yes = 1   No = 0   ☐   ☐

      Present: ☐   ☐

      If yes, specify: _____

(20)

(21–22)

(23–24)

(25)

(26–27)

(28–29)

(30–31)

(32–35)

(36–37)

(38)

(39)

FORM B. PHYSICAL EXAMINATION
(To be completed by the physician)

Family name: _____

First name, other initials: _____

Card serial number: _____

Study number, Subject identity number:_____

Examining body:_____

DATA CARD 5

5   (1–2)

(3–6)

(7–9)

463

Date of examination*_____/_____/19_____
day   month   year

Examining physician: _____

Please tick in the appropriate box, or add comments as appropriate.

The coding system should be ignored when recording the results of the physical examination.

(11–15)

(16–18)

23.0   Height (without shoes):_____mm

(19–22)

24.0   Weight (nude, or assessed nude):_____tenths kg

(23–26)

Abnormal = 1   Normal = 0

25.0   Skull: ☐   ☐

(27)

If abnormal, specify: _____

(28–29)

Yes = 1   No = 0   Diagnosis

26.0   Abnormalities of the eyes?   ☐   ☐   _____

(30)

vision   ☐   ☐   _____

(31)

other abnormalities or diseases   ☐   ☐   _____

(32)

27.0   Abnormalities of ears?   ☐   ☐   _____

(33)

28.0   Abnormalities of nose?   ☐   ☐   _____

(34)

29.0   Abnormalities of skin?   ☐   ☐   _____

(35)

30.0   Mouth and throat:

30.1   Tonsils: normal   ☐ = 0
chronic tonsillitis   ☐ = 1
hypertrophy   ☐ = 2
tonsillectomy   ☐ = 3

(36)

30.2   Teeth: healthy   ☐ = 0
decaying, treated   ☐ = 1
decaying, untreated   ☐ = 2
prosthesis   ☐ = 3

(37)

Abnormal = 1   Normal = 0

30.3   Mouth, tongue and gum: ☐   ☐

(38)

If abnormal, diagnosis: _____

31.0   Neck:

Yes = 1   No = 0

31.1   Lymphadenopathy: ☐   ☐

(39)

If yes, describe: _____

Abnormal = 1   Normal = 0

31.2   Thyroid: ☐   ☐

(40)

If abnormal, specify:

Abnormal = 1   Normal = 0

32.0   Chest: ☐   ☐

(41)

If deformities, specify: _____

* See Appendix A.

464

33.0 Respiratory system: Abnormal = 1 Normal = 0
☐ ☐
If abnormal, description/diagnosis: _____
☐ (42)

34.0 Cardiovascular system:

34.1 Palpation*: Apical impulse: normal ☐ = 0
forceful ☐ = 1
not felt ☐ = 2
☐ (43)
☐ (44)

34.2 Thrills:* Yes = 1 No = 0
☐ ☐
If present, location and type: _____

34.3 Auscultation:*
Heart sounds: Abnormal = 1 Normal = 0
☐ ☐
If abnormal, or accentuation, describe: _____
☐ (45)

34.4 Murmurs:*
Systolic: Yes = 1 No = 0
☐ ☐
☐ (46)

Diastolic: ☐ ☐
☐ (47)
If yes, state types, site of maximum intensity, and whether considered as innocent or significant. Add report of cardiologist when possible and if needed.
_____

34.5 Pulse rate (supine, 5 min rest):_____/min
(48–50)
Rhythm: Irregular = 1 Regular = 0
☐ ☐
(51)
If irregular:
Respiratory arrhythmia: Yes = 1 No = 0
☐ ☐
(52)
Premature beats: ☐ ☐
(53)
Atrial fibrillation: ☐ ☐
(54)
Specify other changes: _____

34.6 Blood pressure, (supine, 5 min rest)*
Systolic:_____mm Hg
(55–57)
Diastolic IV (muffling):_____mm Hg
(58–60)
Diastolic V (disappearance):_____mm Hg
(61–63)
34.7 Diagnosis of heart findings: Abnormal = 1 Normal = 0
☐ ☐
(64)
Specify:_____

35.0 Abdomen, liver and spleen: Abnormal = 1 Normal = 0
☐ ☐
If abnormal, description or diagnosis:_____
☐ (65)

* See Appendix D.

	Yes = 1 No = 0	
36.0	Hernia: ☐ ☐	☐ (66)
	If present, describe: _____	

	Yes = 1 No = 0	
37.0	Hemorrhoid: ☐ ☐	☐ (67)

38.0 Spine:
- normal ☐ = 0
- round back ☐ = 1
- exaggerated lumbar lordosis ☐ = 2
- straight back ☐ = 3
- scoliosis ☐ = 4
- other ☐ = 5

☐ (68)

Specify: _____

	Abnormal = 1 Normal = 0	
39.0 Upper extremity:	☐ ☐	☐ (69)

If abnormal, description or diagnosis: _____

	Abnormal = 1 Normal = 0	
40.0 Lower extremity:	☐ ☐	☐ (70)

If abnormal, description or diagnosis: _____

40.1 Pulse on posterior tibial artery?

Right = 1 Left = 2 Both = 3 Neither = 0
☐ ☐ ☐ ☐

☐ (71)

40.2 Pulse on dorsalis pedis?

Right = 1 Left = 2 Both = 3 Neither = 0
☐ ☐ ☐ ☐

☐ (72)

Yes = 1 No = 0
40.3 Varicose veins: ☐ ☐

☐ (73)

If yes, sketch or describe _____

	Yes = 1 No = 0	
40.4 Interdigital epidermophytosis:	☐ ☐	☐ (74)

	Abnormal = 1 Normal = 0	
41.0 Nervous system:	☐ ☐	☐ (75)

If abnormal, describe: _____

	Abnormal = 1 Appears Normal = 0	
42.0 Mental state:	☐ ☐	☐ (76)

If abnormal, describe: _____

	Abnormal = 1 Normal = 0	
43.0 Reproductive system:	☐ ☐	☐ (77)

No = 1 Yes = 0
43.1 Boys: both testicles in scrotum: ☐ ☐

☐ (78)

43.2 Girls: primary and secondary sexual development:

Abnormal = 1 Normal = 0
☐ ☐

☐ (79)

Yes = 1 No = 0
43.3 Hermaphroditism? ☐ ☐

☐ (80)

FORM C. LABORATORY DATA

Card serial number: _____

Study number, Subject identity number: _____

Examining body: _____

		6	(1–2)

(3–6)

(7–9)

44.0 Urinalysis:

44.1 Protein: Yes = 1 ☐ No = 0 ☐
If present, microscopic examination: _____

☐ (11)

44.2 Sugar: Yes = 1 ☐ No = 0 ☐

(12)

(13–16)

(17–20)

45.0 Vital capacity: _____ml (BTPS)

46.0 Forced expiratory volume (1.0 sec) _____ml (BTPS)

47.0 Blood:

47.1 Hemoglobin: _____g% (Method = _____)

(21–22)

47.2 Cholesterol: _____mg% (Method = _____)

(23–25)

47.3 Sedimentation rate: _____mm/hr (Method = _____)

(26–27)

_____mm/2hr (Method = _____)

(28–30)

(31)

47.4 Other determinations: State kind and values: _____

48.0 Electrocardiogram: Abnormal = 1 ☐ Normal = 0 ☐
If abnormal, describe: _____

☐ (32)

49.0 ECG at rest:

Frequency: _____/min
P–Q _____
QRS _____
S–T _____
Findings _____

(33–35)

50.0 ECG during or after exercise: Specify: _____

Frequency: _____/min
P–Q _____
QRS _____
S–T _____
Findings _____

(36–38)

467

51.0   Other laboratory examinations?
Yes = 1   No = 0
□   □

(39)

(40–43)

(44–47)

(48–51)

52.0   Fitness for undertaking physiological and physical performance tests.
(a) May participate freely in all tests: _____
(b) May not participate in the following tests:

_____

(c) May not participate in any stress testing: _____

Signed: _____
(Physician)
Date: _____/_____/19_____

Section 3

PHYSIOLOGICAL MEASUREMENTS AND INDICES

Contents

The Committee

M. Ikai (Chairman), Japan
K. L. Andersen (Chairman), Norway
E. Karvinen (Chairman), Finland
D. Aldubi, Israel
K. Asahina, Japan
D. A. Bailey, Canada
B. Balke, United States
C. C. Bartoleme, Philippines
C. Chintanaseri, Thailand
N. Hanne, Israel

O. Ketusinh, Thailand
B. J. Macnab, Canada
R. Margaria, Italy
Z. Mellorowicz, Germany
L. Morehouse, United States
J. Prie, Israel
L. Samek, Czechoslovakia
G. Schönholzer, Switzerland
E. Schvartz, Israel
C. Wyndham, South Africa

A. General Considerations

53.0. *The Capacity to Perform Maximum Work*

Underlying all physiological tests of physical fitness is the view that the capacity to perform maximum physical work depends upon three basic factors:

1. *Anaerobic power*, also known as maximum oxygen debt capacity, which determines the amount of work possible in an all out effort for a period of approximately 45 sec, through anaerobic release mechanisms.
2. *Aerobic power*, also known as maximum oxygen intake, which determines the amount of work possible for a period of approximately 15–30 min through optimally coordinated circulatory and respiratory adjustments resulting in the maximum delivery of oxygen to active tissue.
3. *Metabolic capacity*, which determines the amount of work possible for a period of approximately 2–3 hr through the amount of energy-yielding substrates maximally available from body stores under conditions of maximum aerobic demands.

53.1. Although the assessment of total work capacity as an index of " physical fitness " requires the measurement of each one of these three factors, one can obtain sufficient and valid information about fitness by determining aerobic power, that is, maximum oxygen intake, alone.

This information is sufficiently valid, moreover, even though the effects of training can increase working capacity somewhat more than might be assumed from measured concomitant changes in aerobic power. It is, of course, not valid if attention is not directed adequately at the problems of ensuring comparable levels of motivation, skills and strategies, and techniques of working.

Although aerobic power is primarily dependent upon the cardiorespiratory function of man, it is also dependent (1) upon the duration and nature of the task, (2) on the mass of muscles involved, (3) on intrinsic individual factors such as physical fatigue, extra demands on temperature regulation and so on, and (4) on intrinsic environmental conditions such as climate, altitude, and so on. However, if test procedures are carefully followed, test-retest values are of the same magnitude and are comparable from one laboratory to another. For comparison of data, the test conditions and procedures should be carefully indicated.

54.0. *The Test Laboratories*

Physiological tests of physical fitness are performed at three general locations that impose clear constraints upon the nature of the tests that can be conducted. These locations may be defined as (1) the base laboratory, (2) the mobile laboratory, and (3) the field.

54.1. The Base Laboratory. This is equipped for experimental studies of a complex and precise nature in which one or a very small number of subjects are thoroughly investigated. The work of the base laboratory is usually directed toward the determination of physiological mechanisms underlying physical performance and adaptation to exercise and of the exact effects of environmental factors.

54.2. The Mobile Laboratory. This consists of a selection of instruments installed in a vehicle that can be moved to remote areas. The tests conducted in a mobile laboratory are usually less complex and better adapted to comparative population studies than those in the base laboratory.

54.3. The Field Laboratory. This employs simplified methods and instruments to facilitate the investigation of large numbers of subjects in fairly remote areas. Accuracy of observations and reliability of measuring devices are assumed. The standardized test procedures will permit comparisons to be made with data obtained in mobile or base laboratories.

Field laboratory tests may be useful in school classrooms, training camps, or other mass situations to aid in teaching and evaluation of educational and special training programs.

55.0. *Environmental Conditions*

Environmental conditions during physiological fitness testing should be recorded because they might influence the physiological functions under study. The following standard measurements of the environment are recommended: barometric pressure, dry bulb temperature, wet bulb temperature, black globe temperature, and wind velocity. Additionally, the hour of the day and physical location (laboratory, indoors, outdoors, and so on) should be noted.

56.0. *Standardization of Tests*

The standardization of physical fitness tests for the assessment of aerobic power is guided by the following principles:

56.1. All test procedures should permit the direct measurement, or the indirect estimation, of maximum oxygen intake (aerobic power) as the most meaningful physiological criterion of physical fitness.

This criterion will be expressed as the maximum $\dot{V}_{O_2}$ in milliliters per kilogram of body weight per minute (ml/kg·min).

56.2. The test procedures basically should be the same for investigations in the laboratory as in the field, with the following specifications:

1. Under laboratory conditions, the aerobic power is to be *directly* assessed through the use of sufficiently sophisticated instrumentation and measurements.

2. In the field, aerobic capacity is to be indirectly assessed from restricted physiological measurements.

56.3. All test procedures should yield comparable results.

56.4. The test procedures should all be capable of administration within a single day, preferably in a continuous session. This is to ensure that the testing and retesting of large population groups can be conducted efficiently with regard to time, facilities, and effort.

56.5. The test procedures should be sufficiently flexible to permit testing populations with great differences in physical fitness, age, sex, habitual activity levels, and so on.

57.0. *The Choice of Apparatus*

The principles of physiological fitness testing outlined above are observed first by the choice of the following items of apparatus:

1. Motor-driven treadmill.
2. Bicycle ergometer.
3. Stepping ergometer.
4. Ancillary equipment, as required, which may be common to all.

57.1. The Motor-Driven Treadmill. This is one of the most versatile but also most expensive instruments. Even the smallest version is sufficiently bulky to prevent its extensive use in the field. It should allow for variations of speed, from 3 to *at least* 8 km/hr (2–5 mph), and of grade, from 0 to 30%. The treadmill "grade" is defined as the vertical rise in percent of the horizontal distance travelled. Distance and vertical rise should be indicated in meters, and speed in meters per second (m/sec) or kilometers per hour (km/hr).

57.2. The Bicycle Ergometer. This is the most adaptable of the three instruments to laboratory and field conditions and is sufficiently versatile to provide an adequate number of different work intensities from minimum to maximum range.

Bicycle ergometers are constructed either with mechanical or with electrical braking systems, the latter activated either from an outside electrical power source or from an electrical current produced from an ergometer-driven generator.

The adjustable mechanical resistance is calibrated in kilogram-meters per minute (kgm/min) or in watts. The conversion of kilogram-meters per minute into watts follows the formula: 1 watt = 6 kgm/min.

The bicycle must have an adjustable seat. For ensuring optimum efficiency, the height of the seat should be adjusted individually to allow for an almost completely stretched leg at the lowest pedal position. On average the seat to pedal length at full stretch should be 109% of leg length.

There are a variety of different bicycle ergometers available. However, the type of ergometer used will not affect results *as long as* the indicated loads, either in watts or kilogram-meters per minute truly represent the total external load.

57.3. The Stepping Ergometer. This is a relatively inexpensive machine with stepping heights adjustable from 0 to 50 cm. It is similar to the bicycle ergometer in its flexibility for use in field and laboratory situations.

57.4. The Three Methods Compared. Each device has advantages and disadvantages in laboratory or field use. Generally, work on the treadmill results in slightly greater maximum V_{O_2} than work on the bicycle ergometer, and the latter provides slightly higher values than the step test.

In work against gravity, the basal as well as working metabolic rates are directly proportional to body weight. Therefore, treadmill and stepping exercises provide the same relative workloads for all individuals at any given vertical lift, that is, on the treadmill for any given speed and slope, on the stepping ergometer for any given stepping frequency and height.

On the other hand, the bicycle ergometer, regardless of sex and age, requires nearly identical energy expenditures for given settings of work intensity.

58.0. *General Remarks about Test Procedures*

The practical application of tests for screening large populations favors simple and short testing procedures. Physiological considerations, however, point to more elaborate and more time-consuming tests. For greatest versatility and utility, therefore, these two conflicting requirements must be optimized.

58.1. Work Intensity. The test must begin with a workload low enough to be sufficiently submaximal for people in very poor physical condition. The adaptive capacity of the cardiovascular and respiratory systems must be evaluated through continuous work at gradually increasing intensities. Thus, the approach of functional limitations should be detectable with sufficient discriminatory accuracy. Practical considerations suggest the use of the basal, or resting, metabolic rate as the unit by which to gauge the energy demands at the various workloads. The initial work intensity and the following stepwise increments will therefore be defined in " Mets," multiples of the metabolic rate at complete rest. The physiological units basic to Mets are either the resting oxygen consumptions in milliliters per minute or their caloric equivalents in kilocalories per minute.

Since direct control of work intensity by Mets or by their oxygen consumption equivalents during a test would require the display of continuous computation of oxygen consumption by complex instrumentation not readily available at present, the estimation of the oxygen requirements for given types and intensities of work from empirical formulae appears most practical. The predicted values of oxygen requirements for treadmill work from speed and slope, and for step-test work from stepping height and rate are in close agreement with the values actually measured and can serve as the physiological equivalent of the physical effort to which all physiological indices measured during the test are correlated.

58.2. Test Duration. For adequate test design, the desire for the shortest possible test procedure poses a problem. Tests of too-short duration wil¹ be lacking in sufficiently discriminatory values, whereas tests of too-long duration will activate thermoregulatory mechanisms that will interfere with the assessment of maximum aerobic power. In the standard procedure recommended, each work intensity level will be maintained for 2 min. The average time of the actual test might then range from about 10 to 16 min.

58.3. Indications for Stopping Exercise. The test should be terminated whenever

1. Pulse pressure declines consistently in spite of increasing work intensity.
2. Systolic blood pressure exceeds 240–250 mm Hg.
3. Diastolic pressure rises to more than 125 mm Hg.
4. Symptoms of distress occur such as increasing chest pain, severe dyspnea, intermittent claudication.
5. Clinical signs of anoxia occur such as facial pallor or cyanosis, staggering, confusion, or unresponsiveness to injuries.
6. The following ECG signs occur—paroxysmal superventricular or ventricular dysrhythmia, a succession of ventricular premature complexes occurring before the end of the T wave, conduction disturbances other than a slight AV block, and R-ST depressions of horizontal or descending type of greater than 0.3 mv.

58.4. Safety Procedures.

58.41. Subject's Health. The subjects should be in a normal state of health as certified by a physician after medical examination. Monitoring the ECG by at least one chest lead is highly desirable in all subjects, but should be compulsory in males beyond the age of 40 years. Regularly repeated blood pressure measurements during the exercise test are a mandatory part of the testing procedure. After termination of the exercise test, the subjects have to be informed about measures preventing dangerous blood pooling in the lower limbs.

58.42. Contraindications to Exercise Tests. Subjects should be rejected from the test on the following criteria:

1. Lack of a physician's permission to take part in maximal exercise testing.
2. Oral temperature in excess of 37.5°C.
3. Heart rate above 100 beats/min at the end of a sufficient rest period.
4. Manifest cardiac failure.
5. Myocardial infarction or myocarditis within the past 3 months, or symptoms and ECG signs showing these conditions, or existing angina pectoris.
6. Evidence of an infectious disease including the common cold.

Menstruation is not considered a contraindication for exercise testing, but in special cases rescheduling the test may be advisable.

B. The Standard Tests

59.0. *Description of the Basic Procedures for the Standard Tests*

Whichever of the three modes of exercise is adopted, and notwithstanding whether a submaximal or maximal test is intended, the basic procedures for the three standard tests are the same.

The subjects report to the laboratory in light gym clothing and rubber-soled shoes, having abstained from food, coffee, tobacco, and so on, for at least 2 hr.

59.1. Rest. A preliminary period of at least 15 min of rest must precede the exercise test. During this period the subject sits comfortably in a chair while physiological baseline measurements are established.

59.2. Accommodation Period. The very first test of any individual as well as all subsequent repeats become sufficiently reliable if the actual test is preceded by a short period of exercise at a low work intensity. This accommodation period, 3 min duration is enough, serves:

1. To familiarize the subject with the equipment and with the type of work required.
2. To pretest the subject's physiological response to a workload of approximately 4 Mets, or an initial heart rate response of approximately 100 beats/min.
3. To hasten the proper physiological adjustments to the actual test work.

59.3. Rest. The accommodation period is followed by 2 min of comfortable rest in a chair while the necessary technical adjustments are effected.

59.4. Test. The test begins with the work intensity employed in the accommodation period, (approximately 4 Mets), and the subject continues to exercise without interruption until the test is completed. At the end of every second minute of work, the workload is increased by the equivalent of approximately 1 Met.

The test stops when any of the three following conditions exist.

1. The subject is unable to proceed.
2. The monitoring of physiological criteria indicates physiological decompensations (see paragraph 58.3).
3. The advanced state of effort permits an extrapolation of maximum aerobic power on the basis of sequential physiological measurements.

59.5. Scoring. Maximum oxygen intake in milliliters per kilogram per minute is determined directly or is assessed. The methods for its determination vary as do the supplementary techniques used to analyze the individual's physiological capacities. These points are pursued more fully in due course.

59.6. Recovery. After the cessation of the test exercise, physiological observations are continued for at least 3 min, with the subject again resting in a chair, preferably with legs slightly raised.

Note: The above basic procedure should provide comparable physiological responses to workloads of the same order of magnitude on the treadmill, bicycle, or stepping ergometer. In the following paragraphs the procedure is specifically outlined for each of the testing devices.

60.0. *The Treadmill Test*

60.1. Apparatus. Motor-driven treadmill and ancillary equipment as required.

60.2. Description. The basic test procedure outlined in paragraph 59.0 is followed carefully.

The speed of the treadmill, with the subject walking on it, is set to 80 m/min (4.8 km/hr or 3 mph). At this speed the energy requirements for walking on the horizontal amount to approximately 3 Mets, and each increment of 2.5% in slope adds one unit of the resting metabolic rate, that is, 1 Met, to the energy expenditure.

At the end of the first 2 min the treadmill slope is quickly increased to 5%, after the next 2 min to 7.5%, then to 10%, 12.5%, and so on. The entire scheme is presented in Table VII-I.

Table VII-1 Standard Treadmill Test

Test Phase	Duration min	Energy Mets	Requirements $\dot{V}_{O_2}$, ml/kg·min	Percent grade at 80 m/min
Rest	10–20	1	3.5	—
Accommodation period	3	4	14.0	2.5
Recovery	2	1	3.5	—
Actual test	2	4	14.0	2.5
	2	5	17.5	5.0
	2	6	21.0	7.5
	2	7	24.5	10.0
	2	8	28.0	12.5
	2	9	31.5	15.0
	2	10	35.0	17.5
	2	11	38.5	20.0
	2	12	42.0	22.5
	2	13	45.5	25.0
	2	14	49.0	27.5
	2	15	52.5	30.0

Note: The fitness rating of the subject rises as he demonstrates his capacity for handling the increasing demands for oxygen. The range shown here is from very poor at $\dot{V}_{O_2} = 14$ ml/kg·min to very good at 52.5 ml/kg·min.

60.3. Scoring. The test score is stated as the maximum $\dot{V}_{O_2}$ in ml/kg·min. It is either measured directly by monitoring the respiratory gas exchanges or estimated by extrapolating the test results. See Table VII-1.

60.4. General Guide and Regulations.

60.41. For the accommodation period, the treadmill inclination is set at 2.5%. The same grade and speed are maintained during the first 2 min of the actual test—unless the physiological response during the accommodation period is indicative of a superior performance potential. In such case the energy requirements at the speed of 80 m/min and a 30% grade (assumed limitation for raising the treadmill grade) would not approach the individual's capacity and the test should be modified accordingly (see Table VII-3).

60.42. In case of existing pathological conditions (coronary heart disease, pulmonary deficiency, convalescence after infectious diseases, and so on) a treadmill test modification as presented in Table VII-2 is recommended.

60.43. In a test employing walking or running on the motor-driven treadmill, any continuous contact of arms or hands with a fixed object (guard post or rails) is prohibited.

61.0. *The Bicycle Ergometer Test*

61.1. Apparatus. Bicycle ergometer, with calibrated load adjustment facilities and ancillary equipment, as required.

61.2. Description. The basic procedure outlined in paragraph 59.0 is carefully followed. During the test the subject pedals at a predetermined steady rate of 50 or 60 rpm without interruption in time with a metronome.

Table VII-2 Substandard Treadmill Test
(For testing pathological cardiorespiratory fitness)

Test Phase	Duration min	Energy, Mets	Requirements $\dot{V}_{O_2}$, ml/kg·min	Percent Grade at 53.5 m/min
Rest	10–20	1	3.5	—
Accommodation period	3	2	7.0	0
Recovery	2	1	3.5	—
Actual test	2	2	7.0	0
	2	2.66	9.3	2.5
	2	3.33	11.7	5.0
	2	4	14.0	7.5
	2	4.66	16.3	10.0
	2	5.33	18.7	12.5
	2	6	21.0	15.0
	2	6.66	23.3	17.5
	2	7.33	25.7	20.0
	2	8	28.0	22.5

Table VII-3 Superstandard Treadmill Test

Test Phase	Duration, min	Energy, Mets	Requirement $\dot{V}_{O_2}$, ml/kg·min	Percent Grade at 100 m/min
Rest	10	1	3.5	—
Accommodation period	3	6	21.0	4
Recovery	2	1	3.5	—
Actual test	1	6	21.0	4
	1	7	24.5	6
	1	8	28.0	8
	1	9	31.5	10
	1	10	35.0	12
	1	11	38.5	14
	1	12	42.0	16
	1	13	45.5	18
	2	14	49.0	20
	2	15	52.5	22
	2	16	56.0	24
	2	17	59.5	26
	2	18	63.0	28
	2	19	66.5	30

The intensity of the workload is increased at 2-min intervals as previously indicated. In order to provide on the bicycle ergometer relative workloads comparable to those on the treadmill or stepping ergometer, the body weight should be used for determining both the initial work intensity and the periodic increments of workload, as follows:

1. Set the initial load to 1 watt (6 kgm) per kilogram of body weight.
2. Set the increments at one third of the body weight in kilograms.

Example Subject A = 75 kg; B = 50 kg; C = 25 kg.

Subject	Weight, kg	Increments, watts	Initial Load, watts	2nd	3rd	4th	
A	75	25	75	100	125	150	...
B	50	17	50	67	84	101	...
C	25	8	25	33	41	50	...

61.3. Scoring. The oxygen costs for any given intensity of work can be determined by use of the following formula:

$$\dot{V}_{O_2} = (kgm \times 1.78) + 1.5 \text{ Mets}$$

where: $\dot{V}_{O_2}$ = oxygen requirement in ml/min.
kgm (or watts × 6) = work intensity/min.
1.78 = ml of oxygen required for 1 kgm of work.

1.5 Mets = the approximate oxygen consumption of the individual sitting on the ergometer and pedaling without any load. With increasing resistance more auxiliary muscles are involved, resulting in a rise of this factor to slightly more than 2 Mets at Watt = 1800 kgm/min.

61.4. General Guide and Regulations. *61.41.* Since total oxygen requirements are nearly identical for all individuals working at any given load on the bicycle ergometer, the $\dot{V}_{O_2}$ in milliliters per kilogram per minute varies considerably in subjects of different weights. In contrast, in work against gravity, treadmill grade walking, and bench stepping, the $\dot{V}_{O_2}$ requirement per unit of weight are the same but total $\dot{V}_{O_2}$ varies with total weight. The existing interrelationships between workload, total oxygen requirement, $\dot{V}_{O_2}$ per kilogram and Mets is illustrated in Figure VII-1 for individuals with body weights of 50, 60, 70, and 80 kg, respectively.

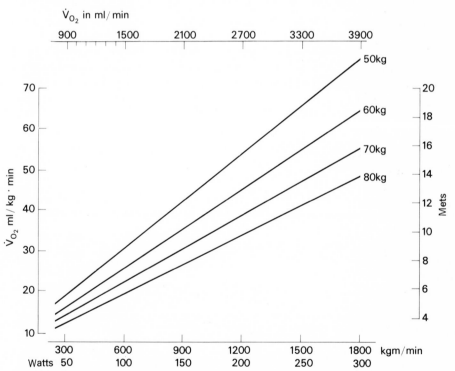

Figure VII-1. Bicycle ergometer. Oxygen requirements (total and per kilogram of body weight) and energy expenditures in Mets (multiples of the resting metabolic rate) for individuals of different body weight, at a wide range of work intensities on the bicycle ergometer.

61.42. The constancy of the pedaling rate should be monitored by a speed indicator, a revolution counter, or by means of a metronome.

61.43. The energy costs of riding the stationary bicycle are well established, provided that the indicated external load is not markedly offset by undue resistances in the pedal bearings and in the drive chain. Every effort, therefore, should be made to keep these moving parts running freely.

61.44. The height of the seat should be adjusted individually to allow for an almost completely stretched leg at the lowest pedal position.

61.45. In case of existing pathological conditions (see paragraph 58.42) the initial settings should be 25 watts or 150 kgm/min. The increments after 2 min at each load should be 12.5 watts or 75 kgm/min.

61.46. For highly trained athletes the standard procedure is applicable with only the modification that, as in the superstandard treadmill test, the first ten increments of work intensity be done in 1-min intervals to reduce total duration of the test. Beyond a load of 275 watts, or 1650 kgm/min, 2-min intervals are used.

61.47. Modifications with regard to body position, such as working in a supine instead of the normal sitting position or cranking instead of bicycling, might be feasible in special situations. However, since efficiency for these types of work is different, the "normal" kilogram-meter per minute oxygen requirement relationship does not apply and the investigators should state precisely the type of modification utilized.

62.0. *The Ergometer Step Test*

62.1. Apparatus. Adjustable height stepping ergometer, multiples of 4.5 cm, and ancillary equipment as selected.

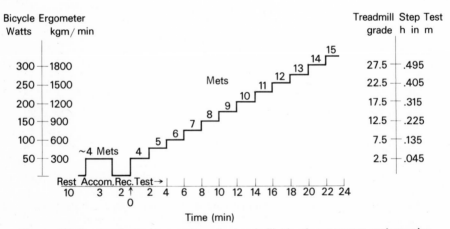

Figure VII-2. Standard test procedures for treadmill, bicycle ergometer, and stepping ergometer.

62.2. Description. The subject, having undertaken the standard rest and warm-up procedure, steps onto and down from the stepping ergometer at the standard rate of 33 mounts/min. This rate, although slightly faster than comfortable, is chosen to keep the stepping heights within tolerable limits at the higher workloads. The initial platform height is 4.5 cm. Each 2 min the height of the ergometer is raised 4.5 cm, as indicated in Figure VII-2 without interruption of the stepping rate. This procedure will permit the steady increase of the workload from very mild to most severe, that is, over an energy expenditure range from 2 to 15 Mets.

62.3. Scoring. The oxygen requirements ($\dot{V}_{O_2}$) in milliliters per kilogram per minute for stepping at the frequency of 33 vertical lifts per minute can be predicted or estimated from the following formula:

$$\dot{V}_{O_2} = (f \times h \times 1.33 \times 1.78) + 10.5$$

where: f = the stepping rate of number of vertical lifts per minute.

h = the height of the step in meters.

1.33 = work involved in the vertical lift plus one third for descending.

10.5 = 10.5 ml/kg·min extra oxygen requirement for the forward and backward stepping additional to the vertical movement.

1.78 = ml of oxygen required for 1 kgm of work.

62.4. General Guide and Regulations. *62.41.* The energy costs in stepping are made up of the following components:

1. Stepping forward and backward on two counts each. At the proposed metronome setting of 132 total counts (132/4 = 33 actual lifts), the energy expenditure for this work is approximately 3 Mets.
2. Lifting the weight of the body to the height of the step level.
3. Descending to the ground. The latter work has been found to be approximately one third of the work of stepping up.

62.42. In Figure VII-2 the stepping ergometer procedure is designed so as to be comparable with the treadmill and bicycle ergometer tests.

62.43. Four counts are taken to complete each up and down stepping cycle: two counts to mount to a completely erect stance on both feet, and two counts to descend to the ground. Frequent changes of the leading leg are encouraged to minimize the development of local muscular fatigue. This can best be accomplished by tapping the descending foot on the floor on the fourth count and immediately lifting it again for the count "one" step-up. With a little practice, especially by establishing a given rhythm, for example, four mounts leading with the left foot and then four with the right, the procedure, which does not require any special skill, quickly becomes automatic.

62.44. As with the treadmill and bicycle ergometer, a great variation of speed (stepping rate) is available. The standard rate of 33 vertical lifts per minute is selected specifically for use with a stepping device like the one described, which has an adjustable vertical range from 0 to 50 cm, to accommodate approximately 90% of any given population.

Holding on to any fixed object during the stepping exercise alters the test results.

62.45. When testing individuals in pathological conditions (see paragraphs 60.42 and 61.45), the following modification will provide nearly the same test loads as the substandard treadmill test:

1. $f = 22$ vertical lifts per minute.
2. Accommodation period and first test load at zero level.
3. All increments at 15 mm as in the standard stepping test.

In this case the formula for predicting or estimating $\dot{V}_{O_2}$ is

$$\dot{V}_{O_2} = (22 \times 1.33 \times 1.7 \times h) + 7 \qquad \text{(see paragraph 62.3)}$$

where h = stepping height in meters; and $7 = 7$ ml/kg·min oxygen required for stepping forward and backward at the rate of $22 \times 4 = 88$ total steps.

C. Measurement Procedures

63.0 *Direct and Indirect Physical Fitness Testing*

The basic procedure for testing maximum aerobic power on the treadmill, bicycle ergometer, or stepping ergometer has been proposed with the idea (1) that it can be applied in the laboratory as well as in the field without modifications and (2) that the test devices should be interchangeable. Differences between direct and indirect assessments of maximum aerobic power only exist because of the complexity of physiological parameters that can be monitored to measure it.

Direct Methods for Measuring Maximum Aerobic Power. It was stated at the beginning of this section that the capacity for maximum aerobic work is related to the capacity of the cardiovascular-respiratory systems to deliver oxygen to the active tissue. Any direct assessment of the maximum aerobic power should, therefore, encompass methods that measure:

1. The capacity of the heart to pump blood through the vascular bed, that is, the maximum cardiac output and its two components—heart rate and stroke volume.
2. The capacity of the respiratory system, including the respiratory processes involved in the gas exchange in the lungs as well as at the tissue level.
3. Actual metabolic processes, that is, the utilization of carbohydrates and fatty acids as energy sources.

4. Properties of the blood essential for gas and foodstuff transport, for the buffering of acid metabolites, for heat transfer, and for temperature regulation.

The relationship between oxygen intake ($\dot{V}_{O_2}$) and cardiac function on one hand, and $\dot{V}_{O_2}$ and respiratory functions on the other hand is expressed by equations (VII-1) and (VII-2)

$$\dot{V}_{O_2} = f_H \times V_s \times (a - V)_{O_2} \qquad\qquad \text{(VII-1)}$$

$$\dot{V}_{O_2} = \dot{V}_E \times (F_{I_{O_2}} - F_{E_{O_2}}) \qquad\qquad \text{(VII-2)}$$

where: $\dot{V}_{O_2}$ = the oxygen intake in ml/min.
f_H = heart rate.
V_s = stroke volume of the heart.
$(a - V)_{O_2}$ = difference of oxygen content between arterial and mixed-venous blood.
$\dot{V}_E$ = pulmonary ventilation (STPD) per minute.
$F_{I_{O_2}}, F_{E_{O_2}}$ = fraction of oxygen in inspired, expired air.

The extent to which the factors that limit maximum aerobic power, such as have been indicated above, are to be studied is left to the discretion of the investigator. Nevertheless a few basic measurements are considered standard requirements for the direct testing of maximum aerobic power. These standards are set out in the following paragraphs.

63.1. Respiratory Function. Since the maximum oxygen intake capacity is considered *the* physiological criterion of "physical fitness," the determination of the respiratory gas exchange at several intervals during the progressive work capacity test is mandatory.

The methods to be used for the determination of the respiratory gas exchange are also left to the discretion of the investigator and depend on the equipment available. Many variations are possible and admissible between (1) the simplest foolproof procedure of collecting expired air in suitable bags for analysis by either chemical or electronic methods in conjunction with volumetric measurement and (2) the most sophisticated continuous electronic determination of all components involved with an automatic computation of the finally desired information. Usually, the analytic labor involved in any of the testing procedures used will determine the number of tests possible within a single day. Considering the limitations of time one encounters, for instance, with the gas analysis according to Haldane, only a limited number of expired air collections are feasible during one test. In such cases it is recommended that these air collections be made not at each level of the stepwise increased work intensities but only at two or three submaximal and three maximal levels; for instance, whenever the heart rate is at 120, 140, and 150–160 beats/min and then three times more at peak loads. It is not feasible to define given heart rates at which these last three collections would have to be made because in different groups of populations maximal heart rates may range from 140 to 200 and more beats per minute.

The continuous monitoring of the respiratory exchange ratio (RER) with a nitrogen meter can facilitate the discovery of the phase at which the aerobic delivery of oxygen begins to become inadequate. By no means, however, is this point a definite indication for the attainment of maximum oxygen consumption.

Respiratory parameters of interest, in addition to the maximum oxygen intake capacity, are

1. The RER at the time of peak oxygen intake.
2. The maximum pulmonary ventilation and its breakdown in respiratory frequency and tidal volumes.
3. The relationship between the maximum $\dot{V}$ during work and the MVV (maximum voluntary ventilation).
4. The ventilation equivalent for oxygen = max $\dot{V}$/max $\dot{V}_{O_2}$.
5. The utilization of the respired oxygen = $F_{I_{O_2}} - F_{E_{O_2}}$.

The Criteria for Attainment of Maximum $\dot{V}_{O_2}$

1. The oxygen consumption ceases to increase linearly with rising work-loads and approaches a plateau, the last two values of $\dot{V}_{O_2}$ agreeing within $\pm 5\%$.
2. In testing maximum aerobic power in "normal" individuals blood lactate concentrations of 90–100 mg/100 ml of blood can be expected 3–5 min after termination of the test.
3. Other respiratory measurements may be used to provide knowledge about an individual's physiological capacities, for example, the diffusing capacity of the lungs for oxygen, carbon monoxide, or carbon dioxide; residual volume and pulmonary nitrogen washout during rest and exercise; maximum voluntary ventilation, and so on. These, however, should be considered to be of supplementary, not primary, value.

63.2. Cardiovascular Function. *63.21.* The most meaningful measure of cardiovascular fitness should be the maximum cardiac output. Most probably limitations in the arterial blood and oxygen supply to the heart muscle itself determine the work capacity of the heart. Unfortunately, measurements of total blood flow and its distribution to the various organs require highly specialized laboratories. The determination of cardiac output by any of the indirect methods suggested should be attempted wherever appropriate techniques and equipment are available.

Of the two components which make up cardiac output, namely heart rate and stroke volume, only the former can be measured readily. A direct measurement of the latter is practically impossible, but relative changes can be estimated with some degree of approximation from changes in the arterial pressure. Since these two readily attainable measures, heart rate and arterial blood pressure, are also essential factors for estimating the work of the heart, they are the two most important directly available measures for the evaluation of cardiac adaptive capacity.

Heart Rate. The heart rate should be continuously monitored by a two-chest-lead electrocardiogram (lead positions just inside the right clavicular-sternal joint and fifth intercostal space in the anterior axillary line), which also serves the purpose, especially in middle-aged and older populations, of detecting deviations fron normal cardiac activity.

In addition, the direct counting of the heart rate, preferably by means of auscultation of the brachial artery, should be standard procedure. Most probably, this would be the only means of measuring heart rates under field conditions. With sufficient practice the differences between heart rates obtained from auscultation and from ECG tracings should not be greater than ± 2 beats/minute. Care should be taken to avoid the quite common mistake of starting the count with " one " at zero time instead of with " zero." In a 15-sec count the error would amount to 4 beats/min.

Arterial Blood Pressure. For routine determination of arterial blood pressure, the traditional auscultation of the brachial artery is the method of choice. With practice and special care for avoiding artificial noises from parts of the measuring devices, sufficiently accurate values of the systolic pressure can be obtained. Their comparison with directly measured intraaortic pressure is good.

At light workloads, the noises created by the test machinery or test mechanics might interfere with the auscultatory detection of the Korotokow sound. Changing the strapped-on stethoscope capsule from the usual position, inward-upward to a place over the artery in the sulcus bicipitalis, might help to obtain clear sounds.

At very high work intensities great variations of systolic pressure may occur from beat to beat. In such cases the highest single pressure, as well as the regularly discernible pressure, should be recorded.

The accurate measurement of *diastolic blood pressures* during exercise is not always possible. On occasion, at more severe workloads, a clear and loud sound can be found at very low or even at zero cuff pressures. This phenomenon is especially observed with individuals trained for high cardiac capacity.

Generally it can be stated that the diagnostic value of the diastolic pressure measured during exercise is negligible, with the exception of one condition—namely, when it continues to rise with increasing work intensities. Such phenomenon should be considered a possible warning signal of approaching cardiovascular decompensation.

Critical Limitation. The combined observation of heart rate and arterial blood pressure during exercise may permit the detection of imminent cardio-vascular limitations. When, for example, diastolic pressure continues to rise without concomitant increments in systolic pressure, or when the systolic pressure begins to decline after a distinct peak has been reached, the investigator should call an end to the test. The heart rate *may* have levelled off at this point but not necessarily so. A further rise in heart rate might, in such cases, not be indicative of a further increase in cardiac output or in oxygen consumption.

A potential index of useful peak oxygen intake is the " oxygen pulse," $\dot{V}_{O_2} : f_H$, calculated from gas exchange and heart rate measurements obtained consecutively during the final stages of the test. Since

$$\dot{V}_{O_2} = f_H \times V_s \times (a - V)_{O_2}$$

then

$$\dot{V}_{O_2} : f_H = V_s \times (a - V)_{O_2}$$

which indicates that changes in the oxygen pulse reflect changes in the product of the stroke volume and $(a - V)_{O_2}$ differences.

A terminal drop from a peak oxygen pulse can be considered a cardio-vascular criterion of maximum aerobic power attained or exceeded.

63.3. Blood Properties. As there are no limitations to the supplementary respiratory and circulatory parameters that might be investigated during the standard tests, any number of desired blood studies can be carried out. However, the following determinations should be considered essential to the direct measurement of aerobic power.

1. Postexercise blood lactic acid in the fifth minute recovery blood sample is useful as an indication of the severity of exertion.
2. Hematocrit and hemoglobin at rest.

D. The Estimation of Maximal Aerobic Power from Submaximal Tests

Situations often arise in which the direct determination of maximum aerobic power by a maximal test is not feasible. In certain individuals, and in some population groups, all-out efforts have to be avoided because of age, functional handicaps of many kinds, or reluctance on the part of testees to exert themselves maximally. In these cases modifications in the tests become essential.

64.0. *The Standard Submaximal Test*

The simplest and most effective method is to conduct the test procedure for one of the standard tests but to end the test when the heart rate of the test subject reaches a level of approximately 80% of its estimated maximal value. The following heart rates can be assumed to represent average maximal values for different age groups:

Age, years	Average maxima, beats/min
10–15	210
16–20	200
21–35	190
36–45	180
46–55	170
56 and older	160

By plotting the heart rates measured during each second minute of the successive work intensity levels, an extrapolation may be made to the assumed maximum heart rate. The oxygen requirement is estimated in milliliters per kilogram per minute for the corresponding load, and it is this value that serves as the criterion of maximum aerobic power.

65.0. *Submaximal Field Step Test*

In testing large groups of people in areas where elaborate equipment is unavailable, and also in a practicing physician's office, the following submaximal step test has been applied with satisfactory results.

65.1. Apparatus. Four steps having a height of 10, 20, 30 and 40 cm (an additional 50 cm step can be added if extraordinary performances are expected); a metronome or pendulum of proper length; stopwatch; blood pressure manometer and cuff; and stethoscope.

65.2. Description. The subject steps for 3 min, at the reduced rate of 30 steps/min at each of the specified step levels, otherwise following the procedure set out under paragraph 62.0. The test may start on the horizontal level or on the 10-cm platform. The transition from one step level to the other should not interrupt the rhythm of the stepping cycle.

65.3. Scoring. The extrapolation procedure described under paragraph 64.0 is followed for assessing the value of maximum V_{O_2}. The energy requirements for the six possible workloads (horizontal stepping, 10, 20, 30, 40, and 50 cm) are 3, 5, 7, 9, 11, and 13 Mets, respectively.

65.4. General Guide and Regulations. Work is terminated when the individual's heart rate reaches a value of approximately 80% of his estimated maximum heart rate (see paragraph 64.0). Other procedures are followed as listed in paragraph 62.0

66.0. *Modified Submaximal Field Step Test for Children Aged* 6–10 *Years*

For children aged between 6 and 10 years the only modifications required to the above test is a reduction in the stepping rate from 30 to 24 lifts/min.

The energy requirements for the five recommended workloads (stepping on the horizontal level, and then progressively up to the 40-cm step maximum) are approximately 2, 3.5, 5, 6.5, and 8 Mets, respectively.

For extrapolation of the heart rate curve, a maximal heart rate of 220 can be assumed for children of this age group.

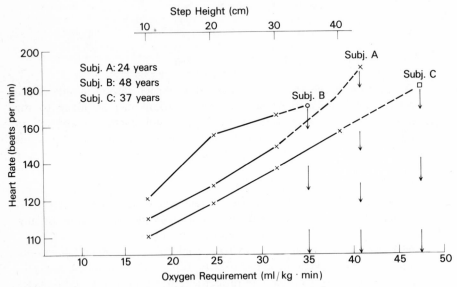

Figure VII-3. Step test. Examples for estimating maximum $\dot{V}_{O_2}$ of three individuals from their heart rate responses to three or four submaximal workloads in a step test ($f = 30$ lifts/min).

67.0. *Estimating Maximum Aerobic Power from Performance*

Where no equipment for the measurement or estimation of maximum aerobic power is available, performance on a 2000-m run, paced at an individual's maximum effort (see Section 5), can be recommended as an excellent substitute. Indeed there are those who argue that such practical performance measurements of aerobic power are always to be preferred to isolated laboratory tests of oxygen uptake capacity and who attack such laboratory tests as being inadequate predictors of performance in the real world. Such arguments, however, usually arise from a confusion about the aims of the two types of test and can usually be resolved when the premises and purposes of the two approaches are clarified.

PHYSIOLOGICAL TESTS WORKSHEET

Name:_____

Study and subject identity number:

1. Check the test criteria met
   - ☐ (a) Physician's permission?
   - ☐ (b) Absence of infectious diseases?
   - ☐ (c) Three months' minimum freedom from myocarditis, myocardial infarction, or angina pectoris.
   - ☐ (d) Absence of ECG aberrations?
   - ☐ (e) Resting heart rate less than 100 beats/min   Rate =_____
   - ☐ (f) Oral temperature less than 37.5°C?   Temp =_____°C
   - ☐ (g) Not short of sleep?
   - ☐ (h) Fully recovered from stress of last severe exercise?
   - ☐ (i) At least 2 hr since last meal? or smoke? or drink?

2. Test stop criteria
   The test is stopped when:
   (a) The subject in the standard test reaches the required maximum $\dot{V}_{O_2}$ plateau (two successive readings not differing by more than 5%).
   (b) The subject in a submaximal test reaches a heart rate that is 80% of the maximum estimated for his age group.

   Additionally the test should be stopped when any of the following are observed, and the exercise reduced to a low, gentle level:
   (a) The subject is unable to proceed because of distress.
   (b) The pulse pressure declines in spite of increasing intensity of work.
   (c) The systolic pressure exceeds 240–250 mm Hg.
   (d) The diastolic pressure exceeds 125 mm Hg.
   (e) Symptoms of distress such as chest pain, severe dyspnea, intermittent claudication.
   (f) Clinical signs of hypoxia, e.g., facial pallor, cyanosis, staggering, confusion, unresponsiveness to inquiries.
   (g) ECG aberrations such as paroxysmal superventricular or ventricular dysrhythmia, successive ventricular premature complexes before the end of the T wave, conduction disturbances other than a slight AV block, S–T depressions of horizontal or descending type greater than 0.3 mv.

3. Data required
   (a) Age (years)_____
   (b) Weight (kg)_____
   (c) Height (cm)_____
   (d) Estimated maximum heart rate for this age group?_____
   (e) Test
      (1) Treadmill: speed (m/min)_____
      (2) Bicycle ergometer: speed (rpm)_____
      (3) Stepping ergometer: speed (steps/min)_____

4. Computations
   The maximum oxygen uptake in milliliters per kilogram per minute ($\dot{V}_{O_2}$) is measured directly for any of the tests as follows:

$$\dot{V}_{O_2} = \dot{V}_E \times (F_{I_{O_2}} - F_{E_{O_2}}) \qquad \text{see Table VII–1}$$

Alternately the maximum oxygen uptake in milliliter per kilogram per minute ($\dot{V}_{0_2}$) may be estimated as follows:
Treadmill

$$\dot{V}_{0_2} = 1.78\, v\left(\frac{g + 7.3}{100}\right)$$

where v = maximum treadmill speed attained in m/min; g = maximum treadmill grade attained as a percent.
Bicycle ergometer

$$\dot{V}_{0_2} = 10.85\, W + 5.3\, w \qquad \text{see Figure VII-1}$$

where W = Watt; w = body weight, kg.
Stepping ergometer

$$\dot{V}_{0_2} = 2.37\, f \times h + 10.5 \qquad \text{see Figure VII-2}$$

5. Results table

Phase	Duration min	W^1 $\%_0^2$ h^3	$f_H{}^4$	Blood Pressure			$\dot{V}_E{}^5$	$F_{E0_2}{}^5$	$\dot{V}_{0_2}{}^5$	Comments
				Sys	Dias	Diff				
Rest	10–20									
Accommodation period	3									
Recovery	2									
Ex. 1										
2										
3										
4										
5										
6										
7										
8										
9										
10										
11										
12										

[1] W = watts if the test is done on the bicycle ergometer.
[2] $\%_0$ = percent grade if test is done on treadmill.
[3] h = height of step if the test is done on the stepping ergometer.
[4] f_H = heart rate measured over 15 sec in the second minute of exercise as soon as the systolic blood pressure has been recorded.
[5] Gas measurements to be corrected to STPD.

PHYSIOLOGICAL FITNESS ASSESSMENT

Family name: _____

First name, other initials: _____
(For other information see Section 1A: Personal Data)

Card serial number: _____ | 7 | (1–2)

Study number, Subject identity number:_____ (3–6)

Examining body:_____ (7–9)

Experimental conditions

Location: base lab = 1; mobile lab = 2;
field station = 3 (11)

Barometric pressure(mm Hg) (13–15)

Dry-bulb temperature(°C) (17–19)

Wet-bulb temperature(°C) (21–23)

Black-globe temperature(°C) (25–27)

Wind velocity—if outdoors(m/sec) (29–30)

Time (24-hr clock) (32–35)

Day of week: Mon = 1, Tues = 2, . . ., Sun = 7 (37)

Date of examination* (39–42)

Exercise mode: Treadmill = 1; bicycle ergometer = 2
step ergometer = 3; other (specify) = 4
Details: _____ (44)

Method: direct $\dot{V}_{o_2} = 1$; indirect $\dot{V}_{o_2} = 2$ (46)

Test data

Height(mm) (48–51)

Weight(kg) (53–56)

Maximum heart rate(beats/min) (58–60)

Maximum pulmonary ventilation at BTPS(liters/min) (62–65)

Maximum $\dot{V}_{o_2}$(ml/kg·min) (67–69)

Maximum systolic blood pressure(mm Hg) (71–73)

Maximum diastolic blood pressure(mm Hg) (75–77)

* See Appendix A.

491

SUPPLEMENTARY PHYSIOLOGICAL TEST DATA

Card serial number: _____

Study number, Subject identity number: _____

Examining body: _____

Respiratory function

Maximum voluntary ventilation(liter/min)

Ratio of max $\dot{V}$ during work to MVV

Respiratory exchange ratio at max $\dot{V}_{O_2}$

Lung diffusion capacity for oxygen(ml/min·mm Hg)

Residual volume(ml)

Cardiovascular function

Resting heart rate(beats/min)

Resting hematocrit(%)

Resting hemoglobin(g%)

Postexercise blood lactic acid (5th minute)(mEq/liter)

8 (1–2)
(3–6)
(7–9)

(11–13)
(15–16)
(18–19)
(21–23)
(25–26)

(28–30)
(32–33)
(35–37)
(39–41)

492

Section 4

PHYSIQUE AND BODY COMPOSITION

Contents

The Committee on Physique and Body Composition

J. Wartenweiler (Chairman), Switzerland
V. Correnti, Italy
H. Friermood, United States
M. Hebbelinck, Belgium
K. Hirata, Japan
M. Ikai (late), Japan

G. D. Maas, Holland
L. P. Novak, United States
V. Novotny, Czechoslovakia
J. M. Tanner, England
M. O. Tsai, Republic of China
T. Watanabe, Japan

The size and geometry of a person's body impose constraints upon his capacity for motor performance. Identifying the extent of these constraints is part of the process of analyzing physical fitness.

Many readers will, of course, have a primary interest in anthropometry for its own sake, seeing intrinsic merit in determining patterns of growth and development. They will no doubt trace with enthusiasm differences that reflect characteristics of culturally and genetically distinctive populations and pursue with vigor investigations into the variations in physique or body composition that arise from the imposition of natural or experimental conditions of environmental stress, exercise regimen, nutritional state, postural habits, and the like. Other readers may be interested only in defining the structure and body type of their subjects in order to establish a referential system within which their results might be better interpreted.

Whatever the nature of the interest, the techniques outlined in the following pages should. be of value. Basic and supplementary techniques are described in part A for measuring the dimensions of the body, that is, lengths, diameters, circumferences and skinfold thicknesses, in part B for determining the sizes of the different body compartments, that is, water, fat, lean body mass, and in part C for estimating maturity in the young.

A number of physique indices based on these measurements have been proposed. Perhaps the most useful of these is the ponderal index (PI) in the form suggested by Hirata (1972)*

$$PI = \sqrt[3]{W}/H \times 1000 \qquad \text{(see Appendix E)}$$

where W is weight (kg) and H is height (cm).

A recording and coding system is again suggested for those who wish to avail themselves of it.

A. Anthropometric Measurements

68.0. *The Basic Measurements*

The following are the basic measurements that might be included in the anthropometric measuring program. From these measurements a general impression of body constitution is obtained.

Weight
Measurements of length
   Standing
      Standing height
      Height of acromial
      Height of radial

---

* K.-I. Hirata: Ponderal index. A paper presented to the International Conference of Sports Sciences, Munich, 1972.

    Height of dactylion
    Height of trochanterion
    Height of tibial
  Sitting
    Sitting height
    Height of suprasternal when seated

Measurement of diameters
  Biacromial diameter
  Bicristal diameter
  Biepicondylar diameter humerus
  Biepicondylar diameter femur

Measurements of circumferences
  Chest circumference (xiphoidal level)
  Upper arm circumference (contracted and uncontracted)
  Thigh circumference

Measurements of skinfold thickness
  Biceps
  Triceps
  Subscapular
  Suprailiac
  Thigh medial
  Thigh lateral

For those wishing to carry out a more extensive program, a series of supplementary measurements have been included. These are marked with an asterisk in the following pages.

69.0. *General Facility Requirements*

An anthropometric laboratory is required where the ambient temperature should be maintained at a level that undressed subjects find comfortable. Privacy should be ensured for the examinee, but the anthropometrist should have an assistant present in the room. This assistant will normally act as a recorder.

70.0. *General Apparatus Requirements for the Anthropometric Measurements*

Weighing scales
Steel anthropometer
Spreading caliper
Sliding caliper
Skinfold caliper

Steel flexible tape or clothed fiberglass tape
Dermographic pencil

71.0. *The Principal Anatomical Landmarks*

Skin markings should be made on the subject, with a dermographic pencil, in the form of a short horizontal line to mark each principal anatomical landmark. These should be completed at the beginning of the session.

Measurements should be made on the *right* side of the body with the subject nude or, at the most, dressed in slips.

71.1. Frankfort Plane. The line from the lowest point of the lower border of the right orbit to the highest point of the upper margin of the right external auditory meatus.

71.2. Vertex. The highest point on the top of the head in the midsagittal plane when the head is in the horizontal Frankfort plane. This point is determined when measuring and does not need to be marked beforehand.

71.3. Suprasternal. The midpoint of the anterior-superior border of the manubrium sterni.

71.4. Mesosternal. The midpoint of the sternum at the height of the fourth costal articulation.

Note: This point can be determined by locating the sternum angle (corresponding with the second sternocostal articulation) and then counting downward two ribs to locate the fourth sternocostal articulation.

71.5. Xiphoidal. The lowest point of the sternum in the midsagittal plane, where it tapers to the xiphoid process.

71.6. Acromial. The most lateral point on the acromion process of the scapula. Mark both the right and the left points.

71.7. Radial. The uppermost point of the border of the radial cup with arm hanging down.

71.8. Stylion. The most distal point of the styloid process of the radius.

71.9. Dactylion. The midpoint of the tip of the middle finger. This point is determined when measuring and does not need to be skin-marked beforehand.

71.10. Iliocristal. The most laterally projecting point of the iliac crest. This point is determined when measuring and does not need to be skin-marked beforehand.

71.11. Trochanterion. The uppermost point of the greater trochanter.

Note: In some subjects (obese men and women) the greater trochanter is difficult to identify. In such cases the subject should be asked to rotate his leg inward and outward, while the measurer places his fingers on the area of the greater trochanter in order to locate it.

71.12. Tibial. The upper border and edge of the inner tuberosity of the head of the tibia, on the highest point of its medial border.

71.13. Sphyrion. The lowest point on the tip of the medial malleolus.

71.14. Midarm. Make the horizontal skin mark on the arm halfway between the acromial and the olecranon (tip of elbow).

71.15. Midthigh. Make the horizontal skin mark on the thigh halfway between the trochanterion and the tibial.

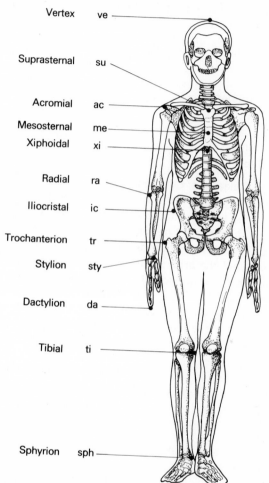

Vertex — ve
Suprasternal — su
Acromial — ac
Mesosternal — me
Xiphoidal — xi
Radial — ra
Iliocristal — ic
Trochanterion — tr
Stylion — sty
Dactylion — da
Tibial — ti
Sphyrion — sph

Figure VII-4. Principal "points" on the human body. ICSPFT anthropometric measurements.

72.0. *Measurement of Weight*

72.1. Apparatus. A beam type weighing scale is to be preferred. The scales should be regularly checked by calibrating them with known weights. A true zero balance should be demonstrated before they are used.

72.2. Description and General Considerations. The subject should be weighed nude. If this is not possible then the weight of his garments should be subtracted afterward. Measurements immediately after a meal or after exercise should be avoided if a reliable " standard " weight is to be recorded.

73.0. Measurements of the Heights of the Reference Points (Standing)

73.1. Apparatus. Anthropometer or stadiometer.

73.2. Description.

73.21. Standing height—measure from vertex to floor
73.22. Height of acromial
73.23. Height of radial
73.24. Height of stylion*
73.25. Height of dactylion
73.26. Height of trochanterion
73.27. Height of tibial
73.28. Height of sphyrion*

73.3. General Guide and Comments. In measuring the heights of the above points the arm of the anthropometer should be brought down successively to each one in turn and the height read off. Throughout the procedure the subject should stand on a horizontal flat platform, barefoot, with his heels together, and stretched upward to his fullest extent. The shoulders should be relaxed and the arms stretched straight downward. The marked Frankfort plane should be horizontal.

Care must be taken to ensure that the anthropometer does not deviate from the perpendicular. The time of day when the measurements are taken should be noted so that due account might be taken subsequently of diurnal variation.

74.0. Measurements of Height of Selected Reference Points (Sitting)

74.1. Apparatus. Anthropometer or stadiometer, flat-topped table or bench of known height, and foot rest of appropriate height.

74.2. Description.

74.21 Sitting height—measured from vertex to table top.
74.22 Height of suprasternal

74.3. General Guide and Comments. The considerations outlined in paragraph 73.3 apply equally to these measurements, with the following modifications. The subject sits on the table top or bench with his legs hanging down and stretches up to his fullest extent. His relaxed arms should rest on his thighs. If necessary the feet should be supported on a foot rest so that hip,

---

* All items marked with an asterisk are supplementary items. They should be added to the basic anthropometric measurement program as required.

knee, and ankles form right angles. Contraction of the buttock muscles should be avoided.

Measurements should either be taken directly from the table top with the upper two sections of the anthropometer, care being exercised to maintain the vertical alignment of the anthropometer, or be taken from the floor and the height of the table top subtracted.

75.0. *Calculations of Limb and Segment Lengths*

The lengths of the upper and lower extremities of the related limb segments can be calculated by subtraction as follows:

75.1. Total Upper Extremity Length. Subtract measurement 73.25 from 73.22.

75.2. Upper Arm Length. Subtract measurement 73.23 from 73.22.

75.3. Forearm Length.* Subtract measurement 73.24 from 73.23.

75.4. Total Lower Extremity Length. Height of trochanterion.

75.5. Thigh Length. Subtract measurement 73.27 from 73.26.

75.6. Lower Leg Length.* Subtract measurement 73.28 from 73.27.

76.0. *Measurements of Diameter*

76.1. Apparatus. Anthropometer, upper section only, with straight and recurved arms, spreading caliper, standard and large size, and sliding caliper, standard and large size.

76.2. Description.

76.21. Biacromial Diameter (Anthropometer). Distance between left and right acromial.

76.22. Bicristal Diameter (Anthropometer). Distance between left and right iliocristal. Pressure is applied to the anthropometer blades so as to push aside any fat covering the bone at the fixed point of the iliac crests.

*76.23. Transverse Chest Width** (Anthropometer with recurved arms, or large spreading caliper). The measurement is taken at the end of normal expiration, at the level of the mesosternal mark in a horizontal plane. The caliper is brought into contact with the outermost points of the ribs on this level.

*76.24. AP Chest Depth** (Anthropometer with recurved arms, or large spreading caliper.) The measurement is taken at the level of the mesosternal mark in a horizontal plane. The posterior point should be on the tip of a vertebral spine, the anterior point on the mesosternal mark.

76.25. Biepicondylar Diameter Humerus (Spreading or sliding caliper). The subject's elbow is bent at a right angle and the width across the outermost parts of the condyles of the humerus is taken. This measurement is usually oblique since the inner condyle of the humerus is lower than the outer one.

76.26. Biepicondylar Diameter Femur (Spreading or sliding caliper). The subject's knee is bent at a right angle and the maximum width between the lateral and the medial epicondyles of the femur is measured.

76.3. General Guide and Comments. A convenient technique for using the large caliper or anthropometer is to take hold of the caliper, one pointer in each hand so that the fingertips are used to palpate the bony reference points and guide the pointers into position.

77.0. *Measurements of Circumferences*

77.1. Apparatus. Steel flexible tape, or clothed fiber glass tape, and dermographic pencil.

77.2. Descriptions

77.21. Chest at Xiphoidal Level

77.211. CHEST CIRCUMFERENCE. Measure in the horizontal plane with the tape placed on the xiphoidal. The measurement is taken at the end of normal expiration.

77.212. MAXIMUM CHEST CIRCUMFERENCE.* At the point of maximal inspiration.

77.213. MINIMUM CHEST CIRCUMFERENCE.* At the point of maximal expiration.

*77.22. Chest at Mesosternal Level**

77.221. CHEST CIRCUMFERENCE.* The measurement is taken at the end of normal expiration with the tape in the horizontal plane at mesosternal level.

77.222. MAXIMUM CHEST CIRCUMFERENCE.* At the point of maximal inspiration.

77.223. MINIMUM CHEST CIRCUMFERENCE.* At the point of maximal expiration.

77.23. Upper Arm

77.231. UPPER ARM CIRCUMFERENCE UNCONTRACTED. Measured horizontally at the marked level halfway between acromial and olecranon (elbow tip) with the subject's arm hanging freely, slightly abducted. Skin mark the level of the top of the tape at the time the measurement is taken as a guide to the location of the site for the appropriate skinfold thickness.

77.232. UPPER ARM CIRCUMFERENCE CONTRACTED. Maximum circumference of the upper arm with the muscles fully contracted. An assistant pulls the subject's wrist to straighten the elbow and the subject resists the pulling strain.

*77.24. Forearm Circumference.** Maximum circumference of the forearm is measured immediately distal to the elbow joint with the subject's arm hanging freely. Skin-mark the level of the top of the tape at the time the measurement is taken as a guide to the location of the site for the appropriate skinfold thickness.

77.25. Thigh Circumference. Measured horizontally at the marked level halfway between trochanterion and tibial at the previously marked site while the subject is standing, both feet slightly apart, with his legs straight. The measurement point, half way between trochanterion and tibial must be located precisely for the thigh circumference changes greatly a few centimeters upward or downward.

*77.26. Calf Circumference.** Maximum circumference measured horizontally with the subject in the same position as in 77.25. Skin-mark the level of the top of the tape at the time this measurement is taken as a guide to the location of the site for the subsequent skinfold thickness measurement.

77.3. General Guide and Comments. In all the above measurements of circumference care is required to avoid deforming the contours of the skin when tightening the tape into position.

78.0. *Measurements of Skinfold Thickness*

78.1. Apparatus. Skinfold caliper, with standard constant pressure jaws of 10 g/mm².

78.2. Description. Pick up the skinfold between the thumb and forefinger about 1 cm above the skin-marks, with the crest of the fold following the alignment specified, and apply the caliper jaws to the exact site. Release the spring handles fully. When the pointer on the dial has steadied, read off the measurement in tenths of millimeters.

78.21. Skinfold over Triceps. The skinfold is located on the dorsum of the right upper arm (over the triceps), at the marked level half way between acromial and olecranon. In measuring the skinfold, the arm should hang freely. The crest of the skinfold is parallel to the long axis of the upper arm.

78.22. Skinfold over Biceps. The skinfold is located on the ventral side of the upper arm (over the biceps), at the marked level half way between acromial and olecranon. The crest of the skinfold is parallel to the long axis of the upper arm.

*78.23. Forearm Skinfold.** The forearm skinfold is measured at the marked level on the lateral side of the forearm. (See forearm circumference measurement 77.24.) The crest of the skinfold is parallel to the long axis of the forearm.

78.24. Subscapular Skinfold. The subscapular skinfold is measured about 1 cm below the lower angle of the right scapula with the subject standing in a relaxed position. The crest of the skinfold is medially upward and laterally downward at about 45°.

78.25. Suprailiac Skinfold. The fold is measured about 3 cm above the iliocristal. The crest of the skinfold is vertical.

78.26. Thigh Skinfold on Medial Side. The medial side thigh skinfold is measured at the marked level (77.25) half way between the trochanterion and tibial. The subject's right leg should be slightly flexed at the knee. The crest of the skinfold is parallel to the long axis of the thigh.

78.27. Thigh Skinfold on Lateral Side. The lateral side thigh skinfold is measured at the same marked level as the medial side measurement but on the outside of the thigh. The crest of the skinfold is again parallel to the long axis of the thigh.

*78.28. Calf Skinfold.** The calf skinfold is measured at the marked level (77.26) on the medial side of the calf while the subject is standing with his right foot resting on a low stool. The crest of the skinfold is parallel to the long axis of the calf.

78.3. General Guide and Comments. *78.31.* Taking accurate and repeatable skinfold measurements relies upon accurate location of the site of measurement, forming the skinfold *prior* to the application of the caliper jaws, the standardization of the alignment of the skinfold crest, and the complete release of the spring handles of the caliper so that the full standard pressure of the jaws is applied to the soft tissues being measured.

78.32. The pointer on the dial of the skinfold caliper should be allowed to steady and the drift cease, before measurements are read off.

78.33. Precise measuring and marking of the level of the skinfold (see 77.27) are necessary because subcutaneous fat thicknesses over the surfaces being measured vary substantially as the site of measurement changes.

BASIC ANTHROPOMETRIC DATA

Family name: ————————————————————

First name, other initials: ————————————————

	DATA CARD 9 (Basic)

Card serial number: ——————————————
Study number, Subject identity number:——————————
Examining body/investigator: ——————————————

9 (1–2)
(3–6)
(7–9)

Time of examination (24-hr clock)
Date of examination*

(11–14)
(15–19)

Sex: Male = 1; Female = 2

(21)

Age (decimal years*)

(23–26)

Ethnic group†:   Mongoloid = 1; Negroid = 2
                 Caucasian = 3; Mixed = 4

(28)

Country of origin————————

(30–32)

Major sport————————

(34–36)

Weight(kg/10)

(38–41)

Height standing(mm):   vertex

(43–46)

acromial

(48–51)

radial

(53–56)

dactylion

(58–61)

trochanterion

(63–66)

tibial

(68–70)

Upper limb length (acromial – dactylion)(mm)

(72–74)

Upper arm length (acromial – radial)(mm)

(75–77)

Thigh length (trochanterion – tibial)(mm)

(78–80)

* See Appendix A.
† See Appendix C.

503

DATA CARD 10 (Basic)

Card serial number: ————————————

Study number, Subject identity number:————————

| | 1 | 0 | (1–2) |
| | | | (3–6) |

Height sitting(mm):   vertex   (11–14)

                suprasternal   (16–18)

Biacromial diameter(mm)   (20–22)

Bicristal diameter(mm)   (24–26)

Biepicondylar diameter — humerus(mm/10)   (28–31)

Biepicondylar diameter — femur(mm/10)   (33–36)

Chest circumference(mm)   (38–41)

Upper arm circumference—uncontracted(mm)   (43–45)

             —contracted(mm)   (47–49)

Thigh circumference(mm)   (51–53)

Skinfold(mm/10):   triceps   (55–57)

              biceps   (59–61)

              subscapular   (63–65)

              suprailiac   (67–69)

              medial thigh   (71–73)

              lateral thigh   (75–77)

ANTHROPOMETRIC DATA—LONG FORM

Family name: ————————————

First name, other initials: ————————————

DATA CARD 9 (Long)

Card serial number: ————————————

Study number, Subject identity number:————————

Examining body/investigator: ————————————

		9	(1–2)
			(3–6)
			(7–9)

Time of examination (24-hr clock)   (11–14)

Date of examination*   (15–19)

Date of birth*   (20–24)

Age (subtraction)   (25–28)

Sex: Male = 1; Female = 2   (29)

Ethnic group†:   Mongoloid = 1; Negroid = 2   (30)
Caucasian = 3; Mixed = 4

Country of origin: _____   (31–34)
Note: For other personal details see Section 1.

Weight(kg/10)   (36–39)

Height, standing(mm):   vertex   (41–44)

acromial   (46–49)

radial   (51–54)

‡*stylion*   (56–59)

dactylion   (61–64)

trochanterion   (66–69)

tibial   (71–73)

‡*sphyrion*   (75–77)

* See Appendix A.
† See Appendix C.
‡ Supplementary measurements are indicated in italics.

DATA CARD 10 (Long)

Card serial number: _____ | 1 | 0 | (1–2)

Study number, Subject identity number:_____   (3–6)

Height, sitting(mm):   vertex   (11–14)

suprasternal   (16–18)

Calculate(mm):	upper limb length (acromial − dactylion)			(20–22)
	upper arm length (acromial − radial)			(24–26)
	**forearm length* (radial − dactylion)			(28–30)
	thigh length (trochanterion − tibial)			(32–34)
	**lower leg length* (tibial − sphyrion)			(36–38)
Diameter(mm):	biacromial			(40–42)
	bicristal			(44–46)
	**transverse chest*			(48–50)
	**A–P chest depth*			(52–54)
	biepicondylar humerus(mm/10)			(56–59)
	biepicondylar femur(mm/10)			(61–64)
Circumference(mm):	chest xiphoidal level, normal			(66–69)
	**chest maximum* (*inspiration*)			(71–74)
	**chest minimum* (*expiration*)			(76–79)

DATA CARD 11 (Long)

				1	1	(1–2)
Card serial number: _____						
Study number, Subject identity number:_____						(3–6)

Circumference(mm):	**chest mesosternal level*, *normal*			(11–14)
	**chest maximum* (*inspiration*)			(16–19)
	**chest minimum* (*expiration*)			(21–24)
	upper arm uncontracted			(26–28)
	upper arm contracted			(30–32)
	**forearm*			(34–36)
	thigh			(38–40)
	**calf*			(42–44)
Skinfold(mm/10):	triceps			(46–48)
	biceps			(50–52)
	subscapular			(54–56)
	suprailiac			(58–60)
	medial thigh			(62–64)
	lateral thigh			(66–68)

* Supplementary measurements indicated in italics.

B. Analysis of Body Compartments

79.0. *Total Body Fat*

79.1. Apparatus

Waterfilled tank, or a swimming pool if the water is sufficiently warm and quite still.

Underwater weighing system, suspension system preferred.

Weighing scale, calibrated from 0 to 15 kg in grams, and damped to reduce oscillations below 20-g stability.

Thermometer, water temperature to be held at 35–36°C, for an accuracy of ± 5% of total body fat.

Weight belt.

Equipment for residual volume determination (for example, helium dilution, nitrogen washout, oxygen or hydrogen rebreathing).

Spirometer, if residual volume is to be estimated from vital capacity.

79.2. Description.
The total body volume is determined by the hydrostatic weighing technique, using the Archimedian principle, where the volume of the body is determined from its displacement in water.

The subject's weight on land, nude, is determined and recorded.

The hydrostatic weighing technique is fully explained to alleviate any apprehension and such trial runs are given as are necessary or feasible. The subject, nude, then assumes his position in the previously weighed suspension apparatus and is lowered partway into the water, wearing the standard weighing belt. His body is then scrubbed thoroughly to dislodge gas bubbles on the skin and in the hair.

In position with shoulders submerged the residual volume is measured by an appropriate dilution or wash-out technique or, alternatively, the vital capacity readings are taken. If preferred these measurements can be taken with the subject out of the water, but some loss of accuracy then occurs. During these measurements a nose clip, which is checked to prevent leakage, should be worn.

When ready for submersion the subject, after two or three quick forced breaths, makes a maximal expiration, exactly as he did when the residual volume was measured, and then quietly lowers his head under the surface by flexing at the neck.

In this position, and when the dial oscillations have ceased, the scale is read off to the nearest 10 g. The subject is then signalled by a touch on the head and surfaces simply by raising his head.

The test is repeated at least three times or until the *heaviest* reading is consistently recorded.

79.3. Score. *79.31.* The following data must be secured:

1. Water temperature, which should be 35–36°C.
2. Weight of the subject in air, in grams (W_{BA}).
3. Total submerged weight of the subject plus equipment, in grams.
4. Weight of the submerged equipment alone, in grams.
5. Residual volume of the subject, in milliliters (RV).
6. Gastrointestinal gas (see *Note* to paragraph 79.47) estimated at 100 ml (V_{gi}).

The following values are then derived.

7. The density of water (D_W) at the water temperature specified.
8. The weight of water displaced by the total body gas volume, in grams per milliliter ($RV + V_{gi}$).
9. The corrected body weight in water of the subject (W_{BW})

$$W_{BW} = 3 - (4 + 8) \qquad \text{(numerals refer to list above)}$$

10. The volume of the subject (V_B).

$$V_B = \frac{W_{BA} - W_{BW}}{D_W}$$

From these values body density (D_B) can be determined.

$$D_B = \frac{W_{BA}}{V_B}$$

79.32. Estimating Body Fat from Body Density. From cadaver analysis by several investigations, the density of the lean body mass and fat tissues have been determined for a "standard reference man." Knowing these densities and assuming them to be relatively constant from person to person, body fat may be estimated from body density.

The determination of the proportional masses of these two components, body fat and lean body mass, can be calculated* as:

$$M_1 = \frac{1}{D_B} \times \frac{(d_1)(d_2)}{(d_2 - d_1)} - \frac{d_1}{d_2 - d_1}$$

where M_1 = mass of fat tissue, expressed as a fraction of the total body mass; D_B = body density; d_1 = density of the fat tissue; and d_2 = density of the lean body tissue.

* *Note:* There are several equations for estimating body fat from body density, but a single equation is recommended for the sake of uniformity. This formula has been shown to be applicable in individuals in whom the body weight has been free from large recent fluctuations.

With the introduction of the assumed densities for the reference man, this calculation becomes

$$F_B = \frac{4.570}{D_B} - 4.142$$

where F_B = body fat as a fraction of body weight; D_B = body density; and 4.570 and 4.142 = constants.

79.4. General Guide and Comments. *79.41.* The principle of the estimation of body fat from calculations based on measurements of body density depends upon the following assumptions:

1. That the separate densities of the body components are additive.
2. That the densities of the constituents of the body are relatively constant from person to person.
3. That an individual differs from a "standard reference man" only in the amount of adipose tissue he possesses.

79.42. The difference between the body weight in air and the body weight completely immersed in water is the weight of the displaced volume of water. Knowing the water density, the volume displaced, or body volume, can be calculated. The density of the whole body (D_B) is determined by dividing the total body weight in air (W_{BA}) by the body volume (V_B).

$$D_B = \frac{W_{BA}}{V_B}$$

79.43. D_W. The density of the water can be determined from standard tables if the temperature is known and water is adequately mixed and free of air bubbles.

79.44. It is necessary to maintain a water temperature at mean body temperature value (35–36°C) because extremes in water temperature could induce changes in mean body temperature.

79.45. In order to eliminate the effect of the variable amount of residual air in the lungs from subject to subject, the gross body volume under water must be corrected for the air in the lungs and respiratory passages.

79.46. RV. Residual volume is defined as the volume of air remaining in the lungs at the end of a maximal expiration. The residual volume may be determined

1. Simultaneously with the density determination for greater accuracy.
2. Prior to or following the weighing procedure with some loss of accuracy.
3. Estimated from known lung volumes as

   (a) 20% of the total lung capacity.
   (b) 30% of the vital capacity.

If the residual volume is assumed, the effect of age, sex, and posture must be considered.

79.47. The volume of gas in the gastrointestinal tract (V_{gi}) has been estimated most accurately at 100 ml (BTPS) in the postabsorptive state.

79.48. Precautions. In addition to errors arising from variations in the above measurements, gas bubbles adhering to the skin and hair on the body surface must be removed. If the subject is not weighed in the nude, air may also be trapped in the bathing suit or bathing cap. These sources of error must be eliminated as much as possible, the bathing suit being wetted fully and allowances made for its weight, the hair washed, the cap removed, the body scrubbed, and so on.

Density should be determined while the subject is in a postabsorptive state to reduce the amount of gastrointestinal gas to a minimum.

The water temperature (in °C) is recorded following each weighing. The barometric pressure is recorded at the beginning and end of each session.

The weight of the submerged apparatus is recorded before and after each subject's weighing is completed.

80.0. *Total Body Water*

80.1. Apparatus. Mass spectrometer and reduction train, deuterium oxide (D_2O) (99.8%), paper cups, plastic bottles, pipettes, graduated cylinders.

80.2. Description. Total body water can be determined by the dilution principle. The subject empties his bladder before the test starts. He then takes 25 ml of D_2O orally from a paper cup, emptying it totally. A second drink of tap water from the same cup ensures that no residual drops of D_2O are left.

It is explained to the subject that he is not to drink additional water or any liquid from the time the dose was given until the final collection of urine (4 hr later).

At 2 hr after the dose has been given, the subject empties his bladder again into the toilet (about 0.25% of the dose will be lost in this equilibration urine, which in total calculation of total body water will cause a negligible error).

At 3 hr after the dose has been given, the subject is asked to produce the first urine sample. (Mark this bottle with the name of the subject and the number 1.) Measure the total volume of urine, mark it, and place an aliquot into a 5-ml vial and seal.

At 4 hr after the dose has been given, the subject is asked for the second urine sample. (Mark this bottle with the name of the subject and the number 2.) Measure the total volume of urine and record it. Place an aliquot into a 5-ml vial and seal. Send the samples to a mass spectrometer laboratory for analysis.

Both samples analyzed by the mass spectrometer for the ratio $^2H{:}^1H$ should provide identical results. If the result of the samples disagree by more than 5%, equilibrium was not achieved and the 4-hr urine sample should provide the truer volume distribution.

80.3. Score. *80.31. The Final Volume of Body Water (V_F).* This final volume, into which the test substance has diffused at equilibrium, is given by

$$V_F = \frac{C_1 V_1 - C_E V_E}{C_F}$$

where: C_1 = concentration of test substance administered.
V_1 = volume of test substance administered.
C_E = concentration of test substance lost during equilibration time.
V_E = volume of test substance lost during equilibration time.
C_F = final concentration of test substance after equilibration has been achieved.

Because it has been well documented that the loss of D_2O during the time required for equilibration is less than 0.25%, such losses can be omitted from calculations. The formula then reduces to

$$V_F = \frac{C_1 V_1}{C_F}$$

80.32. The Weight of Body Water (Weight H_2O). This value can be calculated as follows. Given

1. Weight of D_2O administered in grams = Weight D_2O.
2. Normal concentration of D_2O in body water = 0.0150 atom % D.
3. Molecular weight of H_2O:^1H = 18.01571.
4. Molecular weight of D_2O:^2H = 20.02836.
5. Ratio of $^2H/^1H$ = 1.1117

then by definition

$$D_2O \text{ mole } \% = \frac{\text{Weight } D_2O/^2H}{(\text{Weight } D_2O/^2H) + (\text{Weight } H_2O/^1H)} \times 100$$

$$= \frac{\text{Moles } D_2O}{\text{Moles } D_2O + \text{Moles } H_2O} \times 100$$

and solving for body water

$$\text{Weight } H_2O = \frac{\text{Weight } D_2O}{1.1117} \times \frac{100}{D_2O \text{ mole } \%} - 1$$

Where -1 can be ignored for low concentrations of D_2O and mole percent D_2O excess value is obtained from the mass spectrometer.

80.33. Lean Body Mass and Fat. These values can also be calculated from total water body water. Lean body mass (*LBM*) can be calculated from the determination of total body water under the assumption that it has a constant amount of water, namely 73.2% and that body fat is practically anhydrous. Then

$$LBM = \frac{TBW\%}{0.732} \quad \text{or} \quad LBM, \text{kg} = \frac{TBW_L}{0.732}$$

where $TBW\%$ is total body water expressed in percent of body weight, TBW_L is total body water expressed in liters, and 0.732 is a constant hydration of lean body mass based on analyses of small laboratory rodents (Pace and Rathbun, 1945).*

Note then that

$$\text{Fat, } \% = 100 - LBM\%$$

and

$$\text{Fat, kg} = \text{Body weight, kg} - LBM, \text{kg}$$

$$\text{Total body solids, kg} = \text{Body weight, kg} - \text{Total body water, kg}$$

$$\text{Fat-free solids, kg} = \text{Total body solids, kg} - \text{Total body fat, kg}$$

80.4. General Guide and Regulations. *80.41.* The accuracy of the dilution techniques for measuring total body water depends upon the qualities of the test substance which should be

1. Diffusable into all the fluid compartments of the body within a short period of time.
2. Capable of reaching a stable and uniform equilibrium rapidly.
3. Not selectively stored, secreted, or metabolized.
4. Completely exchangeable with body water.

80.42. An inherent error of the deuterium method is in the exchange of deuterium atoms with labile hydrogen atoms of organic molecules. This exchange occurs rapidly and therefore represents only a small loss of deuterium. This loss has been estimated as a water equivalent between 0.5 and 2.0% of body weight.

Thus, for an average adult man who has 45 liters of body water, the D_2O method will overestimate his body water by 0.7 to 1 liter, a figure that sets the limits on the accuracy of body water measurements. Corrected volumes can be obtained by averaging downward by about 1%.

80.43. In cases of abnormal hydration, the time for equilibration of D_2O with body water has to be extended at least to 4 hr.

80.44. The lean body mass contains not only the cellular mass but also the extracellular supporting structures such as extracellular water, collagen,

* N. Pace and E. N. Rathbun: Studies on body composition. III. The body water and chemically combined nitrogen content in relation to fat content. *J. Biol. Chem.*, **158**: 685–691 (1945).

and bone mineral. The former has high oxygen consumption, whereas the latter represents low oxidizing tissues. Therefore, lean body mass represents heterogeneous components of the body.

The derivation of lean body mass from total body water is valid only in the normal state, where the relationship of body water to dry lean body tissues remains constant. In pathological states where either extracellular or intracellular water accumulates, this relationship does not hold. However, a correction factor for the excess of the extracellular water has been proposed by Keys and Brožek (1953).*

81.0. Total Body Potassium

81.1. Lean Body Mass. An alternative and sophisticated method for arriving at lean body mass is to measure the naturally occurring radioactivity of the body arising from its ^{40}K content. Such counts can be carried out if access can be gained to an environmental radiation unit or a suitable medical physics laboratory.

A variety of specialist equipment will be available in these centers, but main items include a whole body counter with sodium iodide, plastic or liquid scintillating detectors; two phantoms, one containing a known amount of naturally occurring potassium for calibration and the other an inert substance, for example, water or sugar to allow for the absorption of gamma rays by the body because of its size.

81.2. Description. The fasting subject is counted for ^{40}K prior to the administration of a ^{42}K dose. He then receives 5 μcuries of ^{42}K and is counted at 1, 6, 12, and 24 hours for an adequate period at each time. Between each whole-body counting period, a urine collection is made and the bottles of urine are also counted in order to determine the amount of tracer lost. Subject counts can thus be corrected for urinary loss of ^{42}K.

A phantom, containing a known amount of potassium chloride (KCl) is then substituted for the subject in the whole-body counter and compared to a calibrated quantity of ^{42}K in the same phantom. A count is also taken on an inert phantom of water, or sugar.

81.3. Score. The following data is obtained

a = Weight (kg) and height (cm) of the subject.

b = Counts per second of the subject.

c = Counts per second of the appropriate inert phantom.

d = Counts per second of adult K phantom.

e = Net subject counts per second = $b - c$.

f = Efficiency of daily counting = $0.3619/(d - c + 850)$. (See paragraph 81.47.)

* A. Keys and J. Brožek: Body fat in adult man. *Physiol. Rev.*, **33**:245–325 (1953).

g = Subject efficiency correction derived from ratio weight/height (see paragraph 81.46).

from which total body potassium (TBK) can be calculated

$$TBK = \frac{e \cdot f}{g}$$

Body cell mass (BCM) in grams can then be computed

$$BCM = 8.33\ TBK$$

81.4. General Guide and Comments. *81.41.* The naturally occurring isotope ^{40}K in the body emits beta particles and gamma rays of maximal energy 1.46 Mev. It is in a constant ratio of 0.0119% to the two stable potassiums ^{39}K—93.08%, and ^{41}K—6.91%. These rays are detected and counted by sensitive detectors surrounding the subject.

81.42. The body cell mass is a pure culture of living cells. It consists of the cellular components of the skeletal, cardiac and smooth muscles, viscera (liver, kidney, spleen, lungs, heart), the intestinal tract, blood, glands, reproductive organs (uterus, ovaries, testes), and the cells of the brain.

If one assumes that these cellular tissues have an average potassium-nitrogen ratio of 3 mEq/g and that their total net weight (excluding extracellular water) is equal to their nitrogen content multiplied by the coefficient 25, then the weight of body cell mass can be calculated as follows:

$$BCM, g = \frac{TBK, mEq - \text{Extracellular potassium, mEq}}{3} \times 25$$

Since the correction for extracellular potassium causes negligible error in calculations of body cell mass, it can be omitted and the equation becomes

$$BCM, g = 8.33\ TBK, mEq$$

81.43. In adult humans the potassium concentration of the lean body mass as determined by chemical analysis, averages 68.1 mEq/kg of lean body mass (range 66.6–72.3 mEq). Thus

$$LBM, kg = \frac{\text{Total body potassium, mEq}}{68.1}$$

Fat, kg = Body weight, kg − Lean body mass, kg

However, the potassium concentration in lean body mass of newborns seems to be between 48–50 mEq/kg; at 1 year of age it is approximately 58 mEq/kg; at 10 years of age 60 mEq/kg; at 15 years of age 68.1 mEq/kg.

81.44. Before calculations of total body potassium can be achieved, the whole-body counter has to be calibrated. This is usually done by injecting subjects of various weights with ^{42}K, which has similar maximum energy, 1.52 Mev, to ^{40}K and a conveniently short half-life (12.5 hr).

81.45. The sugar phantom is used to simulate body thickness and to correct for the internal absorption of gamma rays within the body.

81.46. The weight of the subject in kilograms, and his height in centimeters are required in the establishment of the subject efficiency correction factor, which is given by the counts per second per gram of potassium based on the regression line obtained from calibration of the counter with ^{42}K.

81.47. The efficiency of daily counting is equal to 0.3619 cps/g of the known amount of K phantom divided by the daily counts per second per gram of ^{40}K.

$$TBK, g = \text{cps } ^{40}\text{K (man)} \times \frac{\text{K (phantom)}}{\text{cps } ^{40}\text{K (phantom)}} \times \frac{\text{cps } ^{42}\text{K(phantom)}}{\text{cps } ^{42}\text{K(man)}}$$

The relationship of counts per second per gram of potassium to the ratio of weight/height is determined from the regression equation which includes various ranges of weight and height.

$$\text{Log (cps/g K)} = -0.30122 \text{ (weight/height)} + 0.65499$$

The difference in correlation coefficients of log cps/g K and cps/g K is negligible ($r = 0.822$ and $r = 0.815$, respectively) and both are high.

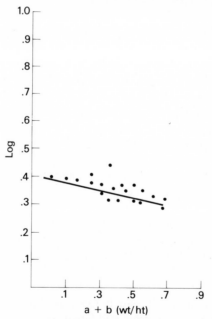

Figure VII-5. The regression relationship between the log cps 1 g K and a + b (wt/ht) for various values of weight/height ratio.

C. Maturation

82.0. *Puberty Ratings*

Some designation of how far a given child has progressed through adolescence is frequently required. A relatively simple and quite practical scheme is to rate the development of secondary sex characteristics. In boys, pubic hair development and genital development is rated; in girls, pubic hair development and breast development. All ratings are carried out separately on a scale from 1 to 5. The pubic hair standard for both sexes is thus comparable.

If a composite sex-character development rating is required, the pubic hair ratings can be averaged with the genital ratings for boys and with the breast ratings for girls. Naturally, the ratings can be assigned with more accuracy if a longitudinal study of a child is available, because they are really based on the occurrence of change from a previous state. However, fair accuracy is attainable even when the child is only seen once. Pubic hair ratings are perhaps easier to give than ratings for genital and breast development under these circumstances. The rating in a longitudinal series refers to the actual time the stage in question is first observed and is not interpolated backward half way to the previous examination, since this would be impossible for ratings given cross-sectionally.

82.1. Pubic Hair Stages

Stage 1. Preadolescent. The vellus over the pubes is not further developed than that over the abdominal wall, that is, no pubic hair.

Stage 2. Sparse growth of long, slightly pigmented downy hair, straight or only slightly curled, appearing chiefly at the base of the penis or along the labia.

Stage 3. Considerably darker, coarser, and more curled. The hair spreads sparsely over the junction of the pubes. It is at this stage that pubic hair is first seen in the usual type of black and white photograph of the entire body; special arrangements are necessary to photograph stage 2 hair.

Stage 4. Hair now resembles adult in type, but the area covered by it is still considerably smaller than in the adult. No spread to the medial surface of the thighs.

Stage 5. Adult in quantity and type with distribution of the horizontal (or classically "feminine") pattern. Spread to medial surface of thighs but not up linea alba or elsewhere above the base of the inverse triangle.

In about 80% of Caucasian men and 10% of the women, the pubic hair spreads further but this takes some time to occur after stage 5 is reached. When it does occur the pubic hair is rated as stage 6, a terminology that retains the uniform rating for male and female over the 5-point scale, and at the same time places this longer-term development, often not completed until the midtwenties or later, beyond the more concentrated period of adolescence.

82.11. Axillary hair may be rated on a 3-point scale: 1 when none is present; 2 for slight growth; and 3 for adult quantity.

82.12. In boys *facial hair* begins to grow at about the time the axillary hair appears. First there is an increase in length and pigmentation of hairs at the corners of the upper lip; this development then spreads medially to complete the moustache. Hair next appears on the upper part of the cheeks, in the midline just below the lower lip, and finally along the sides and lower border of the chin; the actual distribution observed is best recorded.

82.13. The remainder of the body hair appears from about the time of the first axillary hair development up to a considerable period after puberty. The hair on the thigh, calf, abdomen, and forearm usually precedes that on the chest and upper arm.

82.2. Genital Development Stages

Stage 1. Preadolescent. Testes, scrotum, and penis are of about the same size and proportions as in early childhood.

Stage 2. Enlargement of scrotum and of testes. The skin of the scrotum reddens and changes in texture. Little or no enlargement of penis at this stage.

Stage 3. Englargement of penis, which occurs at first mainly in length. Further growth of testes and scrotum.

Stage 4. Increased size of penis with growth in breadth and development of glans. Further enlargement of testes and scrotum; increased darkening of scrotal skin.

Stage 5. Genitalia adult in size and shape. No further enlargement takes place after stage 5 is reached.

82.3. Breast Development Stages

Stage 1. Preadolescent; elevation of papilla only.

Stage 2. Breast bud stage; elevation of breast and papilla as small mound. Enlargement of areolar diameter.

Stage 3. Further enlargement and elevation of breast and areola, with no separation of their contours.

Stage 4. Projection of areola and papilla to form a secondary mound above the level of the breast.

Stage 5. Mature stage; projection of papilla only, due to recession of the areola to the general contour of the breast.

The appearance of the breast bud is as a rule the first sign of puberty in the female, though the appearance of pubic hair may sometimes precede it. The stage 4 development of the areolar mound does not occur in all girls; in probably about a quarter it is absent, and in a further quarter relatively slight. Furthermore, the areolar mound, when it does occur, often persists well into adulthood; it seems to be at least as much a matter of adult physique as a passing stage of adolescent development. Areolar diameter enlargement continues from stage 2 to stage 5 but proceeds faster in the early stages. Accurate breast development ratings on a cross-sectional basis may be difficult, but in longitudinal work the general increase in breast size enables stages 3, 4, and 5 to be assigned fairly confidently.

83.0. Skeletal Age

Skeletal maturity may be determined by x-ray evaluation of the bones of the wrist and hand.*

83.1. Apparatus. X-ray equipment, lead-topped table, lead apron, ancillary equipment, pair of dividers, and rating criteria.

83.2. Description. The palm is placed face downward, in contact with the film, the axis of the middle finger in direct line with the axis of the forearm. The fingers are just not touching, and the thumb is placed in the comfortable natural degree of rotation with its free axis making an angle of about 30° with the first finger. The palm is pressed lightly downward on the film by the subject. If the subject is too young to follow these instructions, the hand is secured in this position with bandage or tape or by other means.

The tube is centered above the head of the third metacarpal, at a tube film distance of 30 in or 76 cm. The exposure with Ilfex or similar film should be about 8 ma-sec at 55 kv for the 8–10-year-old child, with corresponding adjustments for older or younger children.

83.3. Score. All bones of the wrist and hand are examined in comparison with sets of norms* and assigned ratings that contribute toward a skeletal maturity and a skeletal age score. Bone ratings range from A–I(J). A short rating system that considers only the first, third, and fifth fingers and the radius and ulna may be used very satisfactorily. In this case each provides 20% of the final composite score.

83.4. General Guide and Comments. *83.41.* The correct posing of the left hand and wrist is of great importance; unless the x-ray tube is centered properly and the hand and thumb placed as described, the appearance of certain bones will be different from the standardized norms.

Best results in the x-ray are obtained by using double-wrapped films, without cassettes and screens, and by a somewhat lighter than usual development.

83.42. A lead apron pulled well over the child's lap should be used to shield the gonads from radiation. This is in addition to the lead sheeting on the table top.

* J. M. Tanner, R. H. Whitehouse, and M. J. R. Healy, *A New System for Estimating Skeletal Maturity from the Hand and Wrist, with Standards Derived from a Study of 2,600 Healthy British Children.* Paris, International Children's Center, 1962.

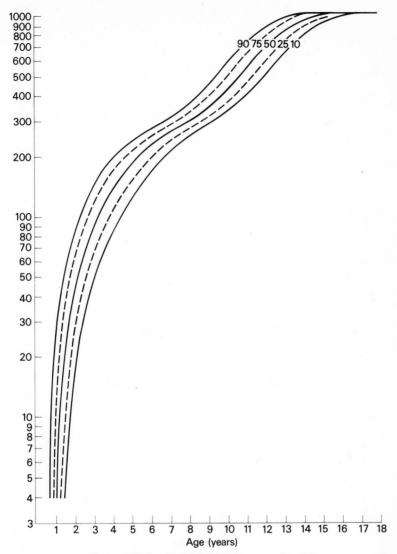

Figure VII-6.   Skeletal maturity scores for girls.

83.43. The assumption is made that maturation is a continuous process in the young and that the appearance of their bones will reflect the stage of maturity they have attained. Under this assumption a single composite skeletal maturity score is developed based on scores assigned to each bone, by simple .addition of ratings.

There are cases where unusually slow development of certain bones reflects some abnormal development.

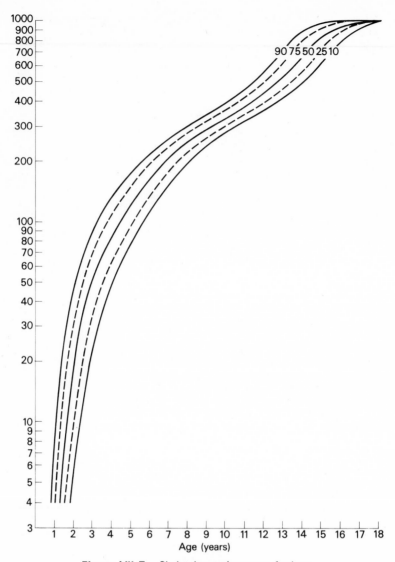

Figure VII-7.   Skeletal maturity scores for boys.

83.44. A log scale is used for maturity scores in order to achieve homogeneous variance scores as age increases. This scale is then converted into percentile scores.

83.45. Skeletal maturity scores can be converted into skeletal age scores by assigning to each score the fiftieth percentile age of children with that score. With British children skeletal age is stated as "adult" at 17 years for girls and 19 years for boys. It could well be that these norms are inappropriate for children in other countries.

83.46. Ratings* for each bone range from A (zero), through B (a single deposit of calcium just detectable at the center of ossification) to I (ossification complete). In the case of the radius of men an additional rating J is occasionally required. These ratings are then converted into skeletal maturity scores by reference to Table VII-4. Weightings have been given to these scores according to their relative importance so that they may all be summed to provide an overall skeletal maturity score.

84.47. Skeletal age can be estimated for given maturity scores for boys by reference to Table VII-5 and for girls in Table VII-6. Growth curves are shown in Figures VII-6 and VII-7.

Table VII-4 Self-Weighting (20 Bone) Maturity Scores

Sum of upper section gives long bone score (out of 500).
Sum of lower section gives round bone score (out of 500).
Total sum gives overall score (out of 1000).

Ratings		A	B	C	D	E	F	G	H	I	J
LONG BONES											
Radius		0	1	2	7	13	26	52	82	98	100
Ulna		0	23	25	28	34	49	81	98	100	
Metacarpal	I	0	2	3	7	11	16	24	30	33	
	III	0	0	1	3	6	10	19	23	25	
	V	0	1	2	4	7	11	19	24	25	
Proximal phalange	I	0	2	3	5	9	16	26	31	33	
	III	0	0	1	3	6	12	19	23	25	
	V	0	0	1	3	7	12	19	23	25	
Middle phalange	III	0	1	2	4	8	13	20	24	25	
	V	0	2	3	5	8	16	21	24	25	
Distal phalange	I	0	0	1	3	8	15	25	28	34	
	III	0	1	2	4	6	11	19	21	25	
	V	0	2	3	5	8	12	20	22	25	
ROUND BONES											
Capitate		0	0	1	4	8	14	20	31	72	
Hamate		0	0	1	6	13	19	25	38	72	
Triquetral		0	4	7	12	18	23	31	46	72	
Lunate		0	9	12	15	19	25	31	48	71	
Navicular		0	13	16	19	23	26	32	51	71	
Great multangular		0	12	15	17	21	26	30	43	71	
Lesser multangular		0	12	14	17	19	24	30	42	71	

Long bone score
Round bone score
Overall score

* Detailed criteria are given, and extensive pictorial guidance presented in the main reference listed.

Physical Fitness Measurements

Table VII-5 Skeletal Ages Corresponding to Skeletal Maturity Scores for Boys

Skeletal Age, years	Skeletal Maturity	Skeletal Age, years	Skeletal Maturity	Skeletal Age, years	Skeletal Maturity
1.0	2	5.7	151	10.4	350
1.1	3	5.8	155	10.5	354
1.2	4	5.9	160	10.6	359
1.3	5	6.0	164	10.7	363
1.4	6	6.1	169	10.8	368
1.5	7	6.2	173	10.9	373
1.6	9	6.3	178	11.0	378
1.7	11	6.4	182	11.1	383
1.8	13	6.5	187	11.2	388
1.9	16	6.6	192	11.3	393
2.0	19	6.7	197	11.4	398
2.1	22	6.8	201	11.5	403
2.2	25	6.9	206	11.6	409
2.3	29	7.0	210	11.7	416
2.4	33	7.1	215	11.8	423
2.5	36	7.2	219	11.9	430
2.6	39	7.3	224	12.0	437
2.7	42	7.4	228	12.1	445
2.8	45	7.5	232	12.2	453
2.9	48	7.6	236	12.3	462
3.0	51	7.7	240	12.4	471
3.1	54	7.8	244	12.5	480
3.2	57	7.9	248	12.6	489
3.3	60	8.0	251	12.7	499
3.4	63	8.1	255	12.8	509
3.5	66	8.2	259	12.9	519
3.6	70	8.3	263	13.0	530
3.7	73	8.4	267	13.1	542
3.8	77	8.5	271	13.2	554
3.9	80	8.6	275	13.3	567
4.0	84	8.7	279	13.4	580
4.1	87	8.8	283	13.5	594
4.2	91	8.9	287	13.6	619
4.3	94	9.0	291	13.7	624
4.4	98	9.1	295	13.8	640
4.5	101	9.2	299	13.9	657
4.6	105	9.3	303	14.0	675
4.7	109	9.4	306	14.1	694
4.8	113	9.5	310	14.2	713
4.9	117	9.6	315	14.3	732
5.0	121	9.7	319	14.4	751
5.1	125	9.8	323	14.5	770
5.2	130	9.9	327	14.6	788
5.3	134	10.0	331	14.7	805
5.4	139	10.1	336	14.8	822
5.5	143	10.2	340	14.9	837
5.6	147	10.3	345	15.0	851

Table VII-5 (*continued*)

Skeletal Age, years	Skeletal Maturity	Skeletal Age, years	Skeletal Maturity	Skeletal Age, years	Skeletal Maturity
15.1	864	16.5	965	17.9	995
15.2	877	16.6	968	18.0	996
15.3	889	16.7	971	18.1	996
15.4	900	16.8	974	18.2	997
15.5	910	16.9	977	18.3	997
15.6	919	17.0	980	18.4	998
15.7	926	17.1	982	18.5	998
15.8	933	17.2	984	18.6	998
15.9	939	17.3	986	18.7	999
16.0	945	17.4	988	18.8	999
16.1	950	17.5	990	18.9	999
16.2	954	17.6	992	Adult	1000
16.3	958	17.7	993		
16.4	962	17.8	994		

Table VII-6 Skeletal Ages Corresponding to Skeletal Maturity Scores for Girls

Skeletal Age, years	Skeletal Maturity	Skeletal Age, years	Skeletal Maturity	Skeletal Age, years	Skeletal Maturity
1.0	5	3.6	116	6.2	235
1.1	7	3.7	120	6.3	239
1.2	11	3.8	125	6.4	243
1.3	15	3.9	130	6.5	247
1.4	19	4.0	135	6.6	251
1.5	23	4.1	140	6.7	254
1.6	27	4.2	145	6.8	258
1.7	31	4.3	150	6.9	261
1.8	35	4.4	154	7.0	264
1.9	39	4.5	159	7.1	267
2.0	43	4.6	164	7.2	270
2.1	47	4.7	168	7.3	273
2.2	52	4.8	173	7.4	276
2.3	56	4.9	178	7.5	279
2.4	61	5.0	183	7.6	282
2.5	65	5.1	187	7.7	285
2.6	70	5.2	191	7.8	288
2.7	74	5.3	196	7.9	291
2.8	79	5.4	200	8.0	295
2.9	83	5.5	205	8.1	299
3.0	88	5.6	209	8.2	303
3.1	92	5.7	214	8.3	307
3.2	97	5.8	218	8.4	311
3.3	102	5.9	222	8.5	315
3.4	106	6.0	226	8.6	320
3.5	110	6.1	231	8.7	325

Table VII-6   (*continued*)

Skeletal Age, years	Skeletal Maturity	Skeletal Age, years	Skeletal Maturity	Skeletal Age, years	Skeletal Maturity
8.8	330	11.6	612	14.4	954
8.9	335	11.7	627	14.5	960
9.0	341	11.8	643	14.6	966
9.1	347	11.9	659	14.7	971
9.2	354	12.0	675	14.8	976
9.3	361	12.1	691	14.9	980
9.4	368	12.2	707	15.0	984
9.5	375	12.3	723	15.1	987
9.6	382	12.4	738	15.2	989
9.7	390	12.5	753	15.3	991
9.8	398	12.6	767	15.4	993
9.9	406	12.7	781	15.5	994
10.0	415	12.8	794	15.6	994
10.1	425	12.9	807	15.7	995
10.2	435	13.0	820	15.8	995
10.3	446	13.1	833	15.9	996
10.4	457	13.2	845	16.0	996
10.5	468	13.3	857	16.1	997
10.6	480	13.4	868	16.2	997
10.7	492	13.5	879	16.3	997
10.8	504	13.6	889	16.4	998
10.9	517	13.7	899	16.5	998
11.0	530	13.8	908	16.6	998
11.1	543	13.9	917	16.7	999
11.2	556	14.0	925	16.8	999
11.3	569	14.1	933	16.9	999
11.4	583	14.2	941	Adult	1000
11.5	597	14.3	948		

Section 5

Basic Physical Performance Tests

Contents

The Committee on Performance Tests

M. Howell (Chairman), Canada
L. C. Arnold, U.S.A.
J. Atha, England
A. Baumann, W. Germany
L. Bollaert, Belgium
W. Campbell, England
S. Celikovsjy, Czechoslavakia
L. Chang, Republic of China
F. H. O. Cords, U.S.A.
E. G. Evans, Wales
M. Fadali, Egypt
D. Herrmann, U.S.A.
P. Hunsicker, U.S.A.
M. Irsan, Indonesia
P. Johnson, Uruguay
A. Kirsch, West Germany

E. Kurimoto, Japan
A. Lage, Spain
L. Larson, U.S.A.
T. Meshizuka, Japan
A. Messinis, Greece
Y. Noguchi, Japan
V. Novotny, Czechoslovakia
H. Ruskin, Israel
C. Schneiter, Switzerland
C. Sierra, Spain
U. Simri, Israel
B. Suvarnabriksha, Thailand
M. Tsai, Republic of China
W. C. Wu, Republic of China
C. J. Yang, Republic of China

83.0 Introduction

The tests have been selected as representing the more important and measurable aspects of physical capacity, for example, speed, power, static strength, flexibility, muscular endurance. The committee realizes that the battery does not test all aspects of physical performance and recognizes that tests of balance, coordination, reaction time, and so on, may be valuable in achieving more complete measurement.

Not all tests should be considered mandatory. Administrators are urged to conduct only such tests as are appropriate to their needs, whatever the capabilities of their personnel and facilities.

Administrators desiring a convenient single index should follow the basic test procedures, then scale their results in standard score form before averaging them. An alternative method, namely, arbitrarily weighting the standard scores, can be used to reflect the administrators' belief in the relative importance of the different tests. Additionally the profile method of graphic representation of scores may be used. There are advantages in the latter method, for it should be noted that the use of a single index has the defect of sacrificing the diagnostic values of the individual tests which are obviously masked in a composite score.

84.0. General Remarks

The performance tests that are listed are demanding; that is one of the reasons they have been selected. In consequence, it is important to ensure that those attempting the tests are healthy and sufficiently well prepared to avoid risk of overstrain, particularly for the distance run.

The basic performance test is recommended for ages 6 to 32 years only. Further study is needed for performance tests for other age groups.

The importance of motivation cannot be overemphasized. Attention, interest, and effort all contribute to reliable results. The subject must be fully acquainted with the details of the tests and understand clearly the objectives behind their administration.

Metric scales are used throughout. Conversions between metric and British systems may be found in Appendix E.

It is recommended that the test battery be given on two separate days. When this is done, tests described in paragraphs 85.0, 86.0, and 87.0 (sprint, long jump, and distance run) should be given on one day and tests described in paragraphs 88.0, 89.0, 90.0, 91.0, 92.0, and 93.0 (grip, pull-ups, shuttle run, sit-ups, and trunk forward flexion) on the other. If all the tests are given on one day, the order of testing may be preserved with one exception: the distance run should be conducted last.

The subjects should be in suitable dress, for example, light shorts, vest, and preferably rubber-soled shoes. Bare feet may be permitted. Spiked shoes must not be worn.

Anthropometric differences may be felt to influence some of the test items. To attempt to adjust administrative details to take account of these differences, however, would be impractical. It would involve arbitrary decisions and might not improve the comparability of scores. It is considered more desirable to use balanced judgment in the interpretation of individual or group results along with overall norms of performance.

All testers should be adequately trained in the details of the event prior to the test session. Such training should include demonstrations of the tests and practice trials.

Environmental information should be recorded. Details of this are given in the physiology section.

85.0. 50–Meter Sprint

85.1. Apparatus. Stop watches, tenth-second movement (one per time-keeper); accurately measured 50-m straight course; starter pistol (or visual device which must provide the timekeepers with a clear visual signal precisely coincident with the start); and finishing posts.

85.2. Test Description. On the signal "Take your marks" the subjects stand with their front feet behind the starting line (that is, the crouch start is not to be used). When ready (and still) the starting signal is given. The subjects sprint the required distance, avoiding any tendency to decelerate in anticipation of the finish.

85.3. Score. Time, to the nearest tenth of a second.

85.4. General Guide and Comments. *85.41.* A regulation starting pistol should be used for the start. Where this is impractical, a visual signal should be made to coincide precisely with the starting signal so that the timekeepers, standing at the finishing post, can react to the visual cue. It must be realized of course, that this procedure may introduce gross errors.

85.42. One attempt only is allowed.

85.43. Subjects run in groups of two or more, but each runner should be timed by a stop watch. (*Note:* An alert and experienced timekeeper may be able to time two runners at the same time using a split-hand watch if he is assigned to two runners of markedly different ability.)

85.44. The course should be flat, straight, in reasonable condition, and be subdivided into separate lanes.

85.45. The weather should be such as to ensure normal, comparable results, that is, relatively windless, and with no extremes of temperature.

86.0. Standing Long Jump

86.1. Apparatus. A flat nonslip surface with a marked take-off line, tape measure, and large T-square. (Fasten the tape measure to the floor, immediately adjacent to the nonslip surface, so that the distance jumped can be read off directly.)

86.2. Test Description. The subject stands with toes just behind the take-off line and jumps when ready. After making a preparatory backward swing with both arms, he swings his arms forward vigorously, springing from both feet simultaneously to jump as far forward as possible.

86.3. Score. The score is the distance jumped, in centimeters, in the better of two attempts.

86.4. General Guide and Comments. *86.41.* The distance jumped is measured from the start line to the rearmost point of contact of the heels. If the subject should happen to overbalance backward and touch the floor with some other part of his body, the trial becomes void and a fresh attempt should be given.

86.42. The feet must remain in contact with the ground behind the start line until the moment of take-off.

87.0. Distance Run

87.1. Apparatus. Stop watches, one for each timekeeper, and an accurately measured course. (Measure the course along a line 15 cm from the innermost edge of the lane.)

87.2. Test Description. This test differs for men, women, and children in only one respect—the distance to be run. In all other ways it is identical.

Distances: Men and boys 12 years and over   2000 or 1000 m
             Women and girls 12 years and over   1500 or 800
             Children under 12 years   600 m

On the signal, "Take your marks" the subjects stand with their front feet behind the starting line. When ready and motionless they are given the command, "Go" and run the required distance in the fastest time possible. Walking is permitted when necessary.

87.3. Score. The score is the time, to the nearest second, needed to complete the course.

87.4. General Guide and Comments. *87.41.* The run should be timed, preferably with a stop watch. Alternatively, reliable results can be secured with the mass testing techniques described in Appendix G.

87.42. The track should be flat and in reasonable, firm condition.

87.43. Weather conditions should ensure normal, comparable results. Extremes of conditions should be avoided.

87.44. The runs conducted over the longer distances have the greater significance as physiological tests of aerobic power if they are performed with maximum effort.

88.0. Grip Strength

88.1. Apparatus. Grip dynamometer, block of magnesium chalk, and recorder's table and chair.

88.2. Test Description. The subject, with hand chalked, takes the dynamometer comfortably in the appropriate hand, holding it in line with the forearm and letting it hang down by the thigh. The second joint of the fingers should fit snugly under the handle and take the weight of the instrument. It is then gripped between the fingers and the palm at the base of the thumb. When firmly gripped it is held away from the body and squeezed vigorously, the subject exerting the maximum force of which he is capable.

88.3. Score. The strength is recorded in kilograms.

88.4. General Guide and Comments. *88.41.* Readings should be taken on the preferred hand only.

88.42. Two trials should be allowed, each score being noted. Only the better result counts.

88.43. During the test neither the hand nor the dynamometer must be permitted to contact the body or any other object. If it does so, the trial should immediately be declared void and a fresh trial be given.

88.44. The arm should not be swung or pumped violently. This may spuriously increase the recorded score.

88.45. An adjustable grip dynamometer of a reliable make should be used.

88.46. Motivation is most important. The full and concentrated effort of each subject is required if the scores obtained are to be a true record of his maximum strength at the time of the test.

88.47. Dynamometers should be recalibrated, for example, by hanging known weights from them, before the testing program begins.

89.0. *Pull-Ups*

This test is used for men and boys 12 years of age and over.

89.1. Apparatus. Horizontal beam or bar 2–5 cm diameter, stool, and block of magnesium chalk.

Note: The beam/bar should be set high enough so that the tallest subject will be fully suspended.

89.2. Test Description. The subject steps from an adjacent stool to clasp the horizontal bar with overgrasp (palms facing forward), hands shoulder width apart, hangs at arm's length, feet clear of the floor. When in position and still, the signal "Go" is given. The subject flexes his arms and raises his body until his chin is pulled just above the level of the bar. Without delay the arms are relaxed and the body is lowered back to the starting position until the arms are completely straight. This procedure is repeated continuously as many times as possible.

89.3. Score. The score is the number of times the chin is raised above the bar.

89.4. General Guide and Comments. *89.41.* Each subject is given one trial only.

89.42. The test stops:

1. If the subject pauses for any appreciable time, that is, for 2 sec or more.
2. If the subject fails to raise his chin above the bar on two successive attempts.

89.43. The subject must not be allowed to gain advantage by swinging or kicking the legs. This tendency can be checked if the test administrator holds an outstretched arm across the thighs or stands closely in front of the subject.

89.44. Several subjects may be tested at the same time by using a partner-judge system, as long as overall supervision is adequate and reliable.

90.0. *Flexed-Arm Hang*

This test is used for women, girls, and for children under 12 years of age.

90.1. Apparatus. Horizontal beam or bar 2–5 cm in diameter, stool, and block of magnesium chalk.

Note: The beam/bar should be set high enough so that the tallest subject will be fully suspended.

90.2. Test Description. The subject steps from an adjacent stool to clasp the horizontal bar or beam with overgrasp (palms facing forward), arms fully flexed, with chin just above the bar. When in position and ready, the command "Go" is given and the subject removes the last supporting foot from the stool and hangs with arms flexed. The chin is held just above the bar or beam for as long as possible.

90.3. Score. Time the position is held, in seconds.

90.4. General Guide and Comments. *90.41.* The chin must be kept above and clear of the bar or beam. Once the chin comes to rest on, or passes underneath it, the test finishes.

90.42. The feet must not be in contact with any support.

91.0. *Shuttle Run*

91.1. Apparatus. Stop watch, tenth-second movement; flat course of 10 m measured between two parallel base lines; two 50-cm radius semicircles behind, but with centers on, the base lines; two wood blocks (5 × 5 × 5 cm); and recorder's table and chair.

91.2. Test Description. On the signal "Take your marks" the subject stands with his front foot behind the starting line. When ready, the command "Go" is given, and the subject sprints toward the other line 10 m away, picks up one of the two blocks of wood which are positioned in the circle, and runs back to place the block in the start circle. The block must not be thrown. Without pause, the subject sprints back again and returns with the second block which he grounds in the start circle to end the test.

91.3. Score. Time, to the nearest tenth of a second, when the second block is grounded in the circle.

91.4. General Guide and Comments. *91.41.* Two attempts shall be made and the better time recorded.

91.42. The timekeeper declares the run void if the block is thrown or dropped into the circle. It must be properly grounded. A repeat run should be given.

91.43. The course should be flat and in good condition and should not be slippery.

92.0. 30-*Sec Sit-Ups*

92.1. Apparatus. Stop watch; mat; and partner.

92.2. Test Description. The subject lies on his back on the mat or on a flat surface with feet about 30 cm apart and knees flexed at a right angle. The hands with fingers interlocked are placed on the back of the neck. A partner kneels at the subject's feet and presses down on the subject's insteps to keep the heels in contact with the floor or mat. When ready, the signal "Go" is given and the subject sits up to touch his knees with his elbows. Without pause he returns to the starting position just long enough for his back and hands to touch the mat and immediately sits up again. He repeats the procedure as rapidly as he can for 30 sec.

92.3. Score. The score is the number of sit-ups completed in 30 sec.

92.4. General Guide and Comments. *92.41.* Subjects work in pairs with one partner holding the ankles down, the heels being in contact with the mat or floor at all times.

92.42. The fingers must remain in contact and interlocked behind the back of the neck for the duration of the test.

92.43. The knees must remain bent approximately at a right angle for the duration of the test.

92.44. The back must return each time to its original position so that the locked fingers make contact with the surface. The test is best conducted on a soft surface such as a mat or grass.

92.45. Using an elbow to push up must not be permitted.

92.46. The subject shall try to keep going without pausing, but he should not be disqualified if some pauses are necessary.

92.47. Several subjects may be tested at the same time by using a partner-judge system as long as overall supervision is adequate and reliable.

93.0. *Trunk Forward Flexion* (*Sitting*)

93.1. Apparatus. A fixed vertical footrest, 35 cm high, set at least 50 cm from a wall; a calibrated board, or solid ruler (marked from 0 to 100 cm); and a sliding wooden marker.

93.2. Test Description. The subject sits with knees extended, soles of feet placed flat against the vertical surface of the fixed support. Keeping his knees fully extended (with the assistance of the test administrator if necessary), he bends forward and reaches (without jerking) as far forward as possible. The position of maximum flexion is held for approximately 2 sec. The test is repeated twice.

93.3. Score. The better of the two scores is recorded in centimeters.

93.4. General Guide and Comments. *93.41.* The ruler is placed parallel to the floor with the 50-cm mark level with the anterior face of the vertical support. The zero mark falls near the level of the subject's knees. With this arrangement, greater flexion during testing is associated with higher scores.

93.42. Readings may be made with the aid of a sliding marker on the calibrated board or ruler.

93.43. Any attempt in which the knees flex is void. No jerking movements are allowed. Only the maximum reach that can be held temporarily is recorded as the flexion score.

94.0. *Trunk Forward Flexion (Standing)*

94.1. Apparatus. One platform or chair; a calibrated board, or solid ruler (marked from 0 to 100 cm); and a sliding wooden marker.

94.2. Test Description. The subject stands with his toes on the edge of the platform with his feet together. Keeping his knees fully extended (with the assistance of the test administrator if necessary) he bends forward and attempts to reach as far down as possible. The maximum flexion position is held for approximately 2 sec. The test is repeated twice.

94.3. Score. The better of the two scores is recorded in centimeters.

94.4. General Guide and Comments. *94.41.* The calibrated board (or ruler) is attached perpendicular to the platform so that the 50-cm mark is level with its top surface. The zero mark of the board then falls near the level of the knees of the subject. With this arrangement greater flexion during testing is associated with higher scores.

94.42. Readings may be made with the aid of a sliding marker attached to the calibrated board or ruler.

94.43. Any attempt in which the knees flex is void. No jerking movement is allowed. Only the maximum reach that can be temporarily held is recorded as a score.

PHYSICAL PERFORMANCE TESTS

Family name: _____

First name, other initials: _____

	DATA CARD 12

Card serial number: _____ | 1 | 2 | (1–2)

Study number, Subject identity number:_____ (3–6)

Examining body:_____ (7–9)

Date of examination:_____/_____/19_____ (11–15)

Date of birth:_____/_____/19_____ (16–20)

Age:_____/_____ (21–24)

Sporting Record:_____ (25–27)

_____ (28–30)

(For other details see other sections).

	Trial 1	Trial 2	
50-meter sprint ($\frac{1}{10}$ sec)	_____	_____	(32–33)
Standing long jump (cm)	_____	_____	(35–37)
Distance run (sec) 2000 m		_____	(39–41)
1500 m		_____	(43–45)
1000 m		_____	(47–49)
800 m		_____	(51–53)
600 m		_____	(55–57)
Grip strength (kg)	_____	_____	(59–60)
Pull-ups (number)	_____	_____	(62–63)
Flexed-arm hang (sec)	_____	_____	(65–67)
Shuttle run ($\frac{1}{10}$ sec)	_____	_____	(69–71)
30-sec sit-ups (number)	_____	_____	(73–74)
Trunk flexion (standing)	_____	_____	(76–77)
Trunk flexion (sitting)	_____	_____	(79–80)

Appendices

Appendix A

Table of Decimals of a Year

	1 Jan.	2 Feb.	3 Mar.	4 Apr.	5 May	6 June	7 July	8 Aug.	9 Sept.	10 Oct.	11 Nov.	12 Dec.
1	000	085	162	247	329	414	496	581	666	748	833	915
2	003	088	164	249	332	416	499	584	668	751	836	918
3	005	090	167	252	334	419	501	586	671	753	838	921
4	008	093	170	255	337	422	504	589	674	756	841	923
5	011	096	173	258	340	425	507	592	677	759	844	926
6	014	099	175	260	342	427	510	595	679	762	847	929
7	016	101	178	263	345	430	512	597	682	764	849	932
8	019	104	181	266	348	433	515	600	685	767	862	934
9	022	107	184	268	351	436	518	603	688	770	855	937
10	025	110	186	271	353	438	521	605	690	773	858	940
11	027	112	189	274	356	441	523	608	693	775	860	942
12	030	115	192	277	359	444	526	611	696	778	863	945
13	033	118	195	279	362	447	529	614	699	781	866	948
14	036	121	197	282	364	449	532	616	701	784	868	951
15	038	123	200	285	367	452	534	619	704	786	871	953
16	041	126	203	288	370	455	537	622	707	789	874	956
17	044	129	205	290	373	458	540	625	710	792	877	959
18	047	132	208	293	375	460	542	627	712	795	879	962
19	049	134	211	296	378	463	545	630	715	797	882	964
20	052	137	214	299	381	466	548	633	718	800	885	967
21	055	140	216	301	384	468	551	636	721	803	888	970
22	058	142	219	304	386	471	553	638	723	805	890	973
23	060	145	222	307	389	474	556	641	726	808	893	975
24	063	148	225	310	392	477	559	644	729	811	896	978
25	066	151	227	312	395	479	562	647	731	814	899	981
26	068	153	230	315	397	482	564	649	734	816	901	984
27	071	156	233	318	400	485	567	652	737	819	904	986
28	074	159	236	321	403	488	570	655	740	822	907	989
29	077		238	323	405	490	573	658	742	825	910	992
30	079		241	326	408	493	575	660	745	827	912	995
31	082		244		411		578	663		830		997

Jan. 1	Feb. 2	Mar. 3	Apr. 4	May 5	June 6	July 7	Aug. 8	Sept. 9	Oct. 10	Nov. 11	Dec. 12

Age (in decimals) = Date of examination (decimals) − Date of birth (decimals)

Example:

Date of examination: 17th October 1968 = 68.792
Date of birth: 20th July 1946 = 46.548

Age at time of examination = 22.244 years—*to the nearest day*

Appendix B

GUIDE TO THE CLASSIFICATION OF TYPES OF WORK

Classification of Types of Work

Sedentary Work

School work, office work, drawing, weaving, and so on.

Light Work

Housework, laboratory work, panel operators, dispatchers, crane operators, handling of transport means (without loading), assembly work, picking hops by hand, and so on.

Medium-Light to Medium-Heavy Work

Work carried out in industry and agriculture on machines; alternately sitting, standing, and possibly walking for exercise, machine ploughing and harvesting, mechanized work (cutting with power saw), mechanized work in the mines, work on heavier machine tools, assembly of heavy objects, machine forging, transport of medium-heavy loads for a short distance.

Heavy Work

Work carried out by large muscle groups during prolonged periods, loading and transport of heavy loads (for example, carrying meat at the slaughterhouse, carrying of sacks, loading wood by hand) wood cutting in the forest by hand tools, agricultural work in mountain regions, grain harvesting by hand, manual work in the mines, timbering in the mines, work with the pneumatic pick, excavation by hand, and so on.

Appendix C

Guide to the Classification of Ethnic Groups

Item	Mongoloid = 1	Negroid = 2	Caucasian = 3	Mixed = 4
Skin	Clear or slightly yellowish	Dark	White to nut brown	?
Hair	Dark; straight and tough	Dark; curly	Dark or fair; straight to wavy	?
Epicanthus	Present	Absent	Absent	?
Nose	Small to large	Small	Large	?
Lips	Middle to thick	Thick to very thick	Narrow to middle	?
Axis of nostrils	Middle	Transverse	Longitudinal	?
Angle of horizontal profile	Great	Middle	Small	?

Appendix D

GUIDE TO CARDIAC INVESTIGATIONS

1. Auscultation and Palpation of the Heart

The examination should be conducted in a quiet, comfortably warm room with the subject supine, arms, and legs fully supported.

In palpation, the beat may exhibit thrills or changes of force. A forceful apex beat means a heaving heart. A forceful thrust left of the sternum means a forcing precordial pulsation. The thrills may be systolic, diastolic, apical, precordial, pulmonic, or aortic.

In auscultation there may be (1) amplitude changes with first or second sounds too loud or too soft, (2) extra sounds such as galloping, clicking, slapping, or there may be (3) murmurs. The most frequent changes are

1. Accentuated A_2
   Accentuated P_2
   Accentuated M_1
   Accentuated M_1 and P_2
   Diminished or absent A_2
   Diminished or absent P_2
   All sounds dampened

2. Gallop
   Third heart sound
   Opening snap
   Systolic click in pulmonary area
   Systolic click in aortic area

3a. Systolic murmurs
   Maximal intensity—apical
                    midprecordial
                    pulmonic
                    aortic

   Soft (1–2 grades)
   Medium (3–4 grades)
   Very loud (5–6 grades)
   Type—pansystolic
          protosystolic
          mezosystolic
          diamond shaped

3b. Diastolic murmurs
   Maximal intensity—apical
                        midprecordial
                        pulmonic
                        aortic
   Type—protodiastolic
         decrescendo
         middiastolic or
         presystolic
3c. Systolo-diastolic murmurs
    Pulmonic area
    Precordial
    Other

2. Blood Pressure Measurements

Both systolic and diastolic blood pressure should be taken using a mercury manometer.*

With the clothing around the arm and shoulder sufficiently removed, attach the cuff, 14 cm wide, firmly and evenly to either arm about 2 cm above the antecubital space. The rubber bag should be centered over the course of the brachial artery. The inflated cuff should not compress the underlying tissue.

The cuff is rapidly inflated to a point 20–30 mm Hg above the pressure at which the radial pulse is obliterated. The stethoscope is applied immediately below the edge of the cuff over the area where the brachial artery pulse is palpable. Cuff pressure is then permitted to fall at a rate of not more than 2–3 mm Hg per pulse-beat, and the point of first appearance of an audible pulse-beat is recorded as the *systolic pressure*. The cuff pressure is permitted to fall further, and the sound will commonly be noted to become quite suddenly muffled and shortly to disappear. Until it becomes clear which phase more correctly represents the diastolic value both pressures should be recorded as *diastolic pressure*.

3. Heart Volume

Apparatus
Radiographic apparatus
Ancillary equipment

Description
Three variables are necessary for the calculation of cardiac volume. They are obtained by teleroentgenography in the frontal and sagittal planes with the patient in the prone position. (See Figures A, B, and C.)

* World Health Organization Technical Report Series, No. 231, pp. 4–5, 1962.

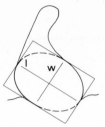

Figure A. Vertical (*l*) and horizontal (*w*) diameters of the heart.

For the film in the frontal plane the cassette is placed close to the heart in front of the sternum; for the sagittal film it is placed directly against the left side of the thorax. The films are exposed in rapid succession, independently, ideally at maximum diastole and in the midinspiratory phase by employing synchronizing electronic double triggering mechanisms. To preclude a Valsalva effect, the subject's mouth remains open. No significant variations in volume occur between the prone and the supine position. In the prone position the frontal area is larger, whereas the anteroposterior diameter is smaller than in the supine position. In the prone position the heart is in broader contact with the anterior chest wall. Its volume, however, is not greater than in the supine position as might be wrongly assumed from the frontal view alone. Therefore, the two required film exposures can be made either in the prone or in the supine position. Before the picture is taken the person will swallow a dose of barium to outline the esophageal mucosa against the posterior border of the heart.

Calculations

The formula for determining heart volume is based on the assumption that the volume of a body of any shape is equal to the sum of the surface area of a parallel projection of the body and its mean linear expansion in the direction of the projection. The surface area is obtained from the ortho-diagram. The mean expansion (depth) in the direction of the projection can only be measured indirectly, as it depends upon the shape of the body. The

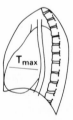

Figure B. The longest anteroposterior diameter (T_{max}).

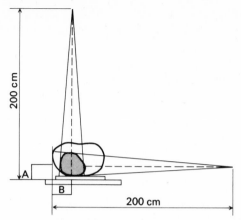

Figure C. The technique used to obtain the radiographs shown in Figures A and B with the heart in the frontal and sagittal planes. In adults the distances assumed for *A* and *B*, respectively, are 10 cm and 20 cm.

mass of the heart is most closely represented by a spheroid body (sphere, ellipsoid) and a constant (K), which is characteristic for the shape of the heart. Thus the Rohrer-Kahlstorf formula is

$$\text{Vol} = K \times Fa \times T_{\max}$$

This means that the heart volume is equal to 0.63 times the product of the area of the frontal (anteroposterior) orthodiagram (*Fa*) and of the greatest depth of the lateral (sagittal) orthodiagram ($T_{\max}$). Heart area can be determined either by planimetry or according to the formula of the area of an ellipse.

$$Fa = \frac{\pi}{4} \times l \times w$$

(where l = the length and w = the width of the area) (Figure A). The difference between the calculated and the planimetrically measured area is less than 3%. On substituting teleroentgenography for the orthodiagraphic method, the projectional error must be corrected. Assuming a focus-to-film distance of 2 m in the frontal and lateral pictures, with a uniform heart-film distance of 10 cm for the frontal, and one of 20 cm for the lateral picture the following formula applies:

$$\text{Vol} = 0.63 \times \frac{\pi}{4} \times \frac{200 - 10}{200} \times l \times w \times \frac{200 - 20}{200} T_{\max}$$

$$= 0.40 \times l \times w \times T_{\max}$$

where l is the length and w is the width of Moritz' cardiac quadrangle, T_{max} is the largest horizontal (depth) diameter of the heart. In children the distance between film and heart is smaller, and therefore the error of the projection larger. The constant (K), for instance, in children 10 years old is 0.42, in children 6 years 0.44.

The relative heart volume is expressed as the ratio of heart volume and body weight: HV/kp.

Example for calculation: Body weight 74 kp, $w = 11.0$, $l = 13.0$ cm, $T_{max} = 14.0$

$$HV = 0.40 \times 11.0 \times 13.0 \times 14.0 = 800.80 \text{ ml}$$
$$HV/kp = 801/74 = 10.8$$

General Guide and Comments

The heart volume measurement allows estimations to be made of the influence of training on the work and load-carrying capacity of men generally and of athletes in particular.

The accuracy of the method has been reexamined several times. Its error in comparative studies is between 3 and 5% in the model, in living subjects, and in cadavers.

Appendix E

Height Conversion Table—Inches to Millimeters

Inches	.0	.1	.2	.3	.4	.5	.6	.7	.8	.9
0	0	3	5	8	10	13	15	18	20	23
1	25	28	30	33	36	38	41	43	46	48
2	51	53	56	58	61	64	66	69	71	74
3	76	79	81	84	86	89	91	94	97	99
4	102	104	107	109	112	114	117	119	122	124
5	127	130	132	135	137	140	142	145	147	150
6	152	155	157	160	163	165	168	170	173	175
7	178	180	183	185	188	190	193	196	198	201
8	203	206	208	211	213	216	218	221	224	226
9	229	231	234	236	239	241	244	246	249	251
10	254	257	259	262	264	267	269	272	274	277
11	279	282	284	287	290	292	295	297	300	302
12	305	307	310	312	315	317	320	323	325	328
13	330	333	335	338	340	343	345	348	351	353
14	356	358	361	363	366	368	371	373	376	378
15	381	384	386	389	391	394	396	399	401	404
16	406	409	411	414	417	419	422	424	427	429
17	432	434	437	439	442	444	447	450	452	455
18	457	460	462	465	467	470	472	475	478	480
19	483	485	488	490	493	495	498	500	503	505
20	508	511	513	516	518	521	523	526	528	531
21	533	536	538	541	544	546	549	551	554	556
22	559	561	564	566	569	572	574	577	579	582
23	584	587	589	592	594	597	599	602	605	607
24	610	612	615	617	620	622	625	627	630	632
25	635	638	640	643	645	648	650	653	655	658
26	660	663	665	668	671	673	676	678	681	683
27	686	688	691	693	696	699	701	704	706	709
28	711	714	716	719	721	724	726	729	732	734
29	737	739	742	744	747	749	752	754	757	759
30	762	765	767	770	772	775	777	780	782	785
31	787	790	792	795	798	800	803	805	808	810
32	813	815	818	820	823	826	828	831	833	836
33	838	841	843	846	848	851	853	856	859	861
34	864	866	869	871	874	876	879	881	884	886
35	889	892	894	897	899	902	904	907	909	912
36	914	917	919	922	925	927	930	932	935	937
37	940	942	945	947	950	953	955	958	960	963
38	965	968	970	973	975	978	980	983	986	988
39	991	993	996	998	1001	1003	1006	1008	1011	1013

Height Conversion (*continued*)

Inches	.0	.1	.2	.3	.4	.5	.6	.7	.8	.9
40	1016	1019	1021	1024	1026	1029	1031	1034	1036	1039
41	1041	1044	1046	1049	1052	1054	1057	1059	1062	1064
42	1067	1069	1072	1074	1077	1080	1082	1085	1087	1090
43	1092	1095	1097	1100	1102	1105	1107	1110	1113	1115
44	1118	1120	1123	1125	1128	1130	1133	1135	1138	1140
45	1143	1146	1148	1151	1153	1156	1158	1161	1163	1166
46	1168	1171	1173	1176	1179	1181	1184	1186	1189	1191
47	1194	1196	1199	1201	1204	1207	1209	1212	1214	1217
48	1219	1222	1224	1227	1229	1232	1234	1237	1240	1242
49	1245	1247	1250	1252	1255	1257	1260	1262	1265	1267
50	1270	1273	1275	1278	1280	1283	1285	1288	1290	1293
51	1295	1298	1300	1303	1306	1308	1311	1313	1316	1318
52	1321	1323	1326	1328	1331	1334	1336	1339	1341	1344
53	1346	1349	1351	1354	1356	1359	1361	1364	1367	1369
54	1372	1374	1377	1379	1382	1384	1387	1389	1392	1394
55	1397	1400	1402	1405	1407	1410	1412	1415	1417	1420
56	1422	1425	1427	1430	1433	1435	1438	1440	1443	1445
57	1448	1450	1453	1455	1458	1461	1463	1466	1468	1471
58	1473	1476	1478	1481	1483	1486	1488	1491	1494	1496
59	1499	1501	1504	1506	1509	1511	1514	1516	1519	1521
60	1524	1527	1529	1532	1534	1537	1539	1542	1544	1547
61	1549	1552	1554	1557	1560	1562	1565	1567	1570	1572
62	1575	1577	1580	1582	1585	1588	1590	1593	1595	1598
63	1600	1603	1605	1608	1610	1613	1615	1618	1621	1623
64	1626	1628	1631	1633	1636	1638	1641	1643	1646	1648
65	1651	1654	1656	1659	1661	1664	1666	1669	1671	1674
66	1676	1679	1681	1684	1687	1689	1692	1694	1697	1699
67	1702	1704	1707	1709	1712	1715	1717	1720	1722	1725
68	1727	1730	1732	1735	1737	1740	1742	1745	1748	1750
69	1753	1755	1758	1760	1763	1765	1768	1770	1773	1775
70	1778	1781	1783	1786	1788	1791	1793	1796	1798	1801
71	1803	1806	1808	1811	1814	1816	1819	1821	1824	1826
72	1829	1831	1834	1836	1839	1842	1844	1847	1849	1852
73	1854	1857	1859	1862	1864	1867	1869	1872	1875	1877
74	1880	1882	1885	1887	1890	1892	1895	1897	1900	1902
75	1905	1908	1910	1913	1915	1918	1920	1923	1925	1928
76	1930	1933	1935	1938	1941	1943	1946	1948	1951	1953
77	1956	1958	1961	1963	1966	1968	1971	1974	1976	1979
78	1981	1984	1986	1989	1991	1994	1996	1999	2002	2004
79	2007	2009	2012	2014	2017	2019	2022	2024	2027	2029

Height Conversion (*continued*)

Inches	.0	.1	.2	.3	.4	.5	.6	.7	.8	.9
80	2032	2035	2037	2040	2042	2045	2047	2050	2052	2055
81	2057	2060	2062	2065	2068	2070	2073	2075	2078	2080
82	2083	2085	2088	2090	2093	2095	2098	2101	2103	2106
83	2108	2111	2113	2116	2118	2121	2123	2126	2129	2131
84	2134	2136	2139	2141	2144	2146	2149	2151	2154	2156
85	2159	2162	2164	2167	2169	2172	2174	2177	2179	2182
86	2184	2187	2189	2192	2195	2197	2200	2202	2205	2207
87	2210	2212	2215	2217	2220	2222	2225	2228	2230	2233
88	2235	2238	2240	2243	2245	2248	2250	2253	2256	2258
89	2261	2263	2266	2268	2271	2273	2276	2278	2281	2283
90	2286	2289	2291	2294	2296	2299	2301	2304	2306	2309
91	2311	2314	2316	2319	2322	2324	2327	2329	2332	2334
92	2337	2339	2342	2344	2347	2349	2352	2355	2357	2360
93	2362	2365	2367	2370	2372	2375	2377	2380	2383	2385
94	2388	2390	2393	2395	2398	2400	2403	2405	2408	2410
95	2413	2416	2418	2421	2423	2426	2428	2431	2433	2436
96	2438	2441	2443	2446	2449	2451	2454	2456	2459	2461
97	2464	2466	2469	2471	2474	2476	2479	2482	2484	2487
98	2489	2492	2494	2497	2499	2502	2504	2507	2510	2512
99	2515	2517	2520	2522	2525	2527	2530	2532	2535	2537
100	2540	2543	2545	2548	2550	2553	2555	2558	2560	2563

Weight Conversion Table—Kilograms to Pounds

Kilograms	.0	.1	.2	.3	.4	.5	.6	.7	.8	.9
0	0.0	0.2	0.4	0.7	0.9	1.1	1.3	1.5	1.8	2.0
1	2.2	2.4	2.6	2.9	3.1	3.3	3.5	3.7	4.0	4.2
2	4.4	4.6	4.9	5.1	5.3	5.5	5.7	6.0	6.2	6.4
3	6.6	6.8	7.1	7.3	7.5	7.7	7.9	8.2	8.4	8.6
4	8.8	9.0	9.3	9.5	9.7	9.9	10.1	10.4	10.6	10.8
5	11.0	11.2	11.5	11.7	11.9	12.1	12.3	12.6	12.8	13.0
6	13.2	13.4	13.7	13.9	14.1	14.3	14.6	14.8	15.0	15.2
7	15.4	15.7	15.9	16.1	16.3	16.5	16.8	17.0	17.2	17.4
8	17.6	17.9	18.1	18.3	18.5	18.7	19.0	19.2	19.4	19.6
9	19.8	20.1	20.3	20.5	20.7	20.9	21.2	21.4	21.6	21.8
10	22.0	22.3	22.5	22.7	22.9	23.1	23.4	23.6	23.8	24.0
11	24.3	24.5	24.7	24.9	25.1	25.4	25.6	25.8	26.0	26.2
12	26.5	26:7	26.9	27.1	27.3	27.6	27.8	28.0	28.2	28.4
13	28.7	28.9	29.1	29.3	29.5	29.8	30.0	30.2	30.4	30.6
14	30.9	31.1	31.3	31.5	31.7	32.0	32.2	32.4	32.6	32.8
15	33.1	33.3	33.5	33.7	34.0	34.2	34.4	34.6	34.8	35.1
16	35.3	35.5	35.7	35.9	36.2	36.4	36.6	36.8	37.0	37.3
17	37.5	37.7	37.9	38.1	38.4	38.6	38.8	39.0	39.2	39.5
18	39.7	39.9	40.1	40.3	40.6	40.8	41.0	41.2	41.4	41.7
19	41.9	42.1	42.3	42.5	42.8	43.0	43.2	43.4	43.7	43.9
20	44.1	44.3	44.5	44.8	45.0	45.2	45.4	45.6	45.9	46.1
21	46.3	46.5	46.7	47.0	47.2	47.4	47.6	47.8	48.1	48.3
22	48.5	48.7	48.9	49.2	49.4	49.6	49.8	50.0	50.3	50.5
23	50.7	50.9	51.1	51.4	51.6	51.8	52.0	52.2	52.5	52.7
24	52.9	53.1	53.4	53.6	53.8	54.0	54.2	54.5	54.7	54.9
25	55.1	55.3	55.6	55.8	56.0	56.2	56.4	56.7	56.9	57.1
26	57.3	57.5	57.8	58.0	58.2	58.4	58.6	58.9	59.1	59.3
27	59.5	59.7	60.0	60.2	60.4	60.6	60.8	61.1	61.3	61.5
28	61.7	61.9	62.2	62.4	62.6	62.8	63.1	63.3	63.5	63.7
29	63.9	64.2	64.4	64.6	64.8	65.0	65.3	65.5	65.7	65.9
30	66.1	66.4	66.6	66.8	67.0	67.2	67.5	67.7	67.9	68.1
31	68.3	68.6	68.8	69.0	69.2	69.4	69.7	69.9	70.1	70.3
32	70.5	70.8	71.0	71.2	71.4	71.6	71.9	72.1	72.3	72.5
33	72.8	73.0	73.2	73.4	73.6	73.9	74.1	74.3	74.5	74.7
34	75.0	75.2	75.4	75.6	75.8	76.1	76.3	76.5	76.7	76.9
35	77.2	77.4	77.6	77.8	78.0	78.3	78.5	78.7	78.9	79.1
36	79.4	79.6	79.8	80.0	80.2	80.5	80.7	80.9	81.1	81.3
37	81.6	81.8	82.0	82.2	82.5	82.7	82.9	83.1	83.3	83.6
38	83.8	84.0	84.2	84.4	84.7	84.9	85.1	85.3	85.5	85.8
39	86.0	86.2	86.4	86.6	86.9	87.1	87.3	87.5	87.7	88.0

Weight Conversion (*continued*)

Kilograms	.0	.1	.2	.3	.4	.5	.6	.7	.8	.9
40	88.2	88.4	88.6	88.8	89.1	89.3	89.5	89.7	89.9	90.2
41	90.4	90.6	90.8	91.0	91.3	91.5	91.7	91.9	92.2	92.4
42	92.6	92.8	93.0	93.3	93.5	93.7	93.9	94.1	94.4	94.6
43	94.8	95.0	95.2	95.5	95.7	95.9	96.1	96.3	96.6	96.8
44	97.0	97.2	97.4	97.7	97.9	98.1	98.3	98.5	98.8	99.0
45	99.2	99.4	99.6	99.9	100.1	100.3	100.5	100.8	101.0	101.2
46	101.4	101.6	101.9	102.1	102.3	102.5	102.7	103.0	103.2	103.4
47	103.6	103.8	104.1	104.3	104.5	104.7	104.9	105.2	105.4	105.6
48	105.8	106.0	106.3	106.5	106.7	106.9	107.1	107.4	107.6	107.8
49	108.0	108.2	108.5	108.7	108.9	109.1	109.3	109.6	109.8	110.0
50	110.2	110.5	110.7	110.9	111.1	111.3	111.6	111.8	112.0	112.2
51	112.4	112.7	112.9	113.1	113.3	113.5	113.8	114.0	114.2	114.4
52	114.6	114.9	115.1	115.3	115.5	115.7	116.0	116.2	116.4	116.6
53	116.8	117.1	117.3	117.5	117.7	117.9	118.2	118.4	118.6	118.8
54	119.0	119.3	119.5	119.7	119.9	120.2	120.4	120.6	120.8	121.0
55	121.3	121.5	121.7	121.9	122.1	122.4	122.6	122.8	123.0	123.2
56	123.5	123.7	123.9	124.1	124.3	124.6	124.8	125.0	125.2	125.4
57	125.7	125.9	126.1	126.3	126.5	126.8	127.0	127.2	127.4	127.6
58	127.9	128.1	128.3	128.5	128.7	129.0	129.2	129.4	129.6	129.9
59	130.1	130.3	130.5	130.7	131.0	131.2	131.4	131.6	131.8	132.1
60	132.3	132.5	132.7	132.9	133.2	133.4	133.6	133.8	134.0	134.3
61	134.5	134.7	134.9	135.1	135.4	135.6	135.8	136.0	136.2	136.5
62	136.7	136.9	137.1	137.3	137.6	137.8	138.0	138.2	138.4	138.7
63	138.9	139.1	139.3	139.6	139.8	140.0	140.2	140.4	140.7	140.9
64	141.1	141.3	141.5	141.8	142.0	142.2	142.4	142.6	142.9	143.1
65	143.3	143.5	143.7	144.0	144.2	144.4	144.6	144.8	145.1	145.3
66	145.5	145.7	145.9	146.2	146.4	146.6	146.8	147.0	147.3	147.5
67	147.7	147.9	148.1	148.4	148.6	148.8	149.0	149.3	149.5	149.7
68	149.9	150.1	150.4	150.6	150.8	151.0	151.2	151.5	151.7	151.9
69	152.1	152.3	152.6	152.8	153.0	153.2	153.4	153.7	153.9	154.1
70	154.3	154.5	154.8	155.0	155.2	155.4	155.6	155.9	156.1	156.3
71	156.5	156.7	157.0	157.2	157.4	157.6	157.8	158.1	158.3	158.5
72	158.7	159.0	159.2	159.4	159.6	159.8	160.1	160.3	160.5	160.7
73	160.9	161.2	161.4	161.6	161.8	162.0	162.3	162.5	162.7	162.9
74	163.1	163.4	163.6	163.8	164.0	164.2	164.5	164.7	164.9	165.1
75	165.3	165.6	165.8	166.0	166.2	166.4	166.7	166.9	167.1	167.3
76	167.5	167.8	168.0	168.2	168.4	168.7	168.9	169.1	169.3	169.5
77	169.8	170.0	170.2	170.4	170.6	170.9	171.1	171.3	171.5	171.7
78	172.0	172.2	172.4	172.6	172.8	173.1	173.3	173.5	173.7	173.9
79	174.2	174.4	174.6	174.8	175.0	175.3	175.5	175.7	175.9	176.1

Weight Conversion (*continued*)

Kilograms	.0	.1	.2	.3	.4	.5	.6	.7	.8	.9
80	176.4	176.6	176.8	177.0	177.2	177.5	177.7	177.9	178.1	178.4
81	178.6	178.8	179.0	179.2	179.5	179.7	179.9	180.1	180.3	180.6
82	180.8	181.0	181.2	181.4	181.7	181.9	182.1	182.3	182.5	182.8
83	183.0	183.2	183.4	183.6	183.9	184.1	184.3	184.5	184.7	185.0
84	185.2	185.4	185.6	185.8	186.1	186.3	186.5	186.7	187.0	187.2
85	187.4	187.6	187.8	188.1	188.3	188.5	188.7	188.9	189.2	189.4
86	189.6	189.8	190.0	190.3	190.5	190.7	190.9	191.1	191.4	191.6
87	191.8	192.0	192.2	192.5	192.7	192.9	193.1	193.3	193.6	193.8
88	194.0	194.2	194.4	194.7	194.9	195.1	195.3	195.5	195.8	196.0
89	196.2	196.4	196.7	196.9	197.1	197.3	197.5	197.8	198.0	198.2
90	198.4	198.6	198.9	199.1	199.3	199.5	199.7	200.0	200.2	200.4
91	200.6	200.8	201.1	201.3	201.5	201.7	201.9	202.2	202.4	202.6
92	202.8	203.0	203.3	203.5	203.7	203.9	204.1	204.4	204.6	204.8
93	205.0	205.2	205.5	205.7	205.9	206.1	206.4	206.6	206.8	207.0
94	207.2	207.5	207.7	207.9	208.1	208.3	208.6	208.8	209.0	209.2
95	209.4	209.7	209.9	210.1	210.3	210.5	210.8	211.0	211.2	211.4
96	211.6	211.9	212.1	212.3	212.5	212.7	213.0	213.2	213.4	213.6
97	213.8	214.1	214.3	214.5	214.7	214.9	215.2	215.4	215.6	215.8
98	216.1	216.3	216.5	216.7	216.9	217.2	217.4	217.6	217.8	218.0
99	218.3	218.5	218.7	218.9	219.1	219.4	219.6	219.8	220.0	220.2
100	220.5	220.7	220.9	221.1	221.3	221.6	221.8	222.0	222.2	222.4
101	222.7	222.9	223.1	223.3	223.5	223.8	224.0	224.2	224.4	224.6
102	224.9	225.1	225.3	225.5	225.8	226.0	226.2	226.4	226.6	226.9
103	227.1	227.3	227.5	227.7	228.0	228.2	228.4	228.6	228.8	229.1
104	229.3	229.5	229.7	229.9	230.2	230.4	230.6	230.8	231.0	231.3
105	231.5	231.7	231.9	232.1	232.4	232.6	232.8	233.0	233.2	233.5
106	233.7	233.9	234.1	234.3	234.6	234.8	235.0	235.2	235.5	235.7
107	235.9	236.1	236.3	236.6	236.8	237.0	237.2	237.4	237.7	237.9
108	238.1	238.3	238.5	238.8	239.0	239.2	239.4	239.6	239.9	240.1
109	240.3	240.5	240.7	241.0	241.2	241.4	241.6	241.8	242.1	242.3
110	242.5	242.7	242.9	243.2	243.4	243.6	243.8	244.0	244.3	244.5
111	244.7	244.9	245.2	245.4	245.6	245.8	246.0	246.3	246.5	246.7
112	246.9	247.1	247.4	247.6	247.8	248.0	248.2	248.5	248.7	248.9
113	249.1	249.3	249.6	249.8	250.0	250.2	250.4	250.7	250.9	251.1
114	251.3	251.5	251.8	252.0	252.2	252.4	252.6	252.9	253.1	253.3
115	253.5	253.7	254.0	254.2	254.4	254.6	254.9	255.1	255.3	255.5
116	255.7	256.0	256.2	256.4	256.6	256.8	257.1	257.3	257.5	257.7
117	257.9	258.2	258.4	258.6	258.8	259.0	259.3	259.5	259.7	259.9
118	260.1	260.4	260.6	260.8	261.0	261.2	261.5	261.7	261.9	262.1
119	262.3	262.6	262.8	263.0	263.2	263.4	263.7	263.9	264.1	264.3
120	264.6	264.8	265.0	265.2	265.4	265.7	265.9	266.1	266.3	266.5

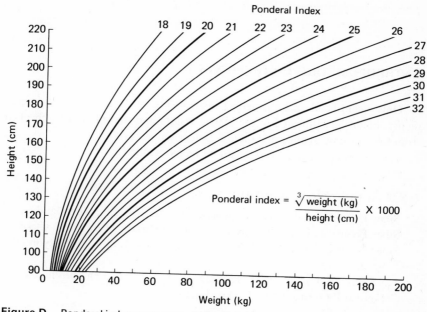

Figure D. Ponderal index nomogram. (After K.-I. Hirata : Ponderal index. A paper read at the International Conference of Sports Sciences, Munich, 1972.)

Appendix F

ANTHROPOMETRIC INSTRUMENTS

Only scientifically acknowledged instruments are to be used. All instruments should be calibrated in the metric system and they should be checked from time to time against a standard caliper gauge.

The following manufacturers can be recommended:

GPM Anthropological Instruments

Siber Hegner & Co. A.G., Talstrasse 14, 8022 Zurich, Switzerland

Siber Precision, Inc., 450 Barell Avenue, Carlstadt, N.J., 07072 U.S.A.

Siber Hegner & Cie-France S.A., 5, Quai Jean-Moulin, F-69 Lyon (1er) France

Siber Seiko K.K., Shin Kokusai Bldg. 4, Marunouchi 3-chome chiyoda-ku Central P.O. Box 1214, Tokyo, Japan

"Harpenden" and "Holtain" Instruments

Holtain Limited, Brynberian Nr. Crymmych, Pembrokeshire, U.K.

Siber Hegner & Co. A.G., Talstrasse 14, 8022 Zurich, Switzerland

"ABA" Instruments

ABA-Werk GmbH, Mullerstrasse 27-31, D18750 Aschaffenburg, Germany

Skinfold Calipers

Lange: Cambridge Scientific Industries, Inc., Cambridge, Massachusetts, U.S.A.

Prof. Venerardo Correnti: Instituto di Antropologia, Universita di Roma, Italy.

Appendix G

ALTERNATIVE MASS TESTING TECHNIQUES
FOR ENDURANCE RUN

A. Partner-Judge Method

1. Assign a partner-judge to each runner. The partner stands beside the timekeeper, in line with the finishing post.
2. The timekeeper, who has the only watch, counts out the time precisely in seconds. Each judge notes the time of arrival of his runner, and, when called upon to do so, announces this time to the recorder.

B. Funnel Touch Method

1. *Apparatus*

Stop watch
Subject list and timing forms
Pencil (and spare sharpened)
Two 16-m ropes and six high jump poles
One table and two chairs
Numbered index cards (as many as necessary)

2. *Procedure*

2.1. A team of four judges is required, one timekeeper, one recorder, one "toucher" and one scorer (numbers 1, 2, 3 and 4 in the following sketch, respectively).
2.2 A "funnelled" fence of ropes, tied between high jump poles, is installed on the finish line in the following way:

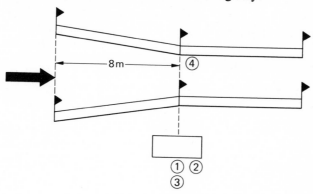

2.3 The timekeeper (No. 1) sits behind a desk at the finish line, about 1–2 m from the bottle neck. He has the only watch, and loudly counts the time precisely in seconds.

2.4 The recorder (No. 2) sits next to the timekeeper in line with the finish line and behind him stands the "toucher" (No. 3) who is facing the line.

2.5 The recorder has a few "timing forms" to record the time of each runner. Each form has four columns, each column represents one minute which is divided into 60 lines for 60 seconds (see example).

2.6 When the recorder sees the first runner approaching the finish line to complete the endurance run, he writes down the number of the minute the timekeeper counts on top of the first column, and then starts to follow with his pencil the "seconds" lines in the same column. If he needs more than 4 min he proceeds on a second form.

2.7 Each time a runner crosses the finish line in the entrance of the "bottle neck," the toucher (No. 3) taps lightly on the shoulder of the recorder. The recorder then makes a "minus" mark in the appropriate "seconds" line, which was reached by the point of his pencil at that moment. This procedure continues until the last runner finishes his run. The number of the "minus" marks should correspond to the number of runners.

2.8 At the same time, the scorer (No. 4), who stands near the finish line with a package of numbered index cards, gives one numbered card to each runner when he crosses the finish line. The first runner gets card No. 1, the second No. 2, and so on, and then they proceed to advance through the "bottle neck" and into a resting enclosure.

2.9 After all the runners complete the run, the recorder writes on the timing forms the order of arrival of the runners in the appropriate column near each minus mark. The first minus mark receives No. 1, the second No. 2 and so on.

2.10 The last step. The recorder calls the runners to present their numbered index cards, writes down on the "Subject list form" (see example) the name of each runner, and adds the appropriate time as it appears on the "timing form." This procedure can be done with the assistance of one of the other judges.

Runners List: Endurance Run

Place No.	Name	Time	Remarks
1			
2			
3			
4			
5			
6			
7			
8			
9			
10			
11			
12			
13			
14			
15			
16			
17			
18			
19			
20			

Timing Form: Endurance Run

Event:_____ Group:_____ Date:_____

Minute_____   Minute_____   Minute_____   Minute_____

Second Mark Place	Second Mark Place	Second Mark Place	Second Mark Place
1	1	1	1
2	2	2	2
3	3	3	3
4	4	4	4
5	5	5	5
6	6	6	6
7	7	7	7
8	8	8	8
9	9	9	9
⋮	⋮	⋮	⋮
47	47	47	47
48	48	48	48
49	49	49	49
50	50	50	50
51	51	51	51
52	52	52	52
53	53	53	53
54	54	54	54
55	55	55	55
56	56	56	56
57	57	57	57
58	58	58	58
59	59	59	59
60	60	60	60

Appendix H

Country	Name	Address
Australia	Corrigan, B.	1 Look-out Av., Dee way Sydney, Australia
Austria	Prokop, L.	Vienna 9, Kolingasse 6/34, Austria
Belgium	Bollaert, L. M.	10 Collegelaan Borgerhout, Belgium
	*Hebbelinck, M.	A. Buyllaan, 105 Bruxelles 5, Belgium
	Metivier, C.	Laboratoire de L'Effort 28, Ave. Paul Heger, Bruxelles 5, Belgium
Bulgaria	*Mateeff, D.	51 Skobelev Bvd. Sofia, Bulgaria
Burma	*Mya-Tu, M.	Burma Medical Research Institute 5, Zafar Shah Road, Dagon P.O. Rangoon, Burma
Canada	Alderman, R. B.	11756 35A Ave., Edmonton Alberta, Canada
	*Bailey, D. A.	School of Physical Education University of Saskatchewan Saskatoon, Canada
	Brown, S. R.	School of Physical Education and Recreation University of British Columbia, Canada
	Landry, F.	Département d'Education Physique Université LAVAL, Québec, P.Q. Canada
	*Macnab, R. B. J.	Faculty of Physical Education University of Alberta Edmonton, Alberta, Canada
	Yuhasz, M. S.	Department of Physical Education University of Western Ontario Canada
Cuba	Ruiz, R. A.	Calle 5ta, Apto, 6 Vedado, Habana, Cuba
Czechoslovakia	*Čelikovský, S.	Fakulta tělesne vychovy a sportu Karlovy University, Praha 1. Ujezd 450, Czechoslovakia

* Regular Member

	*Král, J.	Fakulta tělesne vychovy a sportu
		Karlovy University, Praha 1.
		Ujezd 450, Czechoslovakia
	Samek, L.	Namesti Kubanské Revoluce 25
		Praha 10, Czechoslovakia
Denmark	*Asmussen, E.	Laboratory for the Theory of Gymnastics
		The University of Copenhagen
		13, Universitetsparken
		2100 Copenhagen, Denmark
England	*Atha, J.	Department of Ergonomics and Cybernetics
		Loughborough University of Technology
		Loughborough, England
	*Campbell, W. R.	St. Lukes College
		Exeter, Devon, England
	Jeffery, J. A.	Physical Education and Industrial Fitness Unit
		The University of Technology
		Loughborough, England
	*Tanner, J. M.	The Hospital for Sick Children
		Great Ormond St.
		London, W.C.1
		England
	Williams, J. G. P.	Farnham Park Rehabilitation Centre
		Farnham Royal, Slough, Bucks
		England
Finland	*Karvinen, E.	Department of Physical Education
		University of Jyväskylä
		Jyväskylä, Finland
	*Karvonen, M. J.	Institute of Occupational Health
		Haartmaninkatu 1
		Helsinki, Finland
France	Plas, F.	18, rue de Grenelle
		Paris 10, France
Germany	*Beuker, F.	Facharzt für Sportmedizia
		Deutsche Hochschule für Korperkultur
		Leipzig, Germany East
	*Hollmann, W.	Institute für Kreislaufforschung und
		Sportmedizin
		5 Köln-Müngersdorf
		Deutsche Sporthochschule, Germany
	*Kirsch, A.	5 Köln-Müngersdorf, Carl-Diem-Weg,
		Postanschrifti Köln 41 Postfach
		450327, Germany
	*Mellerowicz, H.	1 Berlin 33 (Schmargerdorf)
		Forckenbeckstrasse 20, Germany
Greece	*Messinis, A.	51, Niovis St.
		Athens 220, Greece
Holland	Maas, G. D.	arts. FFIMS, van Swietenlaan n°
		Rotterdam 21, Holland

* Regular Member

India	*Sen, R. N.	Industrial Physiology Division, Central Labour Institute Eastern Express Highway, Sion Bombay-22(DD), India
Israel	Aldubi, L. D.	6, Levitan St. Tel-Aviv, Israel
	Hanne-Paparo, N.	Wingate Institute for Physical Education Wingate Post Office, Israel
	*Ruskin, H.	Department of Physical Education and Recreation The Hebrew University Jerusalem, Israel
	Shvartz, E.	Negev Institute for Arid Zone Research Beer-Sheva, Israel
	*Simri, U.	Wingate Institute for Physical Education Wingate Post Office, Israel
Italy	Cavagna, G.	Department of Physiology University of Milan Via Mangialli 32 Milano, Italy
	*Cerretelli, P.	Department of Physiology University of Milano Via Mangialli 32 Milano, Italy
	*Correnti, V.	Instituto di Antropologia Giuseppe Sergi Dell'Universita di Roma, Italy
	*Margaria, R.	Piazza Grandi 9 Milano, Italy
Japan	Hirata, K.	Hirata Institute of Health 2234 Mino-shi, Gifu Prefecture Japan
	*Ikai, M. (late)	School of Education University of Tokyo 3-1, 7-chome, Hongo, Bunkyo-ku, Tokyo, Japan
	*Ishiko, T.	School of Health and Physical Education Juntendo University 4–54, 5-chome, Fujisaki Narashino-shi, Chiba, Japan
	Kurimoto, E.	School of Health and Physical Education Juntendo University 4-54, 5-chome, Fujisaki Narashino-shi, Chiba, Japan
	Kuroda, Y.	College of General Education University of Tokyo 865 Komaba Meguro-ku, Tokyo, Japan

* Regular Member

	Matsuda, I.	Tokyo University of Education 1-40, Nishihara-cho, Shibuya-ku Tokyo, Japan
	*Meshizuka, T.	Laboratory of Physical Fitness College of Science Tokyo Metropolitan University 1-1, 1-chome, Yakumo, Meguro-ku Tokyo, Japan
	Nakamura, M.	4-16-5, Koishikawa, Bunkyo-ku, Tokyo, Japan
	Nakanishi, M.	476-176, Hodokubo, Hinoshi Tokyo, Japan
	Nakayama, J.	106, Kogane-machi the City of Niigata, Japan
	Noguchi, Y.	Kyoto University of Education 1, Fukakusaminamifujimori-cho Fushimi-ku, Kyoto
	Watanabe, T.	1036, 2-chome, Soshigaya Setagaya-ku Tokyo, Japan
Korea	Park, S. K.	112-32, Ahn-Ahm-Dong, Sung-Buck-ku Seoul, Korea
Malaysia	*Ganeshan, V.	Ministry of Culture, Youth and Sports 165 Jalan Ampang Kuala Lumpur, Malaysia
Mexico	Zurita, I.	Plava Langosta #103 Mexico 13 D.F., Mexico
New Zealand	Smithelles, P. A.	School of Physical Education University of Otago Dunedin, New Zealand
Norway	*Andersen, K. L.	Monolistvn, 20 Oslo 3, Norway
Philippines	,Bartolome, C. C.	Philippine Baseball Association Manila, Philippines
	Cailao, A. A.	Department of Physical Education University of Philippines Manila, Philippines
Republic of China	Shiao, P. Y.	Department of Physical Education Taiwan Normal University Taipei, Taiwan
	Tsai, M. O.	7-1, Alley 3, Lane 183, Sec. 1 Hoping E. Rd. Taipei, Taiwan, China
	*Wu, W. C.	Department of Physical Education Taiwan Normal University Taipei, Taiwan
	Yang, C. J.	Department of Physical Education Taiwan Normal University Taipei, Taiwan

* Regular Member

South Africa	C. H. Wyndham	Human Sciences Laboratory
		P.O. Box 809
		Johannesburgh, South Africa
Spain	Sierra, C.	Eduardo Dato
		12-Madrid-10, Spain
Sweden	*Astrand, P. O.	Orrspelsvägen 6
		Näsbypark, Sweden
Switzerland	Schneiter, C.	Hadlaubstrasse 36
		8044 Zurich
		Switzerland
	*Schönholzer, G.	Forschungsinstitut der Eidg.
		Turn- u. Sportschule
		CH 2532 Magglingen, Switzerland
	*Wartenweiler, J.	Eidg. Techn. Hochschule
		Department of Physical Education
		Plattenstr. 26
		8032 Zurich, Switzerland
Thailand	*Ketusinh, O.	Sports Science Center
		Sport Organization of Thailand
		The National Stadium, Rama I Rd.
		Bangkok 5, Thailand
	Suvarnabriksha, B.	328 Ruam Chit Lane
		Nakornchaisri Road
		Bangkok, Thailand
United Arab Republic	*Fadali, M. M.	33 Haroun Street, #601
		Doukki-Giza
		Egypt, U.A.R.
United Soviet Social Republic	*Letunov, S. P.	Central Scientific Institute of Physical Education
		Moscow Kazakova 18, U.S.S.R.
United States	Arnold, L. C.	National Council of YMCAs
		291 Broadway
		New York, N.Y. 10007
		U.S.A.
	Balke, B.	P.O. Box 630
		Aspen, Colo. 81611
		U.S.A.
	Cords, F. H. O.	Pacific Region of the National Council of YMCA
		Suite 1000
		714 W. Olympic Blvd.
		Los Angeles, Calif. 90015
		U.S.A.
	Cureton, T. K., Jr.	213 Huff Gym
		Department of Physical Education for Men
		University of Illinois
		Champaign, Illinois 61822
		U.S.A.

* Regular Member

	Friermood, H. T.	National Council of the YMCA
		291 Broadway
		New York, N.Y. 10001
		U.S.A.
	Green, M. M.	219 Leroy St.
		Dayton, Ohio 45407
	*Howell, Maxwell L.	San Diego State College
		San Diego, Calif. 92115
	*Hunsicker, P. A.	2016 Vinewood Boulevard
		Ann Arbor, Michigan
		U.S.A.
	Jokl, E. F.	University of Kentucky
		Lexington, Kentucky
		U.S.A.
	*Larson, L. A.	The University of Wisconsin School of Education
		Department of Physical Education—Men
		2000 Observatory Drive
		Madison Wisconsin 53706
		U.S.A.
	*Novak, L. P.	4245 Rickover Circle
		Dallas, Texas 75234
		U.S.A.
	Rosandich, T.	Athletic Director
		University of Wisconsin
		Parkside Campus
		Racine, Wisconsin
		U.S.A.
	*Ryan, A. J.	114 Nautilus Drive
		Madison, Wisconsin 53705
		U.S.A.
Uruguay	Johnson, P. K.	Instituto Tecnico
		South American Confederation of YMCAs
		Cosilla 172
		Montevideo, Uruguay
Vietnam	*Hung, V.	53, Truong Cong Dinh
		Saigon, Vietnam
Wales	Evans, E. G.	Sports Hall, University College of Wales
		Penglais, Aberystwyth
		Cardiganshire, Wales.
Yugoslavia	*Medved, R.	Visoka Skola Za Fizicku Kulturu
		Sagreb-Kaciceva 23, Yougoslavia

* Regular member.

Author Index

Subject Index